Adverse Effects of Herbal Drugs 2

Edited by
P.A.G.M. De Smet (Managing Editor)
K. Keller R. Hänsel R.F. Chandler

Contributors
I.H. Bowen D. Corrigan I.J. Cubbin P.A.G.M. De Smet
R. Hänsel U. Sonnenborn J. Westendorf H. Winterhoff
H.J. Woerdenbag

In collaboration with the Pharmaceuticals Programme
of the World Health Organization, Regional Office for Europe

Springer-Verlag
Berlin Heidelberg New York
London Paris Tokyo
Hong Kong Barcelona
Budapest

Dr. PETER A.G.M. DE SMET
Drug Information Center
Royal Dutch Association for the Advancement of Pharmacy
Alexanderstraat 11, 2514 JL The Hague
The Netherlands

Dr. KONSTANTIN KELLER
Institut für Arzneimittel des Bundesgesundheitsamtes
Seestraße 10, 13353 Berlin
Germany

Prof. Dr. RUDOLF HÄNSEL
Westpreußenstraße 71, 81927 München
Germany

Prof. Dr. R. FRANK CHANDLER
College of Pharmacy, Dalhousie University, Halifax B3H 3J5
Canada

ISSN 0942-2242
ISBN-13: 978-3-540-55800-2 e-ISBN-13: 978-3-642-48906-8
DOI: 10.1007/978-3-642-48906-8

Typesetting: Best-Set Typesetter Ltd., Hong Kong
13/3145-5 4 3 2 1 0 – Printed on acid-free paper

Adverse Effects of Herbal Drugs

Volume 2

Editors

P.A.G.M. De Smet (Managing Editor)

K. Keller R. Hänsel R.F. Chandler

To Isolde
A Blue Butterfly in the Delta

Preface

This second volume has the same purpose and set-up as the first one. There is a general introductory chapter on the legislation of herbal remedies in different countries, which is followed by twenty-six plant-oriented monographs. Some of these plants have been selected because of recent concerns about their adverse reaction potential (e. g. Scutellaria species), whereas others have been included because they still have a prominent place in phytotherapy (e. g. Hedera helix). The result is a blend of old and new data, which is precisely what one may expect from a comprehensive coverage.

April 1993 THE EDITORS

Contents

Contributors

Dr. IAN BOWEN
School of Health Sciences,
Sunderland University of Langham Tower, Ryhope Road,
Sunderland SR2 7EE
United Kingdom

Dr. DESMOND CORRIGAN
Department of Pharmacognosy, School of Pharmacy,
Trinity College, 18 Shrewsbury Road, Dublin 4
Ireland

Mr. IAN J. CUBBIN
School of Health Sciences,
SunderlandUniversity of Langham Tower, Ryhope Road,
Sunderland SR2 7EE
United Kingdom

Dr. PETER A.G.M. DE SMET
Drug Information Center,
Royal Dutch Association for the Advancement of Pharmacy,
Alexanderstraat 11,
2514 JL The Hague
The Netherlands

Prof. Dr. RUDOLF HÄNSEL
Westpreußenstraße 71, 81927 München
Germany

Dr. ULRICH SONNENBORN
Fa. Dr. Poehlmann & Co, Loerfelderstraße 20,
58313 Herdecke
Germany

Prof. Dr. JOHANNES WESTENDORF
Institut für Pharmakologie, Universität Hamburg,
Grindelallee 117, 20146 Hamburg
Germany

Dr. HILKE WINTERHOFF
Institut für Pharmakologie und Toxikologie,
Westfälische Wilhelms-Universität Münster,
Domagkstraße 12, 48149 Münster
Germany

Dr. HERMAN J. WOERDENBAG
Department of Pharmacognosy, University Centre for Pharmacy,
University of Groningen,
Antonius Deusinglaan 2, 9713 AW Groningen
The Netherlands

Legislatory Outlook on the Safety of Herbal Remedies

Peter A.G.M. De Smet

Introduction

Just as the first volume of this book series, this second volume starts with an introductory chapter on a general topic. This time the choice has fallen on the legal position of herbal remedies in various countries. The basic consideration is that herbal remedies have gained such an obvious place in our health care system that it has become hard for public health legislators to ignore them. Yet the regulations for herbal remedies vary considerably from country to country, and nations prominent in the field of synthetic drug legislation may be less progressive in the regulation of herbal products. To illustrate this point, the current legislation of herbal remedies in the European Economic Community and in certain individual countries will be discussed. These countries have been selected, either because they have developed special guidelines for the marketing of herbal preparations as drugs (Germany, France, Belgium) or because they have internationally well-respected drug regulatory bodies rooted in the Anglo-Saxon tradition (United Kingdom, United States, Australia, Sweden).

Following these general descriptions, this chapter will present a plant-by-plant review of the herbal remedy decisions in Germany, France, Belgium and Sweden, where health authorities have already evaluated hundreds of botanical preparations. As the outcome of these endeavours provides a wealth of data on the herbal drug market, it is made accessible here for drug information centers and other interested parties.

European Economic Community

Directive 65/65 of the Council of the European Economic Community (EEC) defines a medicinal product as follows: "Any substance or combination of substances presented for treating or preventing disease in human beings or animals. Any substance or combination of substances which may be administered to human beings or animals with a view to making a medical diagnosis or to restoring, correcting or modifying physiological

Adverse Effects of Herbal Drugs, Vol. 2
(ed. by P.A.G.M. De Smet, K. Keller, R. Hänsel, R.F. Chandler)

functions in human beings or in animals is likewise considered a medicinal product" [1]. The Directive subsequently defines a substance as any matter irrespective of origin which may be, inter alia, "vegetable, e.g., micro-organisms, plants, parts of plants, vegetable secretions, extracts, etc." [1].

To place a medicinal product on the EEC drug market, drug manufacturers and license holders must apply for authorization. This application must be accompanied by documents which provide the results of tests and trials carried out on the product concerned. To promote the free movement of medicinal products from one member state of the EEC to another, the Council of the EEC has adopted directives in which uniform application rules for all member states are laid down concerning the tests and trials requested, the compilation of dossiers and the examination of applications. To prevent differences between the member states in the interpretation of this general directive, the Committee for Proprietary Medicinal Products (CPMP) in Bruxelles regularly issues so-called Notes for Guidance, in which specific topics are elucidated. Although these Notes are recommendations, which are not quite as obligatory as the directive itself, they are influential on drug registry procedures throughout the EEC.

One of the CPMP Notes for Guidance concerns the quality of herbal remedies [2]. This Note defines herbal remedies, vegetable drugs and vegetable drug preparations (see Table 1). It deals with several orthodox concerns about the quality of herbal remedies, which have been listed in the introductory chapter of the previous volume of this book series [3] by providing rules for specific problem areas related to the quality assurance of medicinal products of vegetable origin: (a) description of the qualitative and quantitative particulars of the constituents; (b) description of the method of preparation; (c) control of starting materials; (d) control tests carried out at an intermediate stage of the manufacturing process of the finished product; (e) control tests on the finished product; (f) stability tests.

According to section (c), a complete pharmacopoeial monograph (or an equivalent monograph if a pharmacopoeial one is not available) on each vegetable drug should be submitted. When constitutents have known therapeutic activity, assay methods are required and a range of their content should also be included, so as to ensure a reproducible quality of the finished product. As a general rule, vegetable drugs must be tested for microbiological contamination, residues of pesticides and fumigation agents, radioactivity, toxic metals, and adulterants, unless otherwise justified. Furthermore, if the herbal remedy does not contain the vegetable drug itself but a preparation, the monograph on the vegetable drug must be followed by a monograph on the preparation, which gives particulars on identification tests, purity tests, and quantitative determination of characteristic constituents. If the preparation is standardized on constituents with known therapeutic activity, the method of standardization should be specified.

According to section (e), control tests on the finished product should allow qualitative and quantitative determination of the vegetable ingredients

Table 1. EEC definitions of herbal remedies, vegetable drugs and vegetable drug preparations [2]

Herbal remedies (herbal medicines) are medicinal products containing as active ingredients exclusively plant material and/or vegetable drug preparations.

Vegetable drugs are plant material used for a medicinal purpose. A vegetable drug or a preparation thereof is regarded as one active ingredient in its entirety whether or not the constituents with therapeutic activity are known.

Vegetable drug preparations are comminuted or powdered vegetable drugs, extracts, tinctures, fatty or essential oils, expressed juices etc. prepared from vegetable drugs, and preparations whose production involves a fractionation, purification or concentration process. However, chemically defined isolated constituents or their mixtures are not vegetable drug preparations. Other substances such as solvents, diluents, preservatives may form part of vegetable drug preparations. These substances must be indicated.

and their constituents with known therapeutic activity. If constituents with therapeutic activity are unknown, control tests may be specified by using chemically defined constituents of the vegetable ingredient as markers. If ingredients of a herbal remedy cannot be quantitatively determined individually, they may be determined jointly, provided that the need for this procedure is justified.

As the scope of the Note is strictly limited to the pharmaceutical quality of herbal remedies, it does not provide guidance about some other important aspects of herbal remedies, such as:

- The need for adequate quality control of the patient information on herbal products.
- The need for a rational solution of the issue, to which extent traditional empirism is allowed to supplement or replace experimental data in the benefit/risk assessment of well-known medicinal plants with mild pharmacological actions.

Germany [4]

In Germany, the legal requirements for herbal remedies are derived, as for all other drugs, from the Medicines Act of 1976 which came into force in 1978. Plants, plant parts and preparations thereof, whether in a crude or processed state, can be considered as drugs when they are intended to cure, alleviate or prevent diseases, suffering, physical injury or sickness symptoms, or to influence either the nature, the state or the function of the body or mental health conditions. Whether a herbal product is intended for such purposes, can be established on the basis of the herb(s) in question and/or the claimed uses of the product. Isolated constituents of herbal origin (e.g., digoxin) do not qualify as herbal remedies, and a crude herbal ingredient is considered as only one drug substance, even though it is known to consist of many chemical entities.

When a herbal remedy is manufactured industrially and marketed in packages ready for distribution to the consumer, a marketing authorization granted by the "Bundesgesundheitsamt" (BGA or Federal Health Office) is required. This authorization is not needed for pharmacy-made herbal medicines compounded for individual users, as such preparations are not considered to be finished medicines. This exemption is restricted to preparations which are produced in batches up to 100 packages per day, and which are dispensed in the same pharmacy, where they have been prepared.

There are three different ways to market a finished herbal product in Germany:

(1) Via the procedure for evaluation and validation of old medicines

Products already registered in 1978 were given a provisional marketing authorization and could stay on the German market until the end of April 1990. After this date, further marketing was only possible after the product had been approved via the procedure of evaluation and validation of old medicines ("Aufbereitung and Nachzulassung"). This two-step procedure started in 1978, when the Ministery of Health set up an expert committee for the evaluation of herbal remedies, the so-called "Kommission E" (KE). Although this expert committee receives scientific and administrative support from the BGA, it acts as an independent scientific body. It does not evaluate individual products but concentrates on the evaluation of crude herbal drug substances. The result of each evaluation is laid down in a monograph, which conveys either a positive or a negative assessment. When the KE has reached a positive decision, the monograph is structured as a package insert. It then provides concise information about denomination, constituents, uses, contra-indications, side effects, drug interactions, dosage, directions for use, and actions. In the case of a negative judgement, the monograph explains why there are no benefits of the herbal drug or why the claimed virtues are outweighed by potential risks. A KE monograph is first published as a draft, and after the commitee has considered the comments to this draft, a final version appears in the "Bundesanzeiger" (Federal Gazette).* At the time when this review was prepared, the KE had produced about 300 monographs or draft monographs, covering most of the economically important herbal medicines in Germany [5].

Since 1990, suppliers of old herbal medicines (i.e., registered provisionally in 1978) have to apply for prolongation of their provisional marketing authorizations. For each product, they have to present full pharmaceutical and analytical documentation to the BGA as well as proof of a favourable

* Individual issues of this journal should not be ordered from the Bundesgesundheitsamt in Berlin, but from the Bundesanzeiger Verlagsgesellschaft, Postfach 108006, D-5000 Köln 1, Deutschland

benefit/risk ratio. For this latter purpose, the applicant can submit a KE monograph, alone or together with complementary clinical studies. If necessary, bioavailability data or the medical justification of a fixed-combination preparation must also be submitted. When all conditions are satisfied, the procedure of evaluation and validation results in a normal marketing authorization with a regular prolongation period of 5 years.

It should be understood that the KE does not restrict its activities to mildly acting products, but also prepares monographs on potent herbal remedies, such as *Hyoscyamus niger*, *Rauwolfia serpentina* and *Urginea maritima*, all of which should definitely be treated as Prescription Only drugs. In other words, the existence of a KE monograph does not at all imply that the herbal drug is sufficiently harmless to be treated as an over-the-counter product. However, as each monograph outlines the accepted uses and health risks of the herb in question, the work of the KE provides useful information, if one has to assess the safety of individual source plants.

(2) Via individual applications for marketing authorizations

To market a new finished medicinal product, an individual application for approval is necessary. Such an application requires the submission of a complete file comprising analytical, pharmacological/toxicological and clinical documentation. However, it is not always necessary to submit original pharmacological/toxicological and clinical data. When the product contains a drug or a combination of drugs with well-known wanted and unwanted effects, it is sufficient to provide other scientific documentation, such as a KE monograph.

(3) Via reference to a standardized marketing authorization

The BGA can lay down the requirements for the quality of a medicinal product in a general monograph called "Standardzulassung" (SZ or standardized marketing authorization). Such a monograph outlines not only the analytical quality of the product but also specifies the wording of the labelling and the package insert. Many SZ monographs deal with herbal medicines, in particular with herbal teas that are sold by pharmacies and health food stores [6]. A supplier of such a herbal tea does not have to apply for individual marketing authorizations by submitting documentation to the BGA. All that needs to be done is inform the health authorities with reference to the SZ monograph.

In addition to these three ways to obtain marketing authorization for herbal medicines, it is also possible to sell traditional herbal health products in Germany without providing any proof of clinical efficacy. Such products require special labelling on the package, which may only refer to traditional uses (e.g., to tonify or fortify the user). To be acceptable, these traditional uses must be documented and should not be outweighed by health risks.

France [7]

In France, all botanical medicines are subject to general drug regulations. Just as chemical medicines, they can only be granted a marketing licence, when they comply with criteria of efficacy, safety and quality. The French health authorities have acknowledged, however, that it may be difficult or even impossible to demonstrate the efficacy of traditionally used vegetable drugs and preparations in the same rigorous way, in which the efficacy of new synthetic drugs should nowadays be proven. The French Ministry of Health and Social Affairs has therefore defined a process of evaluation, which allows the granting of marketing licences to selected vegetable drugs and preparations on the basis of adapted documentation and an abridged application. The first French guideline that outlined a simplified admission procedure for phytotherapeutical products was issued in 1986 and covered 112 herbal drugs [8]. One year later, it was supplemented by a separate guideline on herbal laxatives, in which about 30 different laxative herbs were included [9]. In 1990, both guidelines were replaced by an adapted and expanded guideline, which listed more than 200 medicinal herbs as non-toxic ingredients of herbal drug preparations [10].

According to the 1990 guideline, the application of a marketing licence for a herbal drug preparation must be accompanied by chemical and pharmaceutical documentation on the composition, method of preparation, control of the raw materials, control of the intermediary products (if necessary), control of the finished product, and stability. Pharmacological and clinical documentation is not necessary, when no other therapeutic uses are recommended than those allowed by the guideline. These allowed uses are specified separately for each herb, and they are selected from a limited list of 35 indications, none of which is so serious that it would be dangerous to refrain from drug treatment with well-proven efficacy. For every indication, the guideline offers a professional description as well as a patient-oriented description. The need to present toxicological documentation depends on the type of preparation. In general, the following preparations are exempt from this requirement (Category 1 preparations):

- Herbal teas, aqueous extracts, and hydroalcoholic extracts prepared with ≤30% v/v alcohol.
- Hydroalcoholic extracts prepared with >30% v/v alcohol and tinctures, provided that their usage is traditional and that they are included in the French and/or European Pharmacopoeia.
- Herbal laxatives, in so far as they have been listed in the guideline.

Submission of experimental data on the acute and subchronic oral toxicity in rats is required, however, for many crude vegetable powders, hydroalcoholic extracts prepared with >30% v/v alcohol and non-traditional tinctures (Category 2 preparations).

The guideline expects that the oral dosage of herbal teas is around

250–1000 ml per day and that corresponding doses are recommended for other forms that have to be dissolved in water before administration. In case of another type of preparation, the applicant has to justify the proposed dosage regimen, whereby he has to take into account traditionally employed doses. Combination of different herbs are permitted, provided that the allowed uses of every ingredient are similar or complementary and that only a single therapeutic domain is claimed for the combination product. Herbal tea mixtures may maximally contain five active and five inactive herbs, whereas other preparations may maximally contain four active and two inactive herbs.

Belgium [11]

In Belgium, the health authorities have introduced a phytotherapeutical policy which resembles the French approach. The Ministry of Public Health and Environment has issued ten lists of source plants, preparations of which may be presented as traditionally used sedatives, laxatives, diuretics, anti-arthritic agents, cough remedies, appetite stimulants, digestive aids, cholagogues, stomatologicals and topical soothing agents, respectively. Special labelling is required.

United Kingdom [12]

In the United Kingdom, there are no special guidelines for the admission of herbal remedies to the drug market. Most herbal remedies are on the so-called General Sale List, which means that they can be sold without prescription and outside pharmacies. To be accepted as a medicinal product, a botanical preparation must comply with the Guidelines on Safety and Efficacy Requirements for Herbal Medicinal Products. Safety may be demonstrated by submitting published literature and/or other supporting data. New animal studies are not normally required. Efficacy may only be documented by general literature data in the case of minor conditions suited for self diagnosis and treatment. For all other conditions, however, evidence from clinical trials with the product is required. Due to the stringency of this latter demand, only few botanical products reach the status of approved drug. A notable example is the drug licensing of preparations containing evening primrose oil (fixed oil obtained from the seed of *Oenothera biennis*) for symptomatic relief of atopic eczema [13] and premenstrual or non-cyclical mastalgia [14].

The efficacy and safety of herbal preparations are strictly evaluated on a product-to-product basis, whereby data on uses, precautions and adverse effects are negotiated between the Department of Health and the individual applicant. This system has the advantage of flexibility, but an inevitable drawback is, of course, that variation and inequality may arise in the assessments of comparable products. Moreover, this approach makes it difficult to obtain an overall picture of British decisions, as the only information available is the actual labelling of reviewed herbal products now on the UK market.

United States

In the United States of America, the regulation of food, drugs and medical devices is the responsibility of the Food and Drug Administration (FDA). The primary mission of this federal agency is to protect the health of the American public by prohibiting commerce in adulterated and misbranded products [15]. The FDA does not recognize a separate regulatory status for herbal medicines. It considers herbal preparations which are marketed for medicinal purposes as drugs, and as such the products must comply with the general requirements of the drug provisions of the federal Food, Drug and Cosmetic Act [16]. This means that rigorous proof of efficacy and safety has to be submitted to the FDA to obtain approval for marketing. To circumvent this tedious process of premarketing clearance and to avoid confiscation of marketed products, suppliers of herbal remedies in the United States usually do not mention medical claims on labels or in package inserts. The resulting information gap is filled by a vast assortment of mostly uncritical herbal booklets and pamphlets, which are available in health food stores [17–19].

With respect to the acceptance of herbal products as drugs, it is noteworthy that in 1972 the FDA set up scientific panels for a class-by-class review of the efficacy of over-the-counter drug ingredients [18]. Several herbs have survived this review process and can now be lawfully labelled with therapeutical claims, but various others have been identified as lacking proof of efficacy [20–22].

In 1975, the FDA completed a toxicological evaluation of herbs which were being offered for sale as herbal teas in health food stores [23]. With consideration to relative toxicity and current or past usage in food or drugs, 171 herbs were arranged in three categories of safety: (i) 27 unsafe herbs; (ii) 53 herbs of undefined safety for food use; (iii) 91 safe herbs. Which herbs were exactly listed by the FDA in the unsafe and safe categories, respectively, is reproduced here in Tables 2 and 3. It should be noted, however, that the FDA no longer uses them as the basis for herbal product seizures, regulatory letters or import detentions. Following criticisms and court case decisions, the FDA adopted the policy to consider action against botanical food products on a case-by-case basis rather than by reliance on toxicological listings. Specific action is only brought, if the herbal product is labeled solely for food use and if there is some valid toxicological concern about the product as a food. Herbal products intended for use as a drug (e.g., preparations labeled with therapeutic claims) must be brought to the

Table 2. Herbs listed as unsafe herbs in a report of the American Food and Drug Administration (FDA) from 1975 [23]

Acorus calamus
Aesculus hippocastanum
Arnica montana
Artemisia absinthium
Atropa belladonna
Conium maculatum
Convallaria majalis
Cytisus scoparius
Datura stramonium
Dipteryx odorata = *Coumarouna odorata*
Dipteryx oppositifolia = *Coumarouna oppositifolia*
Euonymus atropurpureus
Euonymus europaeus
Eupatorium rugosum
Heliotropium europaeum
Hyoscyamus niger
Hypericum perforatum
Ipomoea purga = *Exogonium purga*
Ipomoea purpurea
Lobelia inflata
Mandragora officinarum
Pausinystalia yohimbe = *Corynanthe yohimbe*
Phoradendron flavescens = *Viscum flavescens*
Phoradendron juniperinum
Podophyllum peltatum
Sanguinaria canadensis
Solanum dulcamara
Vinca major
Vinca minor
Viscum album

attention of the Center for Drugs and Biologicals in accordance with the Compliance Program concerning fraudulent drugs and biologicals [19].

Under the provisions of the federal Food, Drug and Cosmetic Act, botanical products can be designated as "Generally Recognized As Safe" (GRAS). This status can only be granted to products marketed for food use and does not apply to drugs [16]. Most of the herbal products with GRAS status belong to the following two categories: (i) spices and other natural seasonings and flavorings; (ii) essential oils, oleoresins (solvent-free), and natural extractives (including distillates). Early 1992, there were 83 items in the former category and 157 items in the latter category. It should be emphasized that the GRAS status of a herbal product only implies general recognition of its safety for the intended use as a spice, seasoning or flavor [24]. It cannot be taken indiscriminately as evidence for the safety of medicinal usage, since the latter may involve another preparation, dosage and/or way of administration. Some examples to underscore this important point are presented in Table 4.

Table 3. Herbs listed as safe herbs in a report of the American Food and Drug Administration (FDA) from 1975 [23]

Acacia senegal or other related African *Acacia* species (gum)
Achillea millefolium
Aloe perryi, *A. barbadensis* (= *A. vera*), *A. ferox*, and hybrids of this species with *A. africana* and *A. spicata*
Alpinia galanga
Alpinia officinarum (root)
Amonum melegueta (seed)
Anethum graveolens (fruit, seed)
Angelica archangelica or other *Angelica* species (root, seed, stem)
Anthemis nobilis (flower)
Brassica species, such as *B. hirta*, *B. juncea* and *B. nigra*
Calendula officinalis
Capsicum annuum and *C. frutescens*
Carica papaya
Cassia acutifolia
Chondrus crispus and *Gigartina mamillosa*
Cinnamomum burmanni (bark), *C. cassia* (bark, leaf), *C. loureirii* (bark, leaf) and *C. zeylanicum* (bark, leaf)
Cola acuminata and other *Cola* species (nut)
Commiphora molmol, *C. abyssinica* and other *Commiphora* species (gum)
Coriandrum sativum
Crocus sativus
Curcuma longa
Erigeron canadensis = *Leptilon canadense*
Eriodictyon californicum
Eucalyptus globulus (leaf)
Ferula assa-foetida and related *Ferula* species
Foeniculum vulgare (seed, fruit) as well as its variety *dulce*
Glycyrrhiza glabra and other *Glycyrrhiza* species (root)
Hedeoma pulegioides and *Mentha pulegium*
Humulus lupulus
Hypericum perforatum (leaf, flower, caulis)*
Hyssopus officinalis
Illicium verum
Inula helenium (rhizome, root)
Iris germanica (including its variety *florentina*) and *I. pallida*
Jasminum officinale and other *Jasminum* species
Juniperus communis (berries)
Laminaria species and *Nereocystitis* species
Laurus nobilis (leaf)
Lavandula officinalis
Levisticum officinale
Lippia citriodora
Majorana hortensis
Majorana onites
Matricaria chamomilla (flower)
Medicago sativa (herb, seed)
Melissa officinalis
Mentha piperita
Mentha spicata
Myristica fragans
Ocimum basilicum and *O. minimum*
Panax ginseng and *P. quinquefolium*

Table 3. *Continued*

Papaver somniferum (seed)
Passiflora incarnata (flower)
Pimpinella anisum
Piper cubeba (berries)
Pogostemon cablin and *P. heyneanus*
Prunus serotina (bark)
Quercus alba
Rosa alba, *R. centifolia*, *R. damascena*, *R. gallica* and varieties of these species (bud, fruit)
Rosmarinus officinalis
Ruta graveolens
Salvia officinalis
Sambucus canadensis and *S. nigra* (flower)
Santalum album
Smilax aristolochiaefolia, *S. regelii*, *S. febrifuga*, or undetermined *Smilax* species
Styrax benzoin, *S. paralleloneurus*, *S. tonkinensis* and other species of the section Anthostyrax of the *Styrax* genus (resin)
Tagetes patula, *T. erecta*, and *T. minuta*
Taraxacum officinale or *T. laevigatum* (root)
Thymus vulgaris
Tilia species (flower, leaf)
Trifolium species
Trigonella foenum-graecum
Tsuga canadensis or *T. heterophylla* (needles, twigs)
Turnera diffusa = *T. aphrodisiaca* (leaf)
Valeriana officinalis (rhizome, root)
Verbascum phlomoides and *V. thapsiforme* (flower)
Verbena officinalis
Viola odorata (leaf)
Zingiber officinale

* This botanical source was also listed in the same FDA report as an unsafe herb (cf. Table 2). Apparently, the classification as a safe herb only applied to the hypericin-free alcohol distillate form [23].

In addition to GRAS recognition, the federal Food, Drug and Cosmetic Act also offers the possibility of designating botanicals as food additives that may be safely used in food as natural flavoring substances or as natural adjuvants used in conjunction with flavors. At the beginning of 1992, this category comprised a total of 130 substances. The general proviso is that the herbs are used in the minimum quantity needed to produce the intended effect. Additional restrictions may be imposed on specific herbs, such as a limitation to the use in alcoholic beverages only (e.g., *Inula helenium*) or the requirement that thujone should be absent in the finished food (e.g., *Artemisia*). Just as in the case of GRAS products, the allowance of herbal products as flavoring substances or adjuvants does not guarantee that their medicinal usage is also safe. On the contrary, the current list includes several botanicals with toxic potential, such as arnica flowers, bryony root and castor oil [24].

Table 4. Risks associated with the medicinal uses of some herbal products given GRAS status

Laurel berries	The oil obtained from the berries is such a potent skin sensitizer due to the presence of allergenic sesquiterpene lactones that topical application must be avoided [25]
Mustard	The external medicinal use of preparations from black mustard has declined because of prominent local reactions [26]
Nutmeg	Large doses of the seed can cause nausea, vomiting, flushing, dry mouth, tachycardia, CNS stimulation possibly with epileptiform convulsions, miosis, mydriasis, euphoria, and hallucinations. The essential oil contains the mutagenic and animal carcinogenic safrol [5]
Oregano	A concentrated dose of oregano oil acts as a gastrointestinal irritant, causing contractions which could stimulate uterine contractions [27].
Sage	The leaf contains 1–2.5% of essential oil consisting for 35–60% of thujone. This compound may produce toxicity, when the herb is taken in overdoses (more than 15 g per dose) or for a prolonged period [5].

Australia [28]

The marketing of therapeutic goods in Australia is regulated by federal laws as well as state laws. The federal laws only cover the importation of therapeutic goods, and cover all substances for which therapeutic claims are made. State laws are more complex but, in general, also cover only the sale of preparations for which therapeutic claims are made. Among the Australian states, Victoria has the strictest legislation covering the use of herbs for medicinal purposes. In this state, any substance for which a therapeutic claim is made (with the exception of terms such as "invigorating") must be registered as a proprietary medicine before it can be sold legally. Registration is granted only if claims of efficacy can be substantiated by adequate scientific evidence and if an appropriate degree of safety can be demonstrated. Usually, specific therapeutic claims (e.g., "for arthritis") are carefully avoided by the manufacturers of herbal preparations, but the intended purpose may be revealed by the retailer, e.g., by selling the preparations on a stand that is labelled with some claim.

To control the importation and distribution of therapeutic substances into Australia, the Department of Community Services & Health has issued guidelines for importers [29]. Attached to these guidelines is a list of prohibited herbs, which may not be imported for therapeutic use. This list is largely composed of herbs with psychotropic or carcinogenic constituents (Table 5). Also attached is a list of restricted herbs, which are the subject of poisons control in some Australian states. This list largely consists of herbs

Table 5. List of prohibited herbs, which may not be imported into Australia for therapeutic use [29]

Abrus precatorius
Acorus calamus
Argyreia nervosa
Aristolochia spp.
Amanita muscaria and related spp.
Anadenanthera colubrina var. *cebil* = *Piptadenia macrocarpa*
Anadenanthera peregrina = *Piptadenia peregrina*
Banisteriopsis caapi and related spp.
Brachyglottis spp.
Cannabis spp.
Catha edulis
Conocybe siligineoides and related spp.
Crotalaria spp.
Cynoglossum officinale
Echium vulgare
Erythroxylum coca
Gymnopilus spp.
Haemadictyon spp.
Heliotropium spp.
Ipomoea burmanni
Ipomoea hederacea
Ipomoea tricolor
Ipomoea violacea
Lithospermum spp.
Lophophora spp.
Opuntia cylindrica
Papaver bracteatum
Papaver somniferum
Peganum harmala
Petasites spp.
Phytolacca americana
Psilocybe spp.
Pteridium aquilinum
Rivea corymbosa
Sassafras albidum
Senecio spp.
Solanum dulcamara
Sophora secundiflora
Stropharia cubensis
Strychnos gaultheriana
Strychnos ignatii
Symphytum spp.
Tussilago farfara

containing toxic alkaloids or cardiac glycosides (Table 6). If an importer wishes to import these restricted herbs, he has to check with his state health authorities to find out, whether he is legally permitted to possess and use these substances.

Table 6. List of restricted herbs, which are the subject of poisons control in some Australian states [29]

Aconitum spp.
Adonis vernalis
Alstonia constricta
Ammi spp.
Apocynum spp.
Areca catechu
Artemisia spp.
Atropa belladonna
Calotropis spp.
Catharanthus spp.
Chondrodendron tomentosum
Chenopodium ambrosoides
Cinchona spp.
Claviceps purpurea
Colchicum autumnale
Conium maculatum
Convallaria majalis
Coronilla spp.
Croton tiglium
Datura spp.
Delphinium spp.
Digitalis spp.
Duboisia spp.
Ephedra spp.
Erysimum canescens
Galanthus nivalus
Gelsemium sempervirens
Hemerocallis flava
Hippomane mancinella
Hyoscyamus spp.
Juniperus sabina
Lobelia spp.
Mandragora officinarum
Nerium oleander
Pausinystalia yohimbe = *Corynanthe yohimbe*
Physostigma venenosum
Pilocarpus spp.
Podophyllum spp.
Rauwolfia spp.
Ricinus communis
Sarothamnus scoparius = *Cytisus scoparius*
Scopolia carniolica
Strophanthus spp.
Strychnos nux-vomica
Tanacetum balsamita
Tanacetum vulgare
Thevetia nereifolia
Thuja occidentalis
Veratrum spp.
Vinca spp.
Xysmalobium undulatum

Sweden [30,31]

In Sweden, basic provisions concerning products of natural origin have been included since 1977 in the Drug Ordinance. These products may be marketed in Sweden as "natural products", when they do not in normal use endanger the health of humans or animals, according to adequate experience. A company wishing to market a natural product must first make an application for registration to the Medical Products Agency. The applicant has to provide information about product formulation, indications, dosage, composition, and documentation showing why the product is judged not to endanger health. For products known from Swedish folk traditions or from similar medical traditions in other countries, references to the scientific literature are often sufficient. The claim of harmlessness is examined by the Agency, but the Agency does not assess whether the product has the claimed medical effect. When the applic ation is accepted, the natural product is exempt from the control regulations concerning pharmaceutical specialities.

Natural products must be marketed with the Swedish text "not tested in accordance with drug regulations" clearly present, both on the package and in other consumer information. Advertisements and other product information must comply with guidelines from the National Board for Consumer Policies governing the claims for medical effects that may be made. These guidelines include a list of approved and non-approved areas of use for natural products.

The regulations for natural products intended for injection differ to some extent from those for other natural products.

Individual Herbal Drugs

In the following pages, the evaluations of the German, French, Belgian and Swedish health authorities of individual herbal remedies are reviewed plant by plant. **It should be noted that these evaluations are generally reproduced here without comments and do not necessarily reflect the personal view of the author of this chapter.**

Each source plant is identified by its major scientific name and other prevailing Latin binomials are listed as synonyms on basis of the consulted regulations and general text book [32–34]. Under each scientific name, the following types of data are listed, in so far as they are available:

VN: *Vernacular Name(s)*
To increase the recognizability of the Latin identifier, common English names (E), German names (G) and French names (F) have been added on basis of the consulted regulations and general text books providing such information [18,32,34–45].

KE: *Kommission E*
This field provides a summary of the safety data in the monograph(s)

of the German "Kommission E" (KE), together with an annotation of the specific reference [5].

SZ: *Standardzulassungen*
This field provides a summary of the safety data, as mentioned in the German "Standardzulassung" (SZ) [6].

FR: *French Guideline*
This field provides a summary of the latest French guideline on phytotherapeutical products [10]. As this guideline only lists the French names of the permitted medicinal plants, it has been used in conjunction with a working document of the French health authorities, which specifies for each vernacular name the particular species which may be used [46]. Between brackets it is specified for every herb, which types of dosage forms require toxicological documentation (Category 2 preparations) and which dosage forms are exempt from this requirement (Category 1 preparations). The following abbreviations are used to identify the different dosage forms: pd = powdered drug; ht = herbal tea; ae = aqueous extract; wa = weakly alcoholic extract; sa = strongly alcoholic extract; ti = tincture.

BE: *Belgian Regulations*
This field provides a summary of the Belgian regulations on phytotherapeutic products [11].

SW: *Swedish Classification*
This field indicates the classification which the herb has received from the Swedish Medical Products Agency: foodstuff, natural product, or drug [31].

AS: *Alternative Source(s)*
This field is used, when a regulation or authoritative text book permits additional source plants and/or when certain subspecies or varieties are specified.

RM: *Remarks*
This field provides additional remarks, in so far as they are considered appropriate in the context.

The fields on foreign regulations apply the following abbreviations to identify different types of drug information: CI = contraindications; AE = adverse effects; I = interactions. It should be noted that, in addition to the CI data which have been systematically reproduced here, the German regulations (KE and SZ) also yield some general cautionary notes concerning:

- *Antidiarrheal remedies*: a physician should be consulted, when diarrhea lasts for more than 3–4 days.
- *Cholagogic/choleretic remedies*: patients with bile-stones should first consult a physician.
- *Diuretic remedies*: Should not be used for edema due to cardiac or renal insufficiency (this warning is evidently based on the fact that the pharmacological profile of herbal diuretics is not comparable to that of

synthetic diuretics, as the latter promote the excretion of salt and water by the kidneys, while the former merely stimulate the excretion of water [47]).

***Abies alba* Mill. = *A. pectinata* DC.**
VN: White spruce (E). Edeltanne; Weißtanne (G). Sapin argenté (F).
FR: Bud permitted for oral use (toxicological categories pd:2 ht/ae/wa:1 sa/ti:1).

***Acacia* spp.**
VN: Acacia (E).
SW: Classified as natural product.

***Achillea millefolium* L.**
VN: Milfoil (E). Gemeine Schafgarbe (G). (Achillée) millefeuille (F).
KE: Herb and flower permitted for oral use. CI: hypersensitivity to milfoil and other Asteraceae. No AE, I [BAnz nr.22a 01.02.90].
SZ: Herb permitted as herbal tea. CI: hypersensitivity to sesquiterpene lactones. AE: rare contact allergy. No I.
FR: Flowering top permitted for oral use (toxicological categories pd:2 ht/ae/wa:1 sa/ti:1).
BE: Herb permitted as traditional topical soothing agent.
SW: Herb classified as natural product.
AS: SW also classifies *Achillea moschata* Jacq. as natural product.

***Aconitum napellus* L.**
VN: Monkshood (E). (Blauer) Eisenhut (G). Casque de jupiter; Napel bleu (F).
KE: Herb and tuber not permitted for therapeutic use. Usefulness is not documented adequately for most advocated uses. Contains the toxic alkaloid aconitine [BAnz nr.193 15.10.87].
SW: Classified as a drug, which must normally be registered as pharmaceutical speciality.

***Acorus calamus* L.**
VN: Sweet flag (E). Kalmus (G). Acore vrai (F).
SW: Classified as a drug, which must normally be registered as pharmaceutical speciality.

***Adhatoda vasica* Nees = *Justicia adhatoda* L.**
VN: Malabar nut (E). Echte Adhatode (G). Noyer des Indes (F).
SW: Classified as natural product.

***Adonis vernalis* L.**
VN: Spring adonis (E). Adonis (G). Adonide de printemps (F).
KE: Herb permitted for oral use. CI, AE, and I of cardiac glycosides [BAnz nr.85 05.05.88].

***Aerva lanata* Juss. = *Achyranthes lanata* L.**
SW: Classified as a drug, which must normally be registered as pharmaceutical speciality.

***Aesculus hippocastanum* L.**
VN: Horse chestnut (E). Roßkastanie (G). Marronier d'Inde (F).
KE: Seed permitted for oral use. No CI, AE, I, except for rare GI-disturbances [BAnz nr.228 05.12.84].
FR: Stem bark permitted for oral use (toxicological categories pd:2 ht/ae/wa:1 sa/ti:1).
Seed permitted for oral use (toxicological categories pd:2 ht/ae/wa:1 sa/ti:2).
SW: Classified as a drug, which must normally be registered as pharmaceutical speciality.

***Agrimonia eupatoria* L.**
VN: Sticklewort (E). Kleiner Odermennig (G). Aigremoine (F).
KE: Herb permitted for oral use. No CI, AE, I [BAnz nr.50 13.03.86].
FR: Flowering top permitted for oral use (toxicological categories pd:2 ht/ae/wa:1 sa/ti:1).
AS: *Agrimonia procera* Wallroth = *Agrimonia odorata* auct. non Mill. [KE].

***Alcea rosea* L. = *Althaea rosea* (L.) Cav.**
VN: Rose mallow (E). Stockmalve (G). Passerose; Rose trémière (F).
KE: Flower not permitted for therapeutic use. Usefulness is not documented adequately. No risks are known, however, and there is no objection to the use as admixture [BAnz nr.43 02.03.89].
FR: Flower and leaf permitted for oral use (toxicological categories pd:2 ht/ae/wa:1 sa/ti:-).

***Alchemilla xanthochlora* Rothm. = *Alchemilla vulgaris* L.**
VN: Lady's mantle (E). Gemeiner Frauenmantel (G). Alchémille commune; Alchémille vulgaire (F).
KE: Herb permitted for oral use. No CI, AE, I [BAnz nr.173 18.09.86].
SZ: Herb permitted as herbal tea. No CI, I. AE: hepatic damage (rarely) due to presence of tannins.
FR: Aerial parts permitted for oral use (toxicological categories pd:2 ht/ae/wa:1 sa/ti:1).
SW: Classified as natural product.

***Allium cepa* L.**
VN: Onion (E). Zwiebel (G). Oignon (F).
KE: Bulb permitted for oral use. No CI, AE, I. When used for several months, the intake of the constituent diphenylamin should not exceed 35 mg/day [BAnz nr.50 13.03.86].

***Allium sativum* L.**

VN: Garlic (E). Knoblauch (G). Ail (commun) (F).
KE: Bulb permitted for oral use. No CI, AE, I, except for foul breath, rare GI-disturbances and allergic reactions [BAnz nr.122 06.07.88].
FR: Bulb permitted for oral use (toxicological categories pd:1 ht/ae/wa:1 sa/ti:1).
SW: Classified as natural product.

***Allium ursinum* L.**

VN: Bear's garlic (E). Bärlauch (G). Ail des ours (F).
SW: Classified as natural product.

***Aloe barbadensis* Miller = *Aloe vera* L.**

VN: Aloe (E). Curaçao-Aloe; Barbados-Aloe (G). Aloès (F).
KE: Juice permitted for oral use. CI, AE and I of anthranoid laxatives [BAnz nr.154 21.08.85].
FR: Juice permitted for short-term oral use (max. 8–10 days) as laxative by adults and children of 12 years and older. CI, AE and I of anthranoid laxatives.
Juice also permitted for external use (toxicological categories pd:- ht/ae/wa:1 sa/ti:1).
SW: Classified as foodstuff and as a drug, which must normally be registered as pharmaceutical speciality.

***Aloe ferox* Miller**

VN: Aloe (E). Kap-Aloe; Aloe, Afrikanische (G). Aloès (F).
KE: Juice permitted for oral use. CI, AE, I of anthranoid laxatives. [BAnz nr.154 21.08.85].
FR: Juice permitted for short-term oral use (max. 8–10 days) as a laxative by adults and children of 12 years and older. CI, AE and I of anthranoid laxatives.
Juice also permitted for external use (toxicological categories pd:- ht/ae/wa:1 sa/ti:1).

***Alpinia officinarum* (L.) Hance**

VN: Galangal (E). Galgant, (echter) (G). Galanga (F).
KE: Rhizome permitted for oral use. No CI, AE, I [BAnz nr.173 18.09.86].
SW: Classified as natural product.

***Althaea officinalis* L.**

VN: Marshmallow (E). (Echter) Eibisch (G). Guimauve (officinale) (F).
KE: Leaf and root permitted for oral use. No CI, AE. I: absorption of other drugs taken simultaneously may be delayed [BAnz nr.43 02.03.89].
SZ: Leaf and root permitted as herbal tea. No CI, AE, I.

FR: Leaf and flower permitted for oral use (toxicological categories pd:2 ht/ae/wa:1 sa/ti:-).
Root permitted for oral use (toxicological categories pd:1 ht/ae/wa:- sa/ti:-).
Leaf, flower and root permitted as laxative.
BE: Leaf, flower and root permitted as traditional stomatological.
SW: Classified as natural product.

***Ammi visnaga* (L.) Lam.**
VN: Khella; Toothpick ammi (E). Bischofskraut; Zahnstocher-Ammei (G). Herbe au cure-dents (F).
KE: Fruit permitted for oral use. No CI, AE, I [BAnz nr.50 13.03.86].

***Anacyclus pyrethrum* DC. = *Anthemis pyrethrum* L.**
VN: Pellitory root (E). Speichelwurzel (G). Pyrèthre officinal (F).
SW: Classified as natural product.

***Anamirta cocculus* (L.) Wight et Arnott. = *Menispermum cocculus* L.**
VN: (Indian) cockles (E). Fischkörner, Kokkelskörner (G). Coque du Levant (F).
SW: Classified as natural product with a dose limitation.
RM: The seed contains the poisonous principle picrotoxin [32].

***Andrographis paniculata* Nees = *Justicia paniculata* Burm.**
VN: Andrographis (E). Andrographis (G).
SW: Classified as natural product.

***Anethum graveolens* L.**
VN: Dill (E). Dill (G). Aneth (odorant) (F).
KE: Herb not permitted for therapeutic use. Usefulness is not documented adequately. No risks are known, however [BAnz nr.193 15.10.87].
Fruit permitted for oral use. No CI, AE, I [BAnz nr.193 15.10.87].
FR: Fruit permitted for oral use (toxicological categories pd:1 ht/ae/wa:1 sa/ti:1).

***Angelica archangelica* L. = *Archangelica officinalis* Hoffm.**
VN: European Angelica (E). Engelwurz (G). Angélique (officinale) (F).
KE: Root permitted for oral use. No CI, I. AE: photosensitivity due to furocoumarins [BAnz nr.101 01.06.90].
Fruit and herb not permitted for therapeutic use. Usefulness is not documented adequately. Contains photosensitizing furocoumarins [BAnz nr.101 01.06.90].
SZ: Root permitted as herbal tea. CI: peptic ulcer. No I. AE: photosensitivity.
FR: Root and fruit permitted for oral use (toxicological categories pd:1 ht/ae/wa:1 sa/ti:1).

SW: Herb and root classified as natural product.
AS: SW also classifies *Angelica sylvestris* L. as natural product.

***Antennaria dioica* (L.) Gaertn. = *Gnaphalium dioicum* L.**
VN: Cat's foot (E). Gemeines Katzenpfötchen (G). Gnaphale dioique; Pied de chat (F).
FR: Flower-head permitted for oral use (toxicological categories pd:2 ht/ae/wa:1 sa/ti:1).

***Anthyllis vulneraria* L.**
VN: Lady's fingers (E). Wundklee (G). Trèfle jaune (F).
SW: Classified as natural product.

***Apium graveolens* L.**
VN: Celery (E). Küchen-Sellerie; Sellerie (G). Ache des marais; Céleri (F).
KE: Herb, root and fruit not permitted for therapeutic use. Usefulness is not documented adequately. Risks: allergic reactions (even anaphylactic shock). Contains phototoxic furanocoumarins [BAnz nr.127 12.07.91].
FR: Root permitted for oral use (toxicological categories pd:1 ht/ae/wa:1 sa/ti:1).

***Arctium lappa* L. = *Arctium majus* Bernh. = *Lappa major* Gaertn.**
VN: Burdock (E). Große Klette (G). Bardane (grande) (F).
KE: Root not permitted for therapeutic use. Usefulness is not documented adequately. No risks are known, however [BAnz nr.22a 01.02.90].
FR: Root and leaf permitted for oral use (toxicological categories pd:1 ht/ae/wa:1 sa/ti:1)
BE: Root permitted as traditional topical soothing agent.
SW: In Sweden, "*Arctium major*" is classified as natural product.
AS: *Arctium minus* (Hill) Bernh. and *A. tomentosum* Mill. [KE].

***Arctostaphylos uva-ursi* (L.) Sprengel**
VN: (Common) bearberry; Redberry (E). Bärentraube (G). Busserole (officinale); Raisin d'ours (F).
KE: Leaf permitted for oral use. No CI. AE: GI-disturbances. I: urinary acidifiers. Should not be used for prolonged period without consulting physician [BAnz nr.228 05.12.84].
SZ: Leaf permitted as herbal tea powder. No CI. AE: GI-disturbances. I: Urinary acidifiers. Should not be used for prolonged period without consulting physician. An alkaline urine should be provided by dietary measure. Additional $NaHCO_3$ use is possible.
FR: Leaf permitted for oral use (toxicological categories pd:2 ht/ae/wa:1 sa/ti:2).
SW: Classified as natural product.

***Areca catechu* L.**
VN: Areca palm tree (E). Betelnußpalme (G). Aréquier (F).
SW: Classified as a drug, which must normally be registered as pharmaceutical speciality.

***Aristolochia clematitis* L.**
VN: Aristolochy, birthwort (E). Osterluzei (G). Aristoloche commune (F).
SW: Classified as a drug, which must normally be registered as pharmaceutical speciality.

***Armoracia rusticana* Ph. Gaertn. = *Cochlearia armoracia* L.**
VN: Horse radish (E). Meerrettich (G). Grand raifort; Raifort sauvage (F).
KE: Root permitted for oral use. CI: GI-ulcer, nephritis, children younger than 4 years. AE: GI-disturbances. No I. [BAnz nr.85 05.05.88].
FR: Root permitted for oral use (toxicological categories pd:1 ht/ae/wa:1 sa/ti:1).

***Arnica montana* L.**
VN: Arnica; Mountain arnica (E). Arnika (G). Arnica (des montagnes) (F).
KE: Flower permitted for external use only. CI: Hypersensitivity. AE: local reactions. No I [BAnz nr.228 05.12.84].
SZ: Flower permitted as tea or tincture for external use only.
CI: Hypersensitivity to sesquiterpene lactones. AE: allergic reactions. The tincture should not be applied in undiluted form.
FR: Flower-head permitted for external use only (toxicological categories pd:- ht/ae/wa:1 sa/ti:1).
SW: Classified as a drug, which must normally be registered as pharmaceutical speciality.
AS: *Arnica montana* is a protected plant species [34]. KE and FR also allow *Arnica chamissonis* Less. ssp. *foliosa* (Nutt.) Maguire as source plant.

***Artemisia absinthium* L.**
VN: Wormwood (E). Wermut (G). Absinthe (grande) (F).
KE: Herb permitted for oral use. No CI, AE, I. The essential oil should not be used as such [BAnz nr.228 05.12.84].
SZ: Herb permitted as herbal tea. CI: GI-ulcer. No AE, I. Beware of the toxicity of high doses.
FR: Leaf and flowering top permitted for oral use (toxicological categories pd:2 ht/ae/wa:1 sa/ti:2).
SW: Classified as a drug, which must normally be registered as pharmaceutical speciality.

***Artemisia dracunculus* L.**
VN: Tarragon (E). Esdragon (G). Estragon (F).
FR: Aerial parts permitted for oral use (toxicological categories pd:1 ht/ae/wa:1 sa/ti:1).

***Artemisia vulgaris* L.**
VN: Mugwort (E). Gemeiner Beifuß (G). Armoise (commune) (F).
KE: Herb and root not permitted for therapeutic use. Usefulness is not documented adequately. An abortive effect and allergic reactions have been described [BAnz nr.122 06.07.88].
FR: Leaf and flowering top permitted for oral use (toxicological categories pd:2 ht/ae/wa:1 sa/ti:2). The level of active constituent has to be limited.

***Ascophyllum nodosum* Le Jol.**
RM: See *Fucus vesiculosus* L.

***Asparagus officinalis* L.**
VN: Asparagus (E). Spargelkraut (G). Asperge (F).
KE: Rhizome permitted for oral use. CI: inflammatory renal diseases. AE: allergic skin reactions (very rarely). No I [BAnz nr.127 12.07.91].
Herb not permitted for therapeutic use. Usefulness is not documented adequately. Allergic reactions occur very rarely [BAnz nr.127 12.07.91].

***Aspidosperma quebracho-blanco* Schlecht.**
VN: Quebracho (E). Quebracho (G). Quebracho (F).
SW: Classified as natural product.

***Asphalatus contaminatus* (Thb.) Druce**
VN: Red bush tea, rooibos tea (E).
SW: Classified as natural product.

***Astragalus gummifer* Labill.**
FR: The gummy exudation from trunk and branches (tragacanth) is permitted as laxative.
AS: Related species [FR].

***Astragalus mongolicus* Bunge**
SW: Classified as a drug, which must normally be registered as pharmaceutical speciality.

***Atropa belladonna* L.**
VN: Belladonna (E). Tollkirsche (G). Belladonne (F).

KE: Leaf and root permitted for oral use. CI, AE, I of belladonna alkaloids [BAnz nr.223 30.11.85].
SW: Classified as a drug, which must normally be registered as pharmaceutical speciality.

***Avena sativa* L.**
VN: Oat (E). (Grüner) Hafer (G). Avoine (cultivée) (F).
KE: Fruit not permitted for therapeutic use. Usefulness is not documented adequately. No risks are known, however, except for rare hypersensitivity to oat's gluten [BAnz nr.85 05.05.88].
Herb not permitted for therapeutic use. Usefulness is not documented adequately. No risks are known, however [BAnz nr.193 15.10.87].
Straw permitted for external use only. No CI, AE, I [BAnz nr.193 15.10.87].
FR: Fruit permitted as laxative.
SW: Classified as natural product.

***Ballota nigra* L. = *Ballota foetida* Lam.**
VN: Black horehound (E). Schwarzer Andorn; Schwarznessel (G).
Ballote fétide; Ballote noire; Marrube noir (F).
FR: Flowering top permitted for oral use (toxicologial categories pd:2 ht/ae/wa:1 sa/ti:1).

***Balsamita major* Desf.**
VN: Balsamite (odorante); Menthe-coq (F).
FR: Leaf and flowering top permitted for oral use (toxicological categories pd:2 ht/ae/wa:1 sa/ti:1).

***Baptisia tinctoria* R. Br.**
VN: Wild indigo (E).
SW: Classified as a drug, which must normally be registered as pharmaceutical speciality.

***Barosma betulina* Bartl.**
VN: Buchu (E). Bucco (strauch) (G). Buchu (F).
KE: Leaf not permitted for therapeutic use. Usefulness is not documented adequately. Contains irritating essential oil with diosphenol and pulegone. No poisonings have been reported, however, and the plant may be used as admixture to herbal teas [BAnz nr.22a 01.02.90].
FR: Leaf permitted for oral use (toxicological categories pd:2 ht/ae/wa:1 sa/ti:1).
SW: Classified as natural product.
AS: *Barosma crenata* Sweet., *Barosma crenulata* Hook., and *Barosma serratifoliata* Willd. [FR].

Berberis vulgaris **L.**

VN: Common barberry (E). Berberitze; Sauerdorn (G). Epine-vinette (F).

KE: Fruit, bark, root bark and root not permitted for therapeutic use. Usefulness is not documented adequately. No risks are known for the fruit, but other plant parts contain the alkaloid berberine, which can be toxic in doses higher than 0.5 g. Actual poisonings have not been reported [BAnz nr.43 02.03.89].

Betula pendula **Roth =** ***Betula alba*** **L. =** ***Betula verrucosa*** **Ehrh.**

VN: Birch (E). Hänge-Birke (G). Bouleau blanc (F).

KE: Leaf permitted for oral use. No CI, AE, I [BAnz nr.50 13.03.86].

SZ: Leaf permitted as herbal tea. CI: Edema due to cardiac or renal insufficiency. No AE, I.

FR: Leaf permitted for oral use (toxicological categories pd:2 ht/ae/wa:1 sa/ti:1).

BE: Leaf permitted as traditional diuretic.

SW: Classified as natural product.

AS: *Betula pubescens* Ehrh. [KE,SZ,FR].

Borago officinalis **L.**

VN: Borage (E). Boretsch (G). Bourrache (F).

KE: Herb and flowers not permitted for therapeutic use. Usefulness is not documented adequately. Risks: borage contains hepatotoxic and carcinogenic pyrrolizidine alkaloids [BAnz nr.127 12.07.91].

FR: Flower permitted for oral use (toxicological categories pd:2 ht/ae/wa:1 sa/ti:1).

SW: Classified as natural product.

Brassica campestris **L.**

VN: Colza (E). Rübsen (G). Colza (F).

SW: Classified as natural product.

Bryonia alba **L.**

VN: Bryony (E). Zaunrübe (G). Bryone officinale (F).

KE: Root not permitted for therapeutic use. The root is a drastic laxative and emetic, while other therapeutic uses are not documented adequately. Contains toxic cucurbitacins [BAnz nr.122 06.07.88].

SW: Classified as a drug, which must normally be registered as pharmaceutical speciality.

AS: *Bryonia cretica* L. ssp. *dioica* (Jacq.) Tutin [KE].

Calamintha officinalis **Moench. =** ***Melissa calamintha*** **L.**

VN: Calamint (E). Bergmelisse; Kalamint (G). Calament (F).

FR: Flowering top permitted for oral use (toxicological categories pd:1 ht/ae/wa:1 sa/ti:1).

***Calendula officinalis* L.**
VN: Goldbloom; Marigold (E). Goldblume; Ringelblume (G). Souci (des jardins) (F).
KE: Flower-head permitted for external use and local use in the mouth. No CI, AE, I [BAnz nr.50 13.03.86].
SZ: Flower-head permitted as herbal tea for local use in the mouth. No CI, AE, I. Also permitted as herbal tea admixture for oral use.
FR: Flower-head permitted for external use (toxicological categories pd:1 ht/ae/wa:1 sa/ti:1). Also permitted as herbal tea admixture for oral use.
BE: Flower-head permitted as traditional topical soothing agent.
SW: Classified as natural product.

***Calluna vulgaris* (L.) Hull. = *Erica vulgaris* L.**
VN: Common heather (E). Heidekraut (G). Callune vulgaire; Fausse bruyère (F).
KE: Herb and flower not permitted for therapeutic use. Usefulness is not documented adequately. No risks are known, however, and there is no objection to the use as an admixture [BAnz nr.101 01.06.90].
FR: Flowering top permitted for oral use (toxicological categories pd:2 ht/ae/wa:1 sa/ti:1).
SW: Classified as natural product.

***Camellia sinensis* (L.) O. Kuntze = *Camellia thea* Link. = *Thea sinensis* L.**
VN: Tea (E). Tee (G). Théier (F).
FR: Leaf permitted for oral use (toxicological categories pd:2 ht/ae/wa:1 sa/ti:1).
BE: Leaf permitted as traditional diurectic.
SW: Classified as foodstuff and as natural product.
AS: FR specifies *Camellia thea* Link. and cultivated varieties.

***Cananga odorata* (Lam.) Hook.f. et Thoms.**
VN: Ylang-ylang (E). Ylang-ylang (G). Ylang-ylang (F).
SW: Classified as foodstuff.

***Capsella bursa-pastoris* (L.) Med.**
VN: Shepherd's purse (E). Hirtentäschel (G). Bourse à pasteur (F).
KE: Herb permitted for oral use. No CI, AE, I [BAnz nr.173 18.09.86].
SZ: Herb permitted as herbal tea. No CI, AE, I. Physician should be consulted when the bleeding continues.
FR: Aerial parts permitted for oral use (toxicological categories pd:2 ht/ae/wa:1 sa/ti:2).
SW: Classified as natural product.

***Capsicum annuum* L.**
VN: Paprika (E). Paprika (G). Paprika (F).

KE: Fruit (low-capsaicin varieties) not permitted for therapeutic use. Usefulness is not documented adequately. No risks are known, however, except for rare hypersensitivity reactions [BAnz nr.80 27.04.89].
SW: Classified as natural product.

***Capsicum frutescens* L.**
VN: Cayenne pepper (E). Cayennepfeffer (G). Piment de Cayenne (F).
KE: Fruit permitted for external use only. CI: damaged skin, hypersensitivity. AE: irritant properties; rarely allergic reactions. No I. Not to be used for more than 2 days [BAnz nr.22a 01.02.90].

***Carex arenaria* L.**
VN: Sandcarex (E). Deutsche Sarsaparilla; Deutsche Sandsegge (G). Laîche des sables; Salsepareille d'Allemagne (F).
KE: Rhizome not permitted for therapeutic use. Usefulness is not documented adequately. Contains irritating saponins [BAnz nr.101 01.06.90].

***Carica papaya* L.**
VN: Melontree (E). Melonenbaum (G). Papayer (commun) (F).
KE: Leaf not permitted for therapeutic use. Usefulness is not documented adequately. There are other more effective agents to treat intestinal infections, but no direct risks are known [BAnz nr.193 15.10.87].
FR: Leaf permitted for oral use (toxicological categories pd:1 ht/ae/wa:1 sa/ti:-).
Fruit juice permitted for oral use (toxicological categories pd:1 ht/ae/wa:- sa/ti:-).
SW: Classified as foodstuff.

***Carum carvi* L.**
VN: Caraway (E). Kümmel (G). Carvi; Cumin des prés (F).
KE: Fruit permitted for oral use. No CI, AE, I [BAnz nr.22a 01.02.90]
Essential oil permitted for oral use. No CI, AE, I for daily doses of 3–6 drops [BAnz nr.22a 01.02.90].
SZ: Fruit permitted as herbal tea. No CI, AE, I.
FR: Fruit permitted for oral use (toxicological categories pd:1 ht/ae/wa:1 sa/ti:1).
SW: Classified as foodstuff and as natural product.

***Cassia angustifolia* Vahl.**
VN: Tinnevelly senna (E). Tinnevelly-Senna (G). Séné de l'Inde; Séné de Tinnevelly (F).
KE: Leaf and fruit permitted for oral use. CI, AE, and I of anthranoid laxatives [BAnz nr.228 05.12.84].

SZ: Leaf and fruit permitted as herbal tea. CI, AE, and I of anthranoid laxatives.
FR: Leaf and fruit permitted for short-term oral use (max. 8–10 days) as a laxative by adults and children of 12 years and older. CI, AE and I of anthranoid laxatives (except for lactation).
BE: Leaf, fruit and dry extracts permitted as traditional laxative. Max. 10 daily doses per package.
SW: Classified as natural product with a dose limitation and as a drug, which must normally be registered as pharmaceutical speciality.

Cassia fistula **L.**
VN: Purging cassia (E). Purgierkassie; Röhrenkassie (G). Casse-muette (F).
FR: Fruit pulp permitted for short-term oral use (max. 8–10 days) as a laxative by adults and children of 12 years and older. CI, AE and I of anthranoid laxatives.

Cassia senna **L. =** ***Cassia acutifolia*** **Del.**
VN: Alexandrian senna (E). Alexandriner-Senna (G). Séné d'Alexandrie; Séné de Khartoum (F).
KE: Leaf and fruit permitted for oral use. CI, AE, and I of anthranoid laxatives [BAnz nr.228 05.12.84].
SZ: Leaf and fruit permitted as herbal tea. CI, AE, and I of anthranoid laxatives.
FR: Leaf and fruit permitted for short-term oral use (max. 8–10 days) as a laxative by adults and children of 12 years and older. CI, AE and I of anthranoid laxatives (except for lactation).
BE: Leaf, fruit and dry extracts permitted as traditional laxative Max. 10 daily doses per package.
SW: Classified as a drug, which must normally be registered as pharmaceutical speciality.

Castanea sativa **Miller =** ***Castanea vulgaris*** **Lam.**
VN: Chestnut (E). Echte Kastanie; Edelkastanie (G). Châtaignier (commun) (F).
KE: Leaf not permitted for therapeutic use. Usefulness is not documented adequately. No risks are known, however [BAnz nr.76 23.04.87].
SW: Classified as natural product.

Centaurea cyanus **L. =** ***Cyanus arvensis*** **Moench.**
VN: Cornflower (E). Blaue Kornblume (G). Bleuet (F).
KE: Flower not permitted for therapeutic use. Usefulness is not documented adequately. No risks are known, however, and there is no objection to the use as admixture [BAnz nr.43 02.03.89].
SZ: Addition of flower to certain herbal tea mixtures is permitted.

FR: Flower-head permitted for external use (toxicological categories pd:- ht/ae/wa:1 sa/ti:-). Also permitted as herbal tea admixture for oral use.
SW: Classified as natural product.

***Centaurium minus* Moench. = *Erythraea centaurium* (L.) Pers.**
VN: European Centaury (E). Tausendgüldenkraut (G). Centaurée (petite); Erythrée (F).
KE: Herb permitted for oral use. No CI, AE, I [BAnz nr.122 06.07.88].
SZ: Herb permitted as herbal tea. CI: GI-ulcer. No AE, I.
FR: Flowering top permitted for oral use (toxicological categories pd:2 ht/ae/wa:1 sa/ti:1).
BE: Flowering top permitted as traditional appetite stimulant.
SW: *Centaurium* species are classified as natural product.

***Centella asiatica* Durban = *Hydrocotyle asiatica* L.**
VN: Gotu Kola; Hydrocotyle; Indian pennywort (E). Asiatischer Wassernabel (G). Hydrocotyle (F).
FR: Entire plant permitted for external use only (toxicological categories pd:- ht/ae/wa:1 sa/ti:1).

***Cephaelis ipecacuanha* A. Rich. = *Uragoga ipecacuanha* (Willd.) Baill.**
VN: Ipecacuanha (E). Ipecacuanha (G). Ipécacuanha (F).
SW: Classified as a drug, which must normally be registered as pharmaceutical speciality.
AS: *Cephaelis acuminata* Karsten [34].

***Ceratonia siliqua* L.**
VN: Carobtree (E). Bockshornbaum (G). Caroubier (F).
FR: Seed and fruit without seed permitted for oral use (toxicological categories pd:1 ht/ae/wa:1 sa/ti:-).
SW: Classified as natural product.

***Cetraria islandica* (L.) Acharius = *Lichen islandicus* L.**
VN: Iceland moss (E). Isländisches Moos (G). Lichen d'Islande; Mousse d'Islande (F).
KE: Thallus permitted for oral use. No CI, AE, I [BAnz nr.43 02.03.89].
SZ: Thallus permitted as herbal tea. No CI, AE, I.
SW: Classified as natural product.
AS: *Cetraria ericetorum* Opiz = *Cetraria tenuifolia* (Retz.) Howe [34].

***Chamaemelum nobile* (L.) All. = *Anthemis nobilis* L.**
VN: Roman Chamomile (E). Römische Kamille (G). Camomille romaine (F).

SZ: Flower-head permitted as herbal tea. No CI, AE, I.
FR: Flower-head permitted for oral use (toxicological categories pd:1 ht/ae/wa:1 sa/ti:1).
BE: Flower-head permitted as traditional digestive aid, as traditional stomatological and as traditional topical soothing agent.
SW: Classified as natural product.

***Chasmanthera palmata* Baill.**
VN: Calumba (E). Kolombo (G). Colombo (F).
FR: Root permitted for oral use (toxicological categories pd:2 ht/ae/wa:1 sa/ti:1).

***Chelidonium majus* L.**
VN: (Greater) celandine (E). Schöllkraut (G). Chélidoine (F).
KE: Herb permitted for oral use. No CI, AE, I [BAnz nr.90 15.05.85].
SW: Classified as a drug, which must normally be registered as pharmaceutical speciality.

***Chenopodium album* L.**
VN: Fat hen; Lamb's-quarters (E). Weißer Gänsefuß (G).
SW: Classified as natural product.

Chlorella ellipsoidea
SW: Classified as natural product.

***Chondrus crispus* (L.) Stack. = *Fucus crispus* L.**
VN: Irish Moss (E). Irländisches Moos; Karrageen (G). Carragaheen; Mousse d'Irlande (F).
FR: Thallus permitted as laxative.

***Chrysanthemum indicum* L.**
SW: Classified as a drug, which must normally be registered as pharmaceutical speciality.

***Chrysanthemum vulgare* (L.) Bernh. = *Tanacetum vulgare* L.**
VN: Common tansy (E). Rainfarn (G). Tanaisie (F).
KE: Flower and herb not permitted for therapeutic use. Usefulness is not documented adequately. Contains essential oil with neurotoxic thujone in such amounts that normal doses may already be toxic [BAnz nr.122 06.07.88].
SW: Classified as natural product.

***Cichorium intybus* L.**
VN: Chicory (E). Cichorie; Wegwarte (G). Chicorée (F).
KE: Herb and root permitted for oral use CI: hypersensitivity to chicory

and other Asteraceae. AE: rare allergic skin reactions. No I [BAnz nr.76 23.04.87]. Patients with bile-stones should first consult a physician [BAnz nr.164 01.09.90].

FR: Root permitted for oral use (toxicological categories pd:1 ht/ae/wa:1 sa/ti:1).

SW: Root classified as natural product.

AS: KE specifies var. *intybus* = *Cichorium intybus* L. var. *sylvestre* Visiani.

***Cimicifuga racemosa* (L.) Nutt. = *Actaea racemosa* L.**

VN: Black snakeroot; Rattleroot (E). Amerikanisches Wanzenkraut; Schwarze Schlangenwurzel (G). Actée à grappes; Herbe au punaise (F).

KE: Rhizome permitted for oral use. No CI, I. AE: occasionally gastric complaints. Not to be used for more than 6 months [BAnz nr.43 02.03.89].

SW: Classified as a drug, which must normally be registered as pharmaceutical speciality.

***Cinchona pubescens* Vahl = *Cinchona succirubra* Pavon**

VN: Cinchona (E). Fieberrinde; (Rote) Chinarinde (G). Quina; Quinquina (F).

KE: Bark permitted for oral use. CI: pregnancy, hypersensitivity. AE: allergic reactions, rarely thrombocytopaenia. I: potentiation of coumarin derivatives [BAnz nr.22a 01.02.90].

SZ: Bark permitted as herbal tea. CI: pregnancy, hypersensitivity, GI-ulcer. AE: allergic skin reactions, fever, rarely thrombocytopaenia. No I. Overdosing or prolonged use may produce toxic effects.

FR: Stem bark permitted for oral use (toxicological categories pd:1 ht/ae/wa:1 sa/ti:1).

AS: Varieties of *Cinchona pubescens* and hybrides with related *Cinchona* species [KE,34]. FR also allows *Cinchona officinalis* and varieties, *Cinchona calisaya* Wedd. and *Cinchona ledgeriana* Moens ex Trim.

RM: SZ also comprises a monograph for composed cinchona tincture with the same CI and AE.

***Cinnamomum aromaticum* Nees = *Cinnamomum cassia* Blume**

VN: Cassia bark (E). Chinesischer Zimtbaum (G). Cannellier de Chine (F).

KE: Bark permitted for oral use. CI: hypersensitivity to cinnamon or Peruviuan balsam; pregnancy. AE: often allergic reactions of skin and mucosae. No I [BAnz nr.22a 01.02.90].
Flower not permitted for therapeutic use. Usefulness is not documented adequately. The flower can be used to correct taste, however. CI: Hypersensitivity to cinnamon or Peruvian balsam, pregnancy. AE: allergic skin reactions and mucosal reactions [BAnz nr.49 11.03.92].

FR: Stem bark permitted for oral use (toxicological categories pd:1 ht/ae/wa:1 sa/ti:1).

***Cinnamomum camphora* (L.) Siebold**

VN: Camphor tree (E). Kampferbaum (G). Camphrier (F).

KE: Camphor is permitted for internal and external use. CI (for external use): damaged skin; camphor preparations should not be applied near the nose of infants and small children. AE: contact eczema. No I [BAnz nr.228 05.12.84].

SW: Classified as natural product.

***Cinnamomum verum* J.S. Presl = *Cinnamomum zeylanicum* Blume**

VN: Cinnamon (E). Zimt (G). Cannelle (F).

KE: Bark permitted for oral use. CI: hypersensitivity to cinnamon or Peruvian balsam. AE: often allergic reactions of skin and mucosae. No I [BAnz nr.22a 01.02.90].

SZ: Bark permitted as herbal tea. CI: GI-ulcer, pregnancy. No AE, I.

FR: Stem bark permitted for oral use (toxicological categories pd:1 ht/ae/wa:1 sa/ti:1).

***Cistanche salsa* (C.A. Mey.) G. Beck**

SW: Classified as a drug, which must normally be registered as pharmaceutical speciality.

***Citrullus colocynthis* (L.) Schrad.**

VN: Colocynth (E). Koloquinthe (G). Coloquinte (F).

KE: Fruit not permitted for therapeutic use. Is a drastic laxative, and usefulness for other purposes is not documented adequately. Contains up to 3% of toxic cucurbitacins [BAnz nr.164 01.09.90].

***Citrus aurantium* L. ssp. *amara* Engler**

VN: Bitter orange (E). Bitterorange; Pomeranzenbaum (G). Bigaradier; Oranger (à fruit) amer (F).

KE: Peel permitted for oral use. No CI, AE, I, except for photosensitivity [BAnz nr.193 15.10.87].

SZ: Peel permitted as herbal tea. CI: GI-ulcer. No AE, I. Addition of the flower to certain herbal tea mixtures is also permitted.

FR: Peel, flower and leaf permitted for oral use (toxicological categories pd:1 ht/ae/wa:1 sa/ti:1).

BE: Flower, leaf, powder and tincture permitted as traditional tranquillizer. Peel permitted as traditional appetite stimulant.

***Citrus aurantium* L. ssp. *dulcis* Pers.**

VN: (Sweet) orange (E). Apfelsine (G). Orange douce; Oranger (à fruit) doux (F).

KE: Peel permitted for oral use. No CI, AE, I [BAnz nr.22a 01.02.90].

FR: Peel, flower and leaf permitted for oral use (toxicological categories pd:1 ht/ae/wa:1 sa/ti:1).

***Claviceps purpurea* Tul.**

VN: Ergot of rye (E). Mutterkorn (G). Ergot de seigle (F).

SW: The sclerotium of this fungus (secale cornutum) is classified as a drug, which must normally be registered as pharmaceutical speciality.

***Clematis vitalba* L.**

VN: Old men's beard; Travellers joy (E). Echte Waldrebe; Gemeine Waldrebe (G). Clématite (F).

SW: Classified as a drug, which must normally be registered as pharmaceutical speciality.

***Cnicus benedictus* L.**

VN: Blessed thistle (E). (Echtes) Benediktenkraut; Karbobenedikten (G). Chardon bénit (F).

KE: Herb permitted for oral use. CI: hypersensitivity to the plant and other Asteraceae. AE: allergic reactions. No I [BAnz nr.193 15.10.87].

***Cochlearia officinalis* L.**

VN: Scurvy grass (E). (Echtes) Löffelkraut (G). Cochléaire; Herbe aux cuillières (F).

FR: Leaf permitted for oral use (toxicological categories pd:1 ht/ae/wa:1 sa/ti:1).

***Coffea arabica* L.**

VN: Coffee (E). Kaffee (G). Café (F).

KE: Coal permitted for oral use. No CI, AE. I: absorption of other drugs taken simultaneously might be reduced [BAnz nr.85 05.05.88].

AS: *Coffea liberica* Bull and *Coffea canephora* Pierre [KE].

***Cola nitida* (Vent.) Schott et Endl.**

VN: Cola (E). Kola (G). Cola; Kolatier (F).

KE: Seed permitted for oral use. CI: gastric and duodenal ulcers. AE: trouble in sleeping, hyperexcitability, nervousness. I: effect enhanced by psychoanaleptic drugs and caffeine-containing beverages [BAnz nr.127 12.07.91].

FR: Seed permitted for oral use (toxicological categories pd:1 ht/ae/wa:1 sa/ti:1).

SW: Classified as natural product.

AS: *Cola acuminata* Schott. et Endl. and related species [KE,FR].

***Colchicum autumnale* L.**

VN: Meadow saffron (E). Herbstzeitlose (G). Colchique (F).

SW: Classified as a drug, which must normally be registered as pharmaceutical speciality.

***Combretum micranthum* G.Don = *Combretum altum* Guill. et Perr. ex DC.**

VN: Combretum (E). Combretum; Kinkeliba (G). Combretum; Kinkéliba (F).

FR: Leaf permitted for oral use (toxicological categories pd:2 ht/ae/wa:1 sa/ti:1).

***Commiphora molmol* Engler**

VN: Myrrh (E). (Echte) Myrrhe (G). Commiphora; Myrrhe (F).

KE: Gum-resin from bark (myrrha) permitted for local use in mouth only. No CI, AE, I [BAnz nr.193 15.10.87].

SZ: Gum-resin from bark (myrrha) permitted as tincture for local use in mouth only. No CI, AE, I. Undiluted tincture may produce burning and local irritation.

FR: Gum-resin permitted for external use only (toxicological categories pd:- ht/ae/wa:- sa/ti:1).

SW: *Commiphora molmol* is classified as natural product, whereas *Commiphora mukul* is classified as a drug, which must normally be registered as pharmaceutical speciality.

AS: The gum-resin of other *Commiphora* species may also be used, when its chemical composition is similar to that of the gum-resin of *C.molmol* [34]. FR also allows *Commiphora abyssinica* Engl. and *Commiphora mukul* Engl.

***Convallaria majalis* L.**

VN: Lily of the valley (E). Maiglöckchen (G). Muguet (F).

KE: Herb permitted for oral use. CI, AE and I of cardiac glycosides [BAnz nr.76 23.04.87].

SW: Classified as a drug, which must normally be registered as pharmaceutical speciality.

***Copaifera reticulata* Ducke**

VN: Copaiba (E). Copaiva (G). Copahu (F).

SW: Balsam is classified as natural product.

***Coriandrum sativum* L.**

VN: Coriander (E). Koriander (G). Coriandre (F).

KE: Fruit permitted for oral use. No CI, AE, I [BAnz nr.173 18.09.86].

SZ: Fruit permitted as herbal tea. No CI, AE, I.

FR: Fruit permitted for oral use (toxicological categories pd:1 ht/ae/wa:1 sa/ti:1).

SW: Classified as natural product.

AS: KE specifies var. *vulgare* Alefeld (= var. *macrocarpum*) and var. *microcarpum* DC.

***Cordyceps sinensis* (Berkeley) Saccardo**

SW: Classified as a drug, which must normally be registered as pharmaceutical speciality.

***Cornus officinalis* Sieb. et Zucc. = *Macrocarpium officinale* Nakai**

SW: Classified as a drug, which must normally be registered as pharmaceutical speciality.

***Corydalis ambigua* Cham. et Schlecht.**

SW: Classified as a drug, which must normally be registered as pharmaceutical speciality.

***Corylus avellana* L.**

VN: Hazel (E). Gemeine Hasel; Haselnußstrauch (G). Coudrier; Noisetier (F).

FR: Leaf permitted for oral use (toxicological categories pd:2 ht/ae/wa:1 sa/ti:1).

SW: Classified as natural product.

***Crataegus oxyacantha* L. = *Crataegus laevigata* (Poir.) DC.**

VN: Hawthorn (E). Weißdorn (G). Aubépine; Épine blanche (F).

KE: Leaf with flower and fruit permitted for oral use. No CI, AE, I [BAnz nr.1 03.01.84].

SZ: Leaf with flower permitted as herbal tea. No CI, AE, I.

FR: Flower and flowering top permitted for oral use (toxicological categories pd:2 ht/ae/wa:1 sa/ti:1).

SW: Classified as natural product.

AS: *Crataegus monogyna* Jacq. [KE,FR] and *Crataegus oxyacanthoides* Thuill. [FR].

***Crocus sativus* L.**

VN: Saffron (E). Safran (G). Safran (F).

KE: Stigma not permitted for therapeutic use. Usefulness is not documented adequately. Up to now, no risks have been documented for daily doses up to 1.5 g. However, 5 g is toxic, 10 g is abortive and 20 g is lethal [BAnz nr.76 23.04.87].

FR: Stigma permitted for external use only (toxicological categories pd:1 ht/ae/wa:1 sa/ti:1).

SW: Classified as foodstuff.

***Cucurbita pepo* L.**

VN: Pumpkin (E). Gartenkürbis; Kürbis (G). Courge; Pépon (F).

KE: Seed permitted for oral use. No CI, AE, I [BAnz nr.223 30.11.85]. As improvement is symptomatic (i.e., no elimination of prostatic hypertrophy), a physician should be consulted regularly [BAnz nr.11 17.01.91].
SZ: Seed permitted as such. No CI, AE, I.
SW: Classified as natural product.
AS: KE also allows cultivars of *C. pepo* L. A German pharmacognostic text book specifies the convar. *citrullina* I. Greb. var. *styriaca* I. Greb. and also mentions *C. maxima* Duch. (Riesenkürbis, Melonenkürbis), *C. moschata* Duch. ex. Poir. (Bisamkürbis, Moschuskürbis), *C. mixta* Pang. and *C. ficifolia* Bouche as potential source plants [34].

***Cupressus sempervirens* L.**
VN: Cypress (E). Immergrüne Zypresse (G). Cyprès (F).
FR: Cone permitted for oral use (toxicological categories pd:- ht/ae/wa:1 sa/ti:1).
SW: Classified as natural product.

***Curcuma domestica* Val. = *Curcuma longa* L.**
VN: Turmeric (E). Gelbwurzel; Kurkuma (G). Curcuma (long); Safran des Indes (F).
KE: Rhizome permitted for oral use. CI: biliary obstruction. No AE, I [BAnz nr.223 30.11.85 and BAnz nr.164 01.09.90].
FR: Rhizome permitted for oral use (toxicological categories pd:1 ht/ae/wa:1 sa/ti:1).
BE: Rhizome permitted as traditional cholagogue.
SW: Classified as natural product.

***Curcuma xanthorrhiza* Roxb.**
VN: Temu lawak (E). Gelbwurz, Javanische (G). Témoé-Lawaq (F).
KE: Rhizome permitted for oral use. CI: biliary obstruction. AE: GI-irritation from continued use. No I [BAnz nr.122 06.07.88 and BAnz nr.164 01.09.90].
SZ: Addition to certain herbal tea mixtures is permitted.
FR: Rhizome was permitted for oral use by the first French phytotherapeutical guideline issued in 1986 [8].
BE: Rhizome permitted as traditional cholagogue.

***Curcuma zedoaria* (Christmann) Rosc.**
VN: Zedoary (E). Zitwer (G). Zédoaire (F).
KE: Rhizome not permitted for therapeutic use. Usefulness is not documented adequately. No risks are known, however [BAnz nr.122 06.07.88].

***Cyamopsis tetragonolobus* L. = *Cyanopsis tetragonoloba* (L.) Taub.**
VN: Guar (E). Guar (G). Cyamopsis; Guar (F).

FR: Seed and gum permitted for oral use (toxicological categories pd:1 ht/ae/wa:- sa/ti:-).
SW: Classified as foodstuff.

***Cymbopogon citratus* (DC.) Stapf.**
KE: Herb and essential oil not permitted for therapeutic use. Usefulness is not documented adequately. Allergic contact dermatitis occurs rarely. There is no objection to the use of low citral herb/oil as admixture [BAnz nr.22a 01.02.90].

***Cymbopogon flexuosus* Stapf.**
SW: Classified as natural product.

***Cymbopogon nardus* Rendle**
KE: Herb not permitted for therapeutic use. Usefulness is not documented adequately. Allergic contact dermatitis occurs rarely. There is no objection to the use of low citral herb as admixture [BAnz nr.22a 01.02.90].
SW: Classified as natural product.

***Cymbopogon winterianus* Jowitt**
KE: Essential oil not permitted for therapeutic use. Usefulness is not documented adequately. Allergic contact dermatitis occurs rarely. There is no objection to the use of low citral oil as admixture [BAnz nr.22a 01.02.90].

***Cynara scolymus* L. = *Cynara cardunculus* L.**
VN: Artichoke (E). Artischocke (G). Artichaut (F).
KE: Leaf permitted for oral use. CI: hypersensitivity to artichoke and other Asteraceae; biliary obstruction. No AE, I [BAnz nr.122 06.07.88 and BAnz nr.164 01.09.90].
FR: Leaf permitted for oral use (toxicological categories pd:2 ht/ae/wa:1 sa/ti:1).
BE: Leaf permitted as traditional diuretic and as traditional cholagogue.
SW: Leaf classified as natural product.

***Cynoglossum officinale* L. = *Cynoglossum clandestinum* Desf.**
VN: Hound's-tongue (E). Hundszunge (G). Cynoglosse (F).
KE: Herb not permitted for therapeutic use. Usefulness is not documented adequately. Risks: high level of hepatotoxic pyrrolizidine alkaloids [BAnz nr.43 02.03.89].

***Datura stramonium* L.**
VN: Thornapple (E). Stechapfel (G). Stramoine (F).

KE: Leaf and seed not permitted for oral use. Usefulness is not documented adequately. Contains toxic belladonna alkaloids [BAnz nr.22a 01.02.90].
SW: Classified as a drug, which must normally be registered as pharmaceutical speciality.

***Daucus carota* L.**
VN: Carrot (E). Karotte; Mohrrübe (G). Carotte (F).
SW: Classified as natural product.

***Delphinium consolida* L. = *Consolida regalis* S.F. Gray**
VN: (Forking) larkspur (E). Rittersporn (G). Dauphinelle consoude; Pied d'alouette (F).
KE: Flower not permitted for therapeutic use. Usefulness is not documented adequately. The plant contains toxic alkaloids, but there are no reliable data on the alkaloid level in the flowers. There is no objection to the use as admixture to herbal teas in levels up to 1% [BAnz nr.80 27.04.89].
SW: Classified as natural product.

***Digitalis purpurea* L.**
VN: Purple foxglove (E). Purpurroter Fingerhut (G). Digitale pourprée (F).
SW: Classified as a drug, which must normally be registered as pharmaceutical speciality.

***Dioscorea* species**
SW: Classified as foodstuff.

***Drosera rotundifolia* L.**
VN: Sundew (E). Sonnentau (G). Drosèra; Rosée du soleil (F).
KE: Herb permitted for oral use. No CI, AE, I [BAnz nr.228 05.12.84].
SW: Classified as a drug, which must normally be registered as pharmaceutical speciality.
AS: *Drosera rotundifolia* and related endemic species are all threatened by extinction and are therefore protected plants. The former DDR therefore allowed the use of *Drosera ramentacea* Burch. ex Harv. et Sond (Madagaskar-Sonnentau) as alternative [34].
KE specifies *Drosera rotundifolia* L., *D. ramentacea* Burch. ex Harv. et Sond., *D. longifolia* L. and *D. intermedia* Hayne as source plants.

***Echinacea angustifolia* DC.**
VN: (Black) Sampson; (Narrow leaved) coneflower (E). Schmallblättriger) Sonnenhut (G). Echinacea (F).

SZ: Root permitted as herbal tea. No CI, AE, I. Does not annihilate a medical need of antibiotics.
SW: Classified as natural product.

***Echinacea purpurea* (L.) Moench**
VN: Purpursonnenhut (G).
KE: Herb permitted for oral use. CI: progressive systemic diseases (e.g., tuberculosis, multiple sclerosis). No AE, I. Should not be used for more than 6 weeks [BAnz nr.43 02.03.89].
SW: Classified as natural product.
AS: According to a German text book, the root of *Echinacea purpurea* is used for the same purposes as the root of *Echinacea angustifolia* (see above); both sources are considered equivalent [34].
RM: KE also permits parenteral use. CI: progressive systemic diseases (e.g., tuberculosis, multiple sclerosis), inclination to hypersensitivity, pregnancy. AE: metabolic worsening in diabetic patients; dose-dependent chills, fever, nausea, vomiting; acute allergic reactions. No I. Not to be used for more than 3 weeks.

***Elettaria cardamomum* (L.) Maton**
VN: Lesser cardamom (E). Kardamompflanze (G). Cardamome plante (F).
KE: Fruit permitted for oral use. No CI, AE, I [BAnz nr.223 30.11.85 and BAnz nr.164 01.09.90].
BE: Fruit permitted as traditional cholagogue.

***Eleutherococcus senticosus* Rupr. ex Max.**
VN: Siberian ginseng (E). Taigawurzel (G). Éleuthérocoque (F).
KE: Root permitted for oral use. CI: hypertension. No AE, I [BAnz nr.11 17.01.91].
FR: Subterranean parts permitted for oral use (toxicological categories pd:1 ht/ae/wa:1 sa/ti:2).
SW: Classified as natural product.
AS: FR also allows related species.

***Elymus repens* (L.) Gould = *Agropyron repens* (L.) Beauv.**
VN: Witch grass (E). Gemeine Quecke (G). Chiendent (petit) (F).
KE: Rhizome permitted for oral use. No CI, AE, I [BAnz nr.22a 01.02.90]. Flower permitted for local thermotherapy only. CI: open wounds, acute rheumatic attacks, acute inflammations. AE: allergic skin reactions (very rarely). No I [BAnz nr.85 05.05.88].
SZ: Rhizome permitted as herbal tea. No CI, AE, I.
FR: Rhizome permitted for oral use (toxicological categories pd:1 ht/ae/wa:1 sa/ti:1).

BE: Rhizome permitted as traditional diuretic.
SW: Classified as natural product.
AS: The source plant of the flower cannot be indicated exactly. *Elymus repens* is just one of the plants that mostly occur in the crude drug [34]. KE describes the source plants of Gramini flos more generally as Poaceae.

Enteromorpha linza L.
SW: Classified as natural product.

***Ephedra sinica* Stapf.**
KE: Herb permitted for oral use. CI, AE, I of the major alkaloid, ephedrin. Not to be used for prolonged period [BAnz nr.11 17.01.91].
SW: *Ephedra* species are classified as drugs, which must normally be registered as pharmaceutical speciality.
AS: *E. shennungiana* Tang and other equivalent spp. [KE].

***Equisetum arvense* L.**
VN: Horsetail; Shave grass (E). Ackerschachtelhalm; Schachtelhalm (G). Prêle (des champs) (F).
KE: Herb permitted for oral use. No CI, AE, I [BAnz nr.173 18.09.86].
SZ: Herb permitted as herbal tea. No CI, AE, I.
FR: Sterile aerial parts permitted for oral use (toxicological categories pd:2 ht/ae/wa:1 sa/ti:1).
BE: Herb permitted as traditional diuretic.
SW: Classified as natural product.

***Erica cinerea* L.**
VN: Bruyère cendrée (F).
FR: Flower permitted for oral use (toxicological categories pd:2 ht/ae/wa:1 sa/ti:1).

***Erica tetralix* L.**
VN: Glockenheide (G).
SW: Classified as natural product.

***Erigeron canadensis* L. = *Conyza canadensis* (L.) Cronq.**
VN: Blood stanch; Butter horse (E). Kanadisches Berufskraut; Kanadische Dürrwurz (G). Vergerette du Canada; Vergerolle (F).
FR: Aerial parts permitted for oral use (toxicological categories pd:2 ht/ae/wa:1 sa/ti:2).

***Eriobothrya japonica* Lind.**
VN: Japanische Mispel (G).
SW: Classified (excl. seed) as natural product.

***Erysimum officinale* L. = *Sisymbrium officinale* (L). Scop.**
VN: Hedge mustard (E). Wegerauke (G). Erysimum; Vélar (F).
FR: Flower and flowering top permitted for oral use (toxicological categories pd:1 ht/ae/wa:1 sa/ti:1).

***Erythroxylum coca* Lam.**
VN: Coca (E). Koka (G). Coca (F).
SW: Classified as a drug, which must normally be registered as pharmaceutical speciality.

***Eschscholtzia californica* Cham.**
VN: California poppy; Eschscholtzia (E). Eschscholtzia; Kalifornischer Goldmohn (G). Eschscholtzia (F).
KE: Aerial parts not permitted for therapeutic use. Usefulness is not documented adequately. Risks: use during pregnancy should be avoided, as the major alkaloid cryptopine shows a stimulating effect on guinea pig uterus in vitro [BAnz nr.178 21.09.91].
FR: Aerial parts permitted for oral use (toxicological categories pd:2 ht/ae/wa:1 sa/ti:2). The level of active constituents has to be limited.

***Eucalyptus globulus* Labill.**
VN: Eucalyptus (E). Eucalyptus (G). Eucalyptus (globuleux) (F).
KE: Leaf and essential oil permitted for oral use. CI: gastrointestinal or biliary inflammation, severe hepatic disease. AE: GI-disturbances. I: hepatic enzyme induction by essential oil. Should not be inhaled by small children [BAnz nr.177a 24.09.86].
SZ: Leaf permitted as herbal tea. CI: gastrointestinal or biliary inflammation, severe hepatic disease. AE: GI-disturbances. No I. Should not be used by children younger than 2 years. The oil is also permitted, but inhalation by small children should be avoided.
FR: Leaf permitted for oral use (toxicological categories pd:1 ht/ae/wa:1 sa/ti:1).
BE: Leaf permitted as traditional cough remedy.
SW: *Eucalyptus globulus* and *Eucalyptus eugenioides* are classified as natural products.
AS: KE specifies *Eucalyptus fructicetorum* F. Von Mueller (syn. *E. polybractea* R.T. Baker) and *E. smithii* R.T. Baker as alternative source plants for the oil.

***Eupatorium cannabinum* L.**
VN: Hemp agrimony (E). Gemeiner Wasserdost; Wasserhanf (G). Chanvrin; Eupatoire commune (F).
SW: Classified as a drug, which must normally be registered as pharmaceutical speciality.

***Eupatorium perfoliatum* L.**

VN: Boneset (E). Durchwachsener Wasserhanf (G). Herbe à la fièvre (F).

SW: Classified as a drug, which must normally be registered as pharmaceutical speciality.

***Fagopyrum vulgare* Hill. = *Polygonum fagopyrum* L.**

VN: Buckwheat (E). Buchweizen (G). Blé sarrasin (F).

SW: Classified as natural product.

***Ficus carica* L.**

VN: Fig (E). Feige (G). Figuier (F).

KE: Fruit not permitted for therapeutic use. Usefulness is not documented adequately. No risks are known, however, and there is no objection to the use as an admixture [BAnz nr. 101 01.06.90].

FR: Fruit permitted as laxative.

***Filipendula ulmaria* (L.) Maxim. = *Spiraea ulmaria* L.**

VN: Meadowsweet (E). (Echtes) Mädesüß (G). Reine des prés; Ulmaire (F).

KE: Herb and flower permitted for oral use. No CI, AE or I, except for hypersensitivity to salicylates as CI for the flower [BAnz nr.43 02.03.89].

SZ: Flower permitted as herbal tea. No CI, AE, I.

FR: Flower and flowering top permitted for oral use (toxicological categories pd:2 ht/ae/wa:1 sa/ti:1).

BE: Flowering top permitted as traditional antiarthritic agent.

SW: Classified as natural product.

***Foeniculum vulgare* Mill.**

VN: Fennel (E). Fenchel (G). Aneth fenouil; Fenouil (doux) (F).

KE: Fruit and essential oil permitted for oral use. No CI for herbal teas (and other preparations providing similar doses of essential oil), but other dosage forms (e.g., the essential oil) should be avoided dring pregnancy. The essential oil should also be avoided in infants and small children. AE: isolated cases of allergic reactions of skin and lungs. No I [BAnz nr.74 19.04.91].

SZ: Fruit permitted as herbal tea. No CI, AE, I.

FR: Fruit and root permitted for oral use (toxicological categories pd:1 ht/ae/wa:1 sa/ti:1).

BE: Fruit permitted as traditional digestive aid.

AS: The 9th edition of the Deutsches Arzneibuch specifies var. *vulgare*, whereas the Pharmacopoea Helvetica VII and the Österreiches Arzneibuch also allow var. *dulce* [34]. FR specifies var. *dulce* DC. as source plant.

***Forsythia suspensa* (Thunb.) Vahl.**
SW: Classified as a drug, which must normally be registered as pharmaceutical speciality.

***Fragaria vesca* L.**
VN: Wild strawberry (E). Walderdbeere (G). Fraisier (F).
KE: Leaf not permitted for therapeutic use. Usefulness is not documented adequately. Hypersensitivity reactions are possible, but there is no objection to the use as an admixture to herbal teas [BAnz nr.22a 01.02.90].
FR: Root and rhizome permitted for oral use (toxicological categories pd:2 ht/ae/wa:1 sa/ti:1).
SW: Classified as natural product.
AS: *Fragaria viridis* Duch. and *F. moschata* Duch. [KE].

***Fraxinus excelsior* L.**
VN: Common ash (E). Gemeine Esche (G). Frêne (élevé) (F).
KE: Leaf and bark not permitted for therapeutic use. Usefulness is not documented adequately. No risks are known, however, and use as an admixture is not excluded categorically [BAnz nr.22a 01.02.90].
FR: Leaf permitted for oral use (toxicological categories pd:1 ht/ae/wa:1 sa/ti:1).
SW: Classified as natural product.
BE: Leaf permitted as traditional antiarthritic agent.

***Fraxinus ornus* L.**
VN: Manna-ash (E). Manna-Esche (G). Frêne à la manne ; Orne à manne (F).
KE: Exudation from stem (manna) permitted for oral use. CI: intestinal obstruction. AE: nausea, flatulence. No I [BAnz nr.22a 01.02.90].
FR: Exudation from stem (manna) permitted as laxative.

***Fucus vesiculosus* L.**
VN: Common seawrack; Sea kelp (E). Fucus; Tang (G). Fucus; Varech vésiculeux (F).
KE: Thallus not permitted for therapeutic use. Usefulness is not documented adequately. There are no risks from daily doses up to 150 μg I per day, but higher doses may induce or exacerbate hyperthyreosis and cause hypersensitivity reactions (rarely) [BAnz nr.101 01.06.90].
FR: Thallus permitted for oral use (toxicological categories pd:1 ht/ae/wa:1 sa/ti:-). The level of active constituent has to be limited.
Thallus permitted as laxative. The adult intake of iodine should not exceed 120 μg per day.
SW: *Fucus vesiculosus* is classified as natural product, and *Ascophyllum nodosum* is classified as foodstuff and as natural product.

AS: KE allows the use of *Ascophyllum nodosum* Le Jol. instead of or together with *Fucus vesiculosus* L.
FR also allows *Fucus serratus* L. and related species.

***Fumaria officinalis* L.**
VN: Fumitory (E). Ackerraute; (Echter) Erdrauch (G). Fiel de terre; Fumeterre (F).
KE: Herb permitted for oral use. No CI, AE, I [BAnz nr.173 18.09.86].
SZ: Herb permitted as herbal tea. No CI, AE, I.
FR: Flowering aerial parts permitted for oral use (toxicological categories pd:2 ht/ae/wa:1 sa/ti:1).

Galeopsis segetum Necker = Galeopsis ochroleuca Lam.
VN: Hemp nettle (E). Bleiche Hanfnessel; Hohlzahn (G). Chanvre bâtard; Galéopside (F).
KE: Herb permitted for oral use. No CI, AE, I [BAnz nr.76 23.04.87].
SW: Classified as natural product.

***Galium odoratum* (L.) Scop. = *Asperula odorata* L.**
VN: Woodruff (E). Waldmeister (G). Aspérule odorante (F).
KE: Herb not permitted for therapeutic use. Usefulness is not documented adequately. No riks are known, however [BAnz nr.193 15.10.87].
FR: Aerial parts permitted for oral use (toxicological categories pd:2 ht/ae/wa:1 sa/ti:1).
SW: Classified as natural product.

***Galium verum* L.**
VN: Lady's bedstraw; Yellow galium (E). Echtes Labkraut, Gelbes Labkraut (G). Gaillet jaune, Caille-lait jaune (F).
FR: Aerial parts permitted for oral use (toxicological categories pd:2 ht/ae/wa:1 sa/ti:1).
SW: *Galium aparine* and other *Galium* species are classified as natural product.
AS: FR merely speaks about "gaillet". In France, four different *Galium* spp. are known under this vernacular name: *Galium aparine* L. (gaillet gratteron); *Galium cruciata* (L.) Scop. (gaillet croisette); *Galium mollugo* L. (gaillet blanc); and *Galium verum* L. (gaillet jaune).

***Gaultheria procumbens* L.**
VN: Wintergreen (E). Wintergrün (G). Thé du Canada (F).
SW: Classified as natural product.

***Gelidium corneum* Lmx. = *Fucus spinosus* L.**
VN: Agar(-agar) (E). Agar(-agar) (G). Agar(-agar) (F).

FR: Polysaccharides obtained by extraction (agar-agar) permitted as laxative.
AS: FR permits *Gelidium* spp., *Euchema* spp. and *Gracilaria* spp. as source plants without specifying which species are exactly allowed.

Gelsemium sempervirens **(L.) Ait.**
VN: Yellow jessamine (E). Gelber Jasmin (G). Jasmin sauvage (F).
KE: Rhizome not permitted for therapeutic use. Usefulness is not documented adequately and serious riks are known. The therapeutic window is narrow and many cases of poisoning, including fatal ones, have occurred. Characteristic symptoms of overdosage are dizziness, loss of speech, dysphagia, dry mouth, visual disturbances, trembling of extremities, muscular rigidity or weakness, and falling of the jaw [BAnz nr.178 21.09.91].
SW: Classified as a drug, which must normally be registered as pharmaceutical speciality.

Genista tinctoria **L.**
VN: Dyers weed (E). Färberginster (G). Genêt de teinturies (F).
SZ: Herb permitted as herbal tea. CI: Hypertension. AE: diarrhoea from overdosing. No I.

Gentiana lutea **L.**
VN: Yellow gentian (E). Gelber Enzian (G). Gentiane (jaune) (F).
KE: Root permitted for oral use. CI: gastric and duodenal ulcer. AE: occasionally headache. No I [BAnz nr.223 30.11.85].
SZ: Root permitted as herbal tea. CI: GI-ulcer. AE: occasionally headache. No I.
FR: Subterranean parts permitted for oral use (toxicological categories pd:1 ht/ae/wa:1 sa/ti:1).
BE: Root permitted as traditional appetite stimulant.
SW: Classified as foodstuff and as natural product.
AS: The Arzneibuch of the former DDR also allowed *Gentiana asclepiadea* L., *G.pannonica* Scop., *G.punctata* L. and *G.purpurea* L. [34].

Geranium robertianum **L.**
VN: Robert herb (E). Robertsgeranium; Ruprechtskraut (G). Géranium (herbe à) Robert; Géranium robertin (F).
FR: Entire plant permitted for oral use (toxicological categories pd:2 ht/ae/wa:1 sa/ti:1).

Geum urbanum **L.**
VN: Herb bennet; Wood avens (E). Nelkenwurz (G). Benoîte (F).
FR: Rhizome permitted for oral use (toxicological categories pd:2 ht/ae/wa:1 sa/ti:1).

***Ginkgo biloba* L.**
VN: Maidenhair tree (E). Ginkgobaum (G). Noyer du Japon (F).
SW: Classified as natural product.

***Glechoma hederacea* L. = *Nepeta glechoma* Benth.**
VN: Ground ivy (E). Gundelrebe (G). Lierre terrestre (F).
FR: Aerial parts permitted for oral use (toxicological categories pd:2 ht/ae/wa:1 sa/ti:1).

***Gleditsia triacanthos* L. = *Gleditschia triacanthos* L.**
VN: Gleditschia (F).
FR: Seed permitted as laxative.

***Glycine max* (L.) Merrill**
KE: Phospholipids obtained from seed (lecithinum ex soja) permitted for oral use. No CI, AE, I [BAnz nr.85 05.05.88].

***Glycyrrhiza glabra* L.**
VN: Licorice; Sweetwort (E). Lakritze; Süßholz (G). Bois doux; Réglisse (F).
KE: Root permitted for oral use. CI: Cholestatic liver diseases, liver cirrhosis, hypertension, hypokalaemia, severe renal insufficiency, pregnancy. As prolonged use/higher doses may give mineralocorticoid AE/I, the root should not be used for more than 4–6 weeks without consulting physician. The use to correct taste in doses providing max. 100 mg of glycyrrhizin per day is also allowed [BAnz nr.90 15.05.85, BAnz nr.50 13.03.90, BAnz nr.74 19.04.91 and BAnz nr.178 21.09.91].
SZ: Root permitted as herbal tea. CI: chronic hepatitis, hepatic cirrhosis, hypertension, hypokalaemia. No AE, I. Should not be used for more than 4–6 weeks, as prolonged use may lead to mineralocorticoid effects (including I with cardiac glycosides).
FR: Subterranean parts permitted for oral use (toxicological categories pd:1 ht/ae/wa:1 sa/ti:1). Maximum dosage: infusion: 8 g of root per day; extract: 3 mg/kg of glycyrrhizin per day; powder: 5 g of root per day. Other sources of licorice (beverages, sweets) should be taken into account. CI: not to be taken by hypertensive patient unless prescribed by physician. I: not to be taken together with corticoid treatment.
BE: Root permitted as traditional cough remedy and as traditional digestive aid.
SW: Classified as foodstuff and as natural product.
AS: SW also classifies *Glycyrrhiza uralensis* Fisch. as natural product. Glycyrrhizinic acid is also present in this species [32].

***Grindelia robusta* Nutt.**
VN: Wild sunflower (E). Grindelia (G). Grindélia (F).

KE: Herb permitted for oral use. No CI, AE or I, except for gastric irritation (rarely) [BAnz nr.11 17.01.91].
FR: Flowering top permitted for oral use (toxicological categories pd:2 ht/ae/wa:- sa/ti:1).
BE: Flowering top permitted as traditional cough remedy.
AS: *Grindelia squarrosa* (Pursh) Dunal [KE,FR], *Grindelia camporum* Green and *Grindelia humilis* Hook et Arn. [FR].

***Guajacum officinale* L.**
VN: Guaiacum (E). Guajak (G). Gayac (F).
KE: Wood permitted for oral use. No CI, AE, I [BAnz. nr.76 23.04.87].
AS: *Guajacum sanctum* L. [KE].
RM: The essential oil called "Guajakholzöl" in German comes from another source plant, *Bulnesia sarmienti* Lorents [KE].

***Guarea rusbyi* (Britt.) Rusby = *Sycocarpus rusbyi* Britt.**
VN: Cocilliana (E). Cocilliana (G).
SW: Classified as natural product.

***Gypsophila paniculata* L.**
KE: Root permitted for oral use. No CI, AE or I, except for gastric irritation (rarely) [BAnz nr.101 01.06.90].
AS: KE does not exclude the use of other *Gypsophila* spp. as source plants.

***Hamamelis virginiana* L.**
VN: Witch hazel (E). Hamamelis; Zauberhasel (G). Hamamélis (de Virginie) (F).
KE: Bark and leaf permitted for oral use. No CI, AE, I [BAnz nr.154 21.08.85].
SZ: Bark and leaf permitted as herbal tea. No CI, I. AE: GI-irritation.
FR: Leaf permitted for oral use (toxicological categories pd:2 ht/ae/wa:1 sa/ti:1).
SW: Classified as natural product.

***Harpagophytum procumbens* (Burch.) DC.**
VN: Devil's claw (E). Teufelskralle (G). Griffe du diable; Harpagophyton (F).
KE: Root permitted for oral use. CI: GI-ulcer. No AE, I [BAnz nr.43 02.03.89 and BAnz nr.164 01.09.90].
FR: Root permitted for oral and external use (toxicological categories pd:1 ht/ae/wa:1 sa/ti:1).
BE: Root permitted as traditional antiarthritic agent.
SW: Classified as natural product.
AS: *Harpagophytum zeyheri* Decne [34].

***Harungana madagascariensis* Lam. ex Poir. = *Haronga madagascariensis* Choisy**

VN: Haronga (G).

KE: Bark with leaf permitted for oral use. CI: acute pancreatitis, severe hepatic dysfunction, bile-stones, biliary obstruction, empyema of gall-bladder, ileus. AE: photosensitivity. No I. Should not be used for more than 2 months [BAnz nr.50 13.03.86].

SW: Classified as natural product.

***Hedera helix* L.**

VN: Common ivy; Woodbind (E). (Gemeiner) Efeu (G). Lierre commun; Lierre grimpant (F).

KE: Leaf permitted for oral use. No CI, AE, I [BAnz nr.122 06.07.88].

FR: Wood permitted for oral use (toxicological categories pd:2 ht/ae/wa:1 sa/ti:1).
Leaf permitted for external use only (toxicological categories pd:- ht/ae/wa:1 sa/ti:1).

SW: Classified as natural product.

***Helianthus annuus* L.**

VN: Sunflower (E). Sonnenblume (G). Hélianthe; Tournesol (F).

SW: Classified as natural product.

***Helichrysum arenarium* (L.) Moench = *Gnaphalium arenarium* L.**

VN: Sandy everlasting; Yellow chaste weed (E). Gelbes Katzenpfötchen; Sand-strohblume (G). Immortelle des sables; Perlière des sables (F).

KE: Flower permitted for oral use. CI: biliary obstruction. No AE, I [BAnz nr.122 06.07.88 and BAnz nr.164 01.09.90].

SZ: Permitted as herbal tea (Ruhrkrautblüten). No CI, AE, I.

SW: Classified as natural product.

***Herniaria glabra* L.**

VN: Flax weed; (Glabrous) rupture wort; (E). Kahles Bruchkraut (G). Herniaire glabre (F).

KE: Herb not permitted for therapeutic use. Usefulness is not documented adequately. No risks are known, however [BAnz nr.173 18.09.86].

AS: *Herniaria hirsuta* L. [KE].

***Hibiscus sabdariffa* L.**

VN: Red sorrel (E). Hibiscus; Karkade (G). Carcade; Karkadé (F).

KE: Flower not permitted for therapeutic use. Usefulness is not documented adequately. No risks are known, however, and there is no objection to the use as admixture [BAnz nr.22a 01.02.90].

FR: Calyx permitted for oral use (toxicological categories pd:1 ht/ae/wa:1 sa/ti:1).

SW: Classified as natural product.
AS: KE specifies the var. *sabdariffa ruber*.
SW also classifies *Hibiscus rosa-sinensis* L. as natural product.

Hieracium pilosella **L.**
VN: Hawkweed; Mouseweed (E). Langhaariges Habichtskraut; Mausohr (G). Oreille de souris; Piloselle (F).
FR: Entire plant permitted for oral use (toxicological categories pd:2 ht/ae/wa:1 sa/ti:1).

Hippophae rhamnoides **L.**
VN: Sea buckthorn (E). Meerdorn; Seedorn (G).
SW: Classified as natural product.

Hordeum sativum **L.**
VN: Barley (E). Gerste (G). Orge (F).
SW: Fruit classified as natural product.

Humulus lupulus **L.**
VN: Hops (E). Hopfen (G). Houblon (F).
KE: Strobile permitted for oral use. No CI, AE, I [BAnz nr.228 05.12.84].
SZ: Strobile permitted as herbal tea. No CI, AE, I.
FR: Female inflorescence permitted for oral use (toxicological categories pd:2 ht/ae/wa:1 sa/ti:1).
BE: Strobile, flowering top, powder, extract, tincture and glandular trichomes (= lupulinum) permitted as traditional tranquillizer.
SW: Classified as natural product.

Hydrastis canadensis **L.**
VN: Goldenseal (E). Goldsiegel; Kanadische Gelbwurzel (G). Hydrastis (F).
SW: Classified as natural product (for external use).

Hyoscyamus niger **L.**
VN: Henbane (E). Bilsenkraut (G). Jusquiame noire (F).
KE: Leaf permitted for oral use. CI, AE, I of belladona alkaloids [BAnz nr.85 05.05.88].
SW: Classified as a drug, which must normally be registered as pharmaceutical speciality.

Hypericum perforatum **L.**
VN: Hardhay; Saint John's wort (E). Hartheu; Johanniskraut (G). Millepertuis (F).
KE: Herb permitted for oral use. No CI, I. AE: photosensitivity [BAnz nr.228 05.12.84].

SZ: Herb permitted as herbal tea. CI, AE: photosensitivity. No I.
FR: Flowering top permitted for external use only (toxicological categories pd:- ht/ae/wa:- sa/ti:1). Not to be used before exposure to sunlight.
SW: Classified as natural product.

Hyssopus officinalis **L.**
VN: Hyssop (E). Ysop (G). Hysope (officinale) (F).
FR: Leaf and flowering top permitted for oral use (toxicological categories pd:2 ht/ae/wa:1 sa/ti:2).
SW: Classified as natural product.

Iberis amara **L.**
VN: Bitter candytuft; Clown's mustard (E). Bauernsenf; Bittere Schleifenblume (G). Téraspic; Thlaspi blanc (F).
SW: Classified as a drug, which must normally be registered as pharmaceutical speciality.

Ilex paraguariensis **St.Hil. =** ***Ilex paraguayensis*** **Lamb.**
VN: Mate (E). Mate (G). Maté; Thé du Paraguay (F).
KE: Leaf permitted for oral use. No CI, AE, I [BAnz nr.85 05.05.88].
FR: Leaf permitted for oral use (toxicological categories pd:1 ht/ae/wa:1 sa/ti:1).
BE: Permitted as traditional diuretic.
SW: Classified as natural product.

Illicium verum **Hooker fil.**
VN: Star anise (E). Sternanis (G). Anis étoilé; Badiane de Chine (F).
KE: Fruit permitted for oral use. No CI, AE, I [BAnz nr.122 06.07.88].
FR: Fruit permitted for oral use (toxicological categories pd:1 ht/ae/wa:1 sa/ti:1).
BE: Fruit permitted as traditional digestive aid.

Inula helenium **L.**
VN: Elfdock; Scabwort (E). Echter Alant (G). Aunée (officinale) (F).
KE: Root not permitted for therapeutic use. Usefulness is not documented adequately. Allergic contact dermatitis is possible, and higher doses produce vomiting, diarrhoea, cramps and paralytic symptoms [BAnz nr.85 05.05.88].
FR: Rhizome and root permitted for oral use (toxicological categories pd:2 ht/ae/wa:1 sa/ti:1).
SW: Classified as natural product.

Iris germanica **L.**
VN: Garden iris (E). Deutsche Schwertlilie (G). Iris d'Allemagne (F).
SW: Classified as natural product.

***Juglans regia* L.**

VN: Walnut tree (E). Walnuß (G). Noyer (royal) (F).

KE: Fruit-shell not permitted for therapeutic use. Usefulness is not documented adequately. Fresh shells contain the naphthoquinone constituent juglone, which is mutagenic and possibly carcinogenic. The juglone, which is mutagenic and possibly carcinogenic. The juglone content of dried shells has not been studied adequately [BAnz nr.101 01.06.90].
Leaf permitted for external use only. No CI, AE, I [BAnz nr.101 01.06.90].

FR: Leaf permitted for oral use (toxicological categories pd:2 ht/ae/wa:1 sa/ti:1).

SW: Classified as natural product.

***Juniperus communis* L.**

VN: Juniper (E). (Gemeiner) Wacholder (G). Genévrier commun (F).

KE: Berry permitted for oral use. CI: pregnancy, nephritis. AE: prolonged use or overdosing may lead to renal damage. No I [BAnz nr.228 05.12.84].

SZ: Berry permitted as herbal tea. CI: pregnancy, nephritis, pyelitis. AE: prolonged use of overdosing can lead to renal damage. No I. Should not be used for more than 4 weeks without consulting a physician.

FR: Female cone permitted for oral use (toxicological categories pd:2 ht/ae/wa:1 sa/ti:2).

SW: Classified as natural product.

***Krameria triandra* Ruiz et Pavon**

VN: Rhatany (E). Ratanhia (G). Ratanhia (F).

KE: Root permitted for local use in the mouth only. No CI, AE or I, except for rare allergic mucosal reactions. Should not be used for more than 2 weeks without consulting a physician [BAnz nr.43 02.03.89].

SZ: Root permitted as herbal tea and tincture for local use in the mouth only. No CI, AE, I. Undiluted tincture may produce burning and local irritation.

FR: Root permitted for oral use (toxicological categories pd:2 ht/ae/wa:1 sa/ti:1).

AS: Related species [FR].

***Lactuca virosa* L.**

VN: Prickly lettuce (E). Giftlattich (G). Laitue vireuse (F).

FR: Leaf permitted for oral use (toxicological categories pd:2 ht/ae/wa:- sa/ti:2).

***Laminaria digitata* Lmx.**

VN: Laminaria (E). Laminaria (G). Laminaire (F).

FR: Stalk permitted as laxative. The adult intake of iodine should not exceed 120 μg per day.
SW: Classified as foodstuff and as natural product.
AS: *Laminaria cloustoni* Le Joly and *Laminaria hyperborea* Foslie [FR]. SW also classifies *Laminaria japonica* Aresch as foodstuff and as natural product.

***Lamium album* L.**
VN: White deadnettle (E). Weiße Taubnessel (G). Lamier blanc; Ortie blanche (F).
KE: Flower permitted for oral use. No CI, AE, I [BAnz nr.76 23.04.87].
SZ: Herb permitted as herbal tea. No CI, AE, I.
FR: Peeled corolla permitted for oral use (toxicological categories pd:2 ht/ae/wa:1 sa/ti:1).
SW: Classified as natural product.

***Larix decidua* Miller**
KE: Balsam (terebinthina laricina) permitted for external use and inhalation. CI: hypersensitivity to essential oils; acute inflammations of respiratory tract (for inhalation). AE: allergic skin reactions. No I [BAnz nr.228 05.12.84].
SW: Classified as natural product.

***Larrea tridentata* (DC.) Coville = *Larrea divaricata* Cav.**
VN: Chaparral; Creosote bush (E).
SW: Classified as a drug, which must normally be registered as pharmaceutical speciality.

***Laurus nobilis* L.**
VN: Laurel (E). Lorbeer (G). Laurier commun; Laurier sauce (F).
FR: Leaf permitted for oral use (toxicological categories pd:1 ht/ae/wa:1 sa/ti:1).
SW: Leaf classified as natural product.

***Lavandula angustifolia* Miller = *Lavandula vera* DC. = *Lavandula officinalis* Chaich.**
VN: Lavender (E). (Echter) Lavendel (G). Lavande (vraie) (F).
KE: Flower permitted for oral use. No CI, AE, I [BAnz nr.228 05.12.84].
SZ: Flower permitted as herbal tea. No CI, AE, I.
FR: Flower and flowering top permitted for oral use (toxicological properties: pd:2 ht/ae/wa:1 sa/ti:2).
BE: Flower, powder and extract permitted as traditional tranquillizer.
SW: Flower classified as natural product.

***Ledum palustre* L.**

VN: Marshtea (E.) Sumpfporst (G). Romarin sauvage (F).

KE: Herb not permitted for therapeutic use. Usefulness is not documented adequately. Contains an essential oil which is a potent irritant of the GI-tract, kidneys and urinary tract; other toxic effects include abortion (CI: pregnancy) [BAnz nr.177a 24.09.86].

***Leonurus cardiaca* L.**

VN: Motherwort (E). (Echtes) Herzgespann (G). Agripaume (F).

KE: Herb permitted for oral use. No CI, AE, I [BAnz nr.50 13.03.86].

FR: Aerial parts permitted for oral use (toxicological categories pd:2 ht/ae/wa:1 sa/ti:1).

SW: Classified as a drug, which must normally be registered as pharmaceutical speciality.

***Levisticum officinale* Koch = *Ligusticum levisticum* L.**

VN: Lovage (E). Liebstöckel (G). Livèche (F).

KE: Root permitted for oral use. CI: acute nephritis, renal insufficiency; look out for photosensitivity, when the root is used for prolonged period. No AE, I [BAnz nr.101 01.06.90].

SZ: Root permitted as herbal tea. CI: nephritis, urinary tract inflammation, renal insufficiency. No AE, I.

***Linum usitatissimum* L.**

VN: Flax (E). Lein; Flachs (G). Lin (F).

KE: Seed permitted for oral use. CI: ileus. I: reduced absorption of other drugs possible. No AE, when used with a sufficient amount of liquid [BAnz nr.228 05.12.84].

SZ: Seed permitted as such. CI: intestinal obstruction. Patients with inflammatory intestinal diseases should only use the seed in swollen state. Abuse of high doses may result in electrolyte losses.

FR: Seed permitted for oral use (toxicological categories pd:1 ht/ae/wa:1 sa/ti:-).
Seed permitted as laxative.

BE: Seed permitted as traditional laxative and as traditional topical soothing agent.

AS: Cultivars of *L. usitatissimum* (L.) Vav. et Ell. [KE].

***Lippia citriodora* (Ort.) H.B.K. = *Aloysia triphylla* (L'Hérit.) Britt. = *Verbena triphylla* L.'Hérit.**

VN: Vervain (E). (Echtes) Verbenenkraut (G). Verveine odorante (F).

FR: Leaf permitted for oral use (toxicological categories pd:2 ht/ae/wa:1 sa/ti:1).

BE: Leaf, powder and extract permitted as traditional tranquillizer.

***Lobelia* species**

SW: Classified as a drug, which must normally be registered as pharmaceutical speciality.

***Lycium chinense* Mill.**

SW: Classified as a drug, which must normally be registered as pharmaceutical speciality.

***Lycopus europaeus* L.**

VN: Wolf's foot (E). Wolfstrapp (G). Lycope; Patte de loup (F).

KE: Herb permitted for oral use. CI: hypothyroidism, goiter without thyroid dysfunction. AE: goiter (rarely), rebound effect. I: thyroid hormones, radioactive iodine [BAnz nr.22a 01.02.90].

AS: *Lycopus virginicus* L. [KE].

***Lythrum salicaria* L.**

VN: Purple loosestrife; Red sally (E). Blutweiderich (G). Lysimaque pourprée; Salicaire (F).

FR: Flowering top permitted for oral use (toxicological categories pd:2 ht/ae/wa:1 sa/ti:1).

***Malpighia punicifolia* L.**

VN: Acerola (E).

SW: Classified as natural product.

***Malva sylvestris* L.**

VN: High mallow (E). Wilde Malve (G). Mauve (sauvage) (F).

KE: Leaf and flower permitted for oral use. No CI, AE, I [BAnz nr.43 02.03.1989].

SZ: Leaf permitted as herbal tea. No CI, AE, I.
The addition of the flower to certain herbal tea mixtures is also permitted.

FR: Leaf and flower permitted for oral use (toxicological categories pd:2 ht/ae/wa:1 sa/ti:-).
Leaf, flower and root are all permitted as laxative.

BE: Leaf, flower and root permitted as traditional stomatological.

SW: Classified as natural product.

AS: KE allows *Malva neglecta* Wallr. as alternative source plant of the leaf and *Malva sylvestris* L. ssp. *mauritiana* (L.) A. et Gr. as alternative source plant of the flower.

RM: Flores Malvae arboreae do not come from *Malva* species, but from *Alcea rosea* L. In the food trade "Malventee" is mostly used for *Hibiscus* flowers [34].

***Marrubium vulgare* L.**

VN: White horehound (E). (Weißer) Andorn (G). Marrube blanc (F).

KE: Herb permitted for oral use. No CI, AE, I [BAnz nr.22a 01.02.90].
FR: Leaf and flowering top permitted for oral use (toxicological categories pd:2 ht/ae/wa:1 sa/ti:1).
BE: Leaf and flowering top permitted as traditional cough remedy.
SW: Classified as natural product.

***Marsdenia cundurango* Reichenb. fil.**
VN: Condurango; Eagle-vine (E). Condurango (G). Condurango (F).
KE: Bark permitted for oral use. No CI, AE, I [BAnz nr.193 15.10.87].
SW: Classified as natural product.

***Matricaria recutita* L. = *Matricaria chamomilla* L. = *Chamomilla recutita* (L.) Rauschert**
VN: German chamomile; Wild chamomile (E). Echte Kamille (G). Camomille (allemande); Matricaire (F).
KE: Flower-head permitted for oral use. No CI, AE, I [BAnz nr.228 05.12.84].
SZ: Flower-head permitted as herbal tea (for oral use or inhalation). No CI, AE, I. Should not be used near the eye.
FR: Flower-head permitted for oral use (toxicological categories pd:2 ht/ae/wa:1 sa/ti:1).
BE: Flower-head permitted as traditional digestive aid, as traditional stomatological and as traditional topical soothing agent.
SW: Classified as foodstuff and as natural product.

***Medicago sativa* L.**
VN: Alfalfa (E).
SW: Classified as natural product.

***Melaleuca leucadendron* L.**
VN: Cajeput tree (E). Kajeputbaum (G). Cajeputier (F).
SW: Classified as natural product (for external use).

***Melilotus officinalis* (L.) Pallas**
VN: Field melilot; Yellow melilot (E). Gelber Steinklee; Honigklee (G). Couronne royale; Mélilot (F).
KE: Herb permitted for oral use. No CI, AE or I, except for headache (rarely) [BAnz nr.50 13.03.86].
FR: Flowering top permitted for oral use (toxicological categories pd:2 ht/ae/wa:1 sa/ti:1).
SW: Classified as a drug, which must normally be registered as pharmaceutical speciality.
AS: FR also allows related species. KE also allows *Melilotus altissimus* Thuill.

***Melissa officinalis* L.**

VN: Balm (E). Melisse (G). Mélisse (officinale) (F).
KE: Leaf permitted for oral use. No CI, AE, I [BAnz nr.228 05.12.84].
SZ: Leaf permitted as herbal tea. No CI, AE, I.
FR: Leaf and flowering top permitted for oral use (toxicological categories pd:1 ht/ae/wa:1 sa/ti:1).
BE: Leaf, powder, tincture and extract permitted as traditional tranquillizer. Herb permitted as traditional digestive aid.
SW: Leaf classified as natural product.

***Mentha arvensis* L. var. *piperascens* Holmes ex C.**

VN: Janpanische Minze (G).
KE: Essential oil permitted for oral use. CI: biliary obstruction, gall-bladder inflammation, severe liver damage. AE: gastric complaints. No I. Not to be inhaled by small children [BAnz nr.177a 24.09.86 and nr.164 01.09.90].

***Mentha × piperita* L.**

VN: Peppermint (E). Pfefferminze (G). Menthe anglaise; Menthe poivrée (F).
KE: Leaf permitted for oral use. No CI, AE, I [BAnz nr.223 30.11.85]. Essential oil also permitted for oral use. CI: biliary obstruction or inflammation, severe liver damage. No AE, I. Should not be inhaled by small children [BAnz nr.50 13.03.86 and BAnz nr.164 01.09.90].
SZ: Leaf permitted as herbal tea. No CI, AE, I.
Essential oil permitted as such. CI: biliary obstruction, gall-bladder inflammation, severe hepatic damage. No AE, I. Should not be inhaled by small children.
FR: Leaf and flowering top permitted for oral use (toxicological categories pd:1 ht/ae/wa:1 sa/ti:1).
BE: Herb permitted as traditional digestive aid.
AS: *Mentha aquatica* L., *Mentha arvensis* L., *Mentha spicata* L. var. *crispa* L. and *M. viridis* L. [8].

***Menyanthes trifoliata* L.**

VN: Buckbean (E). Bitterklee; (Dreiblättriger) Fieberklee (G). Ményanthe; Trèfle d'eau (F).
KE: Leaf permitted for oral use. No CI, AE, I [BAnz nr.22a 01.02.90].
FR: Leaf permitted for oral use (toxicological categories pd:2 ht/ae/wa:1 sa/ti:2).
SW: Classified as natural product.

***Mucuna pruriens* DC. = *Dolichos pruriens* L.**

VN: Cowhage; Cow-itch (E). Juckbohne; Kuhkrätze (G). Pois à gratter; Pois pouillieux (F).
SW: Classified as natural product.

Musa paradisiaca **L.**
VN: Banana (E). Banane (G). Banane (F).
SW: Fruit classified as natural product.

Myristica fragrans **Houttuyn**
VN: Nutmeg tree (E). Muskatbaum (G). Muscadier (F).
KE: Seed and arille not permitted for therapeutic use. Usefulness is not documented adequately. Psychic disturbances by 5 g of seed, atropin-like action by 9 teaspoons of seed powder, abortion by higher doses. The essential oil contains the mutagenic and animal carcinogenic compound safrole. However, the use to correct smell or taste is permitted [BAnz nr.173 18.09.86].
SW: Fruit classified as natural product.

Myroxylon balsamum **(L.) Harms var.** ***balsamum*** **Harms =** ***Myroxylon balsamum*** **var.** ***genuinum*** **(Baill.) Harms**
VN: Tolubalsambaum (G). Arbre de baume de tolu (F).
KE: Balsam (balsamum tolutanum) permitted for internal use. No CI, AE, I [BAnz nr.173 18.09.86].

Myroxylon balsamum **(L.) Harms var.** ***pereira*** **(Royle) Harms**
KE: Balsam (balsamum peruvianum) permitted for external use. CI: allergic disposition. AE: allergic skin reactions. No I. Application on large surfaces max. 10%. Not to be used for more than 1 week [BAnz nr.173 18.09.86].
SW: Peruvian balsam is classified as natural product.

Nasturtium officinale **R. Brown**
VN: Water cress (E). (Echte) Brunnenkresse; Wasserkresse (G). Cresson de Fontaine (F).
KE: Herb permitted for oral use. CI: peptic ulcer, nephritis; not to be used by children younger than 4 years. AE: GI-complaints (rarely). No I [BAnz nr.22a 01.02.90].

Nepeta cataria **L.**
VN: Catmint (E). Echtes Katzenkraut; Katzenminze (G). Cataire (F).
SW: Classified as natural product.

Nerium oleander **L.**
VN: Rose bay; Rose laurel (E). Oleander (G). Laurier rose (F).
KE: Leaf not permitted for therapeutic use. Usefulness is not documented adequately. Accidental and therapeutic use has resulted in partially fatal poisonings [BAnz nr.122 06.07.88].
SW: Classified as natural product.

RM: It is very unclear, why SW has not classified this herb as a drug, which must normally be registered as pharmaceutical speciality.

***Nuphar luteum* (L.) Sibth. et Sm.**

VN: Yellow water-lily (E). Gelbe Teichrose (G). Nénuphar jaune (F).
FR: Rhizome permitted for external use only (toxicological categories pd:- ht/ae/wa:1 sa/ti:1).

***Ocimum basilicum* L.**

VN: (Sweet) basil (E). Basilikum (G). Basilic (doux) (F).
KE: Herb and essential oil not permitted for therapeutic use. Usefulness is not documented adequately. The herb contains up to 0.5% of essential oil, which contains up to 85% of estragole. Estragole is mutagenic following metabolic activation and there is evidence from animal experiments that it may be carcinogenic. The herb and essential oil should not be used during pregnancy and lactation or for prolonged periods. There is no objection to the use of the herb as an admixture in levels up to 5% [BAnz nr.54 18.03.91].
SZ: Herb permitted as herbal tea. No CI, AE, I.
FR: Leaf permitted for oral use (toxicological categories pd:1 ht/ae/wa:1 sa/ti:1).
SW: Classified as natural product.
AS: SW also classifies *Ocimum sanctum* L. as natural product.

***Oenothera biennis* L.**

VN: Evening primrose (E). Gemeine Nachtkerze (G). Herbe aux ânes; Onagre bisanuelle (F).
SW: Classified as natural product.

***Olea europaea* L.**

VN: Olive tree (E). Olivenbaum (G). Olivier (F).
KE: Leaf not permitted for therapeutic use. Usefulness is not documented adequately. No risks are known, however [BAnz nr.11 17.01.91].
Oil not permitted for therapeutic use. Usefulness is not documented adequately. Should not be used in patients with bile-stones because of the risk that a biliary colic is induced. Topical application rarely results in allergic skin reactions [BAnz nr.178 21.09.91].
FR: Leaf permitted for oral use (toxicological categories pd:2 ht/ae/wa:1 sa/ti:1).
Fruit permitted as laxative.

***Ononis spinosa* L.**

VN: Restharrow (E). (Dornige) Hauhechel (G). Arrête-boeuf; Bugrane (épineuse) (F).
KE: Root permitted for oral use. No CI, AE, I [BAnz nr.76 23.04.87].

SZ: Root permitted as herbal tea. No CI, AE, I.
FR: Root permitted for oral use (toxicological categories pd:2 ht/ae/wa:1 sa/ti:1).
SW: Classified as natural product.

***Origanum majorana* L. = *Majorana hortensis* Moench.**
VN: Sweet majoram (E). Gartenmajoran (G). Marjolaine; Origan marjolaine (F).
FR: Leaf and flowering top permitted for oral use (toxicological categories pd:1 ht/ae/wa:1 sa/ti:1).
BE: Leaf and flowering top permitted as traditional cough remedy. Herb permitted as traditional digestive aid.

***Origanum vulgare* L.**
VN: Wild majoram (E). Wilder majoran (G). Marjolaine sauvage; Origan (vulgaire) (F).
KE: Herb not permitted for therapeutic use. Usefulness is not documented adequately. No risks are known, however [BAnz nr.122 06.07.88].
FR: Flowering top permitted for oral use (toxicological categories pd:1 ht/ae/wa:1 sa/ti:1).
BE: Leaf and flowering top permitted as traditional cough remedy. Herb permitted as traditional digestive aid.
SW: Classified as natural product.

***Orthosiphon spicatus* Benth. in DC. = *Orthosiphon stamineus* Benth. in Wall.**
VN: Java tea (E). Javatee; Orthosiphon (G). Orthosiphon; Thé de Java (F).
KE: Leaf permitted for oral use. No CI, AE, I [BAnz nr.50 13.03.86].
SZ: Leaf permitted as herbal tea. No CI, AE, I.
FR: Stalk with leaves permitted for oral use (toxicological categories pd:2 ht/ae/wa:1 sa/ti:1).
BE: Leaf permitted as traditional diuretic.
AS: *Orthosiphon aristatus* Blume Miq. [34].

***Paeonia officinalis* L. emend. Willd.**
VN: Peony (E). Echte Pfingstrose (G). Péone; Pivoine officinale (F).
KE: Flower and root not permitted for therapeutic use. Usefulness is not documented adequately. No risks are known, however, and there is no objection to the use of the flower as an admixture to herbal teas [BAnz nr.85 05.05.88].
SW: Classified as natural product.
AS: *Paeonia mascula* (L.) Mill. [KE].

***Panax ginseng* C.A. Meyer = *Aralia quinquefolia* Decne. et Planch.**
VN: Ginseng (E). Ginseng (G). Ginseng; Panax de Chine (F).
KE: Root permitted for oral use. No CI, AE, I [BAnz nr.11 17.01.91].

FR: Root permitted for oral use (toxicological categories pd:1 ht/ae/wa:1 sa/ti:1). Maximum dosage: 2 g of powder per day for a maximum of 3 months.
SW: Classified as natural product.

***Papaver rhoeas* L.**
VN: Corn poppy (E). Klatschmohn (G). Coquelicot; Pavot rouge (F).
KE: Flower not permitted for therapeutic use. Usefulness is not documented adequately. No risks are known, however, and there is no objection to the use as an admixture to herbal teas [BAnz nr.85 05.05.88].
FR: Petal permitted for oral use (toxicological categories pd:1 ht/ae/wa:1 sa/ti:1).
BE: Flower, powder and extract permitted as traditional tranquillizer.
AS: *Papaver dubium* L. [FR].

***Papaver somniferum* L.**
VN: Opium poppy (E). Schlafmohn (G). Pavot (officinal) (F).
SW: Seed classified as foodstuff.

***Passiflora edulis* Sims**
SW: Classified as natural product.

***Passiflora incarnata* L.**
VN: Maypop; Passion flower (E). Passionsblume (G). Fleur de la passion; Passiflore (F).
KE: Herb permitted for oral use. No CI, AE, I [BAnz nr.223 30.11.85].
SZ: Herb permitted as herbal tea. No CI, AE, I.
FR: Aerial parts permitted for oral use (toxicological categories pd:2 ht/ae/wa:1 sa/ti:1).
BE: Entire plant, powder, tincture, extract permitted as traditional tranquillizer.
SW: Classified as natural product.

***Paullinia cupana* Kunth ex H.B. et K. = *Paullinia sorbilis* Mart.**
VN: Guarana (E). Paullinia (F).
FR: Seed permitted for oral use (toxicological categories pd:1 ht/ae/wa:1 sa/ti:1).
Extract of seed (guarana) permitted for oral use (toxicological categories pd:1 ht/ae/wa:1 sa/ti:-).
SW: Classified as a drug, which must normally be registered as pharmaceutical speciality.

Pausinystalia yohimbe (K. Schum.) Pierre
VN: Yohimbe (E). Yohimbe (G). Yohimbe (F).

KE: Bark not permitted for therapeutic use. Usefulness is not documented adequately. Contains the toxic alkaloid yohimbin [BAnz nr.193 15.10.87].
SW: Classified as a drug, which must normally be registered as pharmaceutical speciality.

***Persea americana* Mill.**
VN: Avocado (E). Avocado (G). Avocat (F).
SW: Classified as natural product.

***Petasites hybridus* (L.) Gaertn., Meyer et Scherb. = *Petasites officinalis* Moench**
VN: Butterbur; Butterfly dock (E). Großblättriger Huflattich; Rote Pestwurz (G). Pétasite (officinale) (F).
KE: Leaf not permitted for therapeutic use. Usefulness is not documented adequately. All plant parts contain hepatotoxic, genotoxic and carcinogenic pyrrolizidine alkaloids (PA) [BAnz nr.138 27.07.90].
Rhizome permitted for oral use. CI: pregnancy, lactation. No AE, I. D: max. 1 μg PA/day for max. 4–6 weeks/year [BAnz nr.138 27.07.90].
SW: Classified as a drug, which must normally be registered as pharmaceutical speciality.
AS: KE speaks more generally of *Petasites* spp. as source plants ot the leaf.

***Petroselinum crispum* (Mill.) Nym. = *Petroselinum hortense* Hoffm. = *Petroselinum sativum* Hoffm. = *Apium petroselinum* L. = *Carum petroselinum* (L.) Benth. et Hook.f.**
VN: Parsley (E). Gartenpetersilie; Petersilie (G). Persil (F).
KE: Herb and root permitted for oral use. CI: pregnancy, nephritis. AE: allergic reactions of skin/mucosae (rarely); phototoxicity. No I. The pure oil is toxic and should not be used [BAnz nr.43 02.03.89].
Fruit not permitted for therapeutic use. Usefulness is not documented adequately. The essential oil and its constituent apiole are toxic [BAnz nr.43 02.03.89].
FR: Leaf, root and fruit permitted for oral use (toxicological categories pd:1 ht/ae/wa:1 sa/ti:1).
SW: Classified as natural product (leaf also classified as foodstuff).

***Peucedanum ostruthium* (L.) Koch. = *Imperatoria ostruthium* L.**
VN: Masterwort; Pellitory of Spain (E). Kaiserwurz; Meisterwurz (G). Benjoin des maléfices; Impératoire (F).
SW: Classified as natural product.

***Peumus boldus* Mol.**
VN: Boldo (E). Boldo (G). Boldo (F).

KE: Leaf permitted for oral use. CI: biliary obstruction, severe liver diseases. No AE, I. Essential oil and destillates should not be used because of their ascaridole content. [BAnz nr.76 23.04.87 and BAnz nr.164 01.09.90].
FR: Leaf permitted for oral use (toxicological categories pd:1 ht/ae/wa:1 sa/ti:1). The level of active constituents has to be limited.
BE: Leaf permitted as traditional cholagogue.
SW: Classified as natural product.
RM: KE specifies the use of preparations which are practically free from ascaridole.

***Phaseolus vulgaris* L.**
VN: Bean; Kidney-bean (E). Bohne; Gartenbohne (G). Haricot (F).
KE: Pericarp (fruit without seed) permitted for oral use. No CI, AE, I [BAnz nr.50 13.03.86].
SZ: Pericarp permitted. No CI, AE, I.
SW: Classified as natural product.

***Phytolacca americana* L. = *Phytolacca decandra* L.**
VN: Poke (E). Kermes (G). Phytolaque (F).
SW: Classified as natural product.

***Picea abies* (L.) Karsten = *Picea excelsa* (Lam.) Link**
KE: Fresh shoot permitted for oral use. No CI, AE, I [BAnz nr.193 15.10.87].
Essential oil permitted for external use and inhalation. CI: asthma bronchiale, whooping-cough. AE: local irritation, exacerbation of bronchospasms. No I [BAnz nr.154 21.08.85].
AS: KE specifies *Abies alba* Miller = *A. pectinata* (Lam.) DC. as alternative source plants for the fresh shoots and *Abies alba* Miller, *A. sachalinensis* (Fr. Schmidt) Masters and *A. sibirica* Ledebour as alternative source plants for the essential oil.

***Pimpinella anisum* L.**
VN: Anise (E). Anis (G). Anis (vert) (F).
KE: Fruit permitted for oral use. CI: Hypersensitivity. AE: allergic reactions (occasionally). No I [BAnz nr.122 06.07.88].
SZ: Fruit permitted as herbal tea. No CI, AE, I.
FR: Fruit permitted for oral use (toxicological categories pd:1 ht/ae/wa:1 sa/ti:1).
BE: Fruit permitted as traditional digestive aid.
SW: Classified as natural product.

***Pimpinella major* (L.) Hudson**
VN: Greater burnet saxifrage; Greater Pimpernel (E). Große Bibernelle (G). Grand boucage; Grande saxifrage (F).

KE: Herb not permitted for therapeutic use. Usefulness is not documented adequately. No risks are known, however [BAnz nr.101 01.06.90]. Root permitted for oral use. No CI, AE, I [BAnz nr.101 01.06.90].
AS: In addition to *Pimpinella major* and *Pimpinella saxifraga*, the related *Pimpinella peregrina* has been suggested as source plant for the root [34].

***Pimpinella saxifraga* L.**
VN: Burnet saxifrage; Pimpernel (E). Kleine Bibernelle (G). Petit boucage (F).
KE: Herb not permitted for therapeutic use. Usefulness is not documented adequately. No risks are known, however [BAnz nr.101 01.06.90]. Root permitted for oral use. No CI, AE, I [BAnz nr.101 01.06.90].
SW: Classified as natural product.
AS: In addition to *Pimpinella major* and *Pimpinella saxifraga*, the related *Pimpinella peregrina* has been suggested as source plant for the root [34].

Pinus flava
SW: Resin classified as natural product.

***Pinus palustris* Miller = *Pinus australis* Mich. fil.**
KE: The purified essential oil (terebinthinae aetheroleum rectificatum) is permitted for external use and inhalation. CI: Hypersensitivity to essential oils; acute inflammation of respiratory tract (inhalation). AE: Toxicity from external use on large surfaces. No I [BAnz nr.90 15.05.85].
AS: *Pinus pinaster* Ait. [KE].

***Pinus sylvestris* L.**
VN: Common pine; Fir tree (E). Gemeine Kiefer; Waldkiefer (G). Pin sauvage; Pin sylvestre (F).
KE: Shoot permitted for oral use. No CI, AE, I [BAnz nr.173 18.09.86]. Essential oil permitted for external use and inhalation. CI: asthma bronchiale, whooping-cough. AE: local irritation, exacerbation of bronchospasms. No I [BAnz nr.154 21.08.85].
FR: Bud permitted for oral use (toxicological categories pd:2 ht/ae/wa:1 sa/ti:1).
SW: Classified as natural product. The resin of *Pinus flava* is also classified as natural product. However, *Pinus nigra* is classified as a drug, which must normally be registered as pharmaceutical speciality.
AS: KE specifies *Pinus mugo* ssp. *pumilio* (Haenke) Franco, *P. nigra* Arnold and *P. pinaster* Soland as alternative source plants for the essential oil.

***Piper methysticum* G. Forster**
VN: Kava-kava (E). Kava-kava; Rauschpfeffer (G). Kava-kava (F).
KE: Rhizome permitted for oral use. CI: pregnancy, lactation, endogenous depression. AE: reversible yellow skin discoloration (prolonged use); allergic skin reactions; visual disturbances. I: CNS depressants. Should not be used for more than 3 months without consulting a physician. Beware of effect on driving ability [BAnz nr.101 01.06.90].
SW: Classified as a drug, which must normally be registered as pharmaceutical speciality.
RM: SW classifies *Piper* species other than *P. methysticum* as foodstuff and as natural product.

***Plantago afra* L. = *Plantago psyllium* L.**
VN: Psyllium (E). Psyllium; Strauchwegerich (G). Plantain des sables; Plantain pucier; Psyllium (F).
KE: Seed permitted for oral use. CI: Esophageal and gastrointestinal stenoses. AE: allergic reactions (rarely). No I [BAnz nr.223 30.11.85].
SZ: Seed permitted as such. CI: Intestinal obstruction. No AE, I.
FR: Seed permitted for oral use (toxicological categories pd:1 ht/ae/wa:1 sa/ti:-).
Seed permitted as laxative.
BE: Seed permitted as traditional laxative.
SW: Classified as natural product.
AS: *Plantago arenaria* Waldst. et Kit. = *Plantago indica* L. [KE, FR].

***Plantago lanceolata* L.**
VN: Leechwort; (Long) plantain (E). Spitzwegerich (G). Plantain lancéolé; plantain (petit) (F).
KE: Herb permitted for oral use. No CI, AE, I [BAnz nr.223 30.11.85].
SZ: Herb permitted as herbal tea. No CI, AE, I.
FR: Leaf permitted for external use only (toxicological categories pd:1 ht/ae/wa:1 sa/ti:-).
Seed permitted as laxative.
BE: Leaf of *Plantago major* permitted as traditional topical soothing agent.
SW: Classified as natural product.
AS: *Plantago major* L. and *Plantago media* L. [FR].
SW also classifies *Plantago major* L. as natural product.

***Plantago ovata* Forsk. = *Plantago ispaghula* Roxb.**
VN: Blond psyllium; Indian plantago (E). Indisches Psyllium; Ispaghula (G). Ispaghul (F).
KE: Seed and seed-shell permitted for oral use. CI: GI-obstruction (ileus); diabetes which is hard to control (as insulin need may be reduced). AE: allergic reactions. I: absorption of other drugs taken simultaneously [BAnz nr.22a 01.02.90 and BAnz nr.74 19.04.91].
SZ: Seed permitted as such. CI: Intestinal obstruction. No AE, I.

FR: Seed and seed-shell permitted as laxative.
SW: Classified as natural product.

***Platycodon grandiflorum* DC. = *Campanula grandiflora* Jacq.**
SW: Classified as a drug, which must normally be registered as pharmaceutical speciality.

***Podophyllum peltatum* L.**
VN: American mandrake; May-apple (E). Amerikanischer Podophyllum; Entenfuß (G). Podophylle américain (F).
KE: Rhizoma and resin permitted for external use only. CI: pregnancy. No AE, I. To be used 1–2 times weekly on skin surfaces not exceeding 25 cm^2 [BAnz nr.50 13.03.86].
SW: *Podophyllum* species are classified as drugs, which must normally be registered as pharmaceutical speciality.

***Polygala senega* L.**
VN: Senega snakeroot (E). Klapperschlangenwurzel (G). Polygala (de Virginie) (F).
KE: Root permitted for oral use. No CI, AE or I, except for GI-irritation from continued use [BAnz nr.50 13.03.86].
FR: Subterranean parts permitted for oral use (toxicological categories pd:2 ht/ae/wa:1 sa/ti:2).
BE: Root permitted as traditional cough remedy.
AS: Related species with the exclusion of species containing podophyllotoxins [FR].

***Polygonatum* species**
SW: *Polygonatum sibiricum* Red. and other *Polygonatum* species are classified as drugs, which must normally be registered as pharmaceutical speciality.

***Polygonum aviculare* L.**
VN: Knotweed (E). Knotgras; Vogelknöterich (G). Renouée des oiseaux (F).
KE: Herb permitted for oral use. No CI, AE, I [BAnz nr.76 23.04.87].
SW: Classified as natural product.

***Polygonum bistorta* L.**
VN: Bistort (E). Wiesenknöterich (G). (Renouée) bistorte (F).
FR: Subterranean parts permitted for oral use (toxicological categories pd:2 ht/ae/wa:1 sa/ti:1).

***Polypodium vulgare* L.**
VN: Adder's fern; Brake-root (E). Engelsüß; Tüpfelfarn (G). Fougère réglisse; Polypode de chêne (F).
SW: Classified as natural product.

***Populus nigra* L.**

VN: Black poplar (E). Schwarzpappel (G). Peuplier noir (F).

KE: Bud permitted for external use only. CI: hypersensitivity to poplar buds, propolis, Peruvian balsam, salicylates. AE: allergic skin reactions (occasionally). No I [BAnz nr.22a 01.02.90].

FR: Bud permitted for oral use (toxicological categories pd:2 ht/ae/wa:- sa/ti:2).
Leaf permitted for oral use (toxicological categories pd:2 ht/ae/wa:1 sa/ti:1).

SW: Classified as natural product.

AS: *Populus balsamifera* L. [FR].
SW also classifies *Populus tremuloides* Michx. as natural product.

***Potentilla anserina* L.**

VN: Argentine; Silverweed (E). Gänse-Fingerkraut; Gänserich (G). Argentine; Potentilla ansérine (F).

KE: Herb permitted for oral use. No CI, AE or I, except for gastric irritation [BAnz nr.223 30.11.85].

SZ: Herb permitted. No CI, I. AE: GI-disturbances.

SW: Classified as natural product.

***Potentilla erecta* (L.) Räuschel = *Potentilla tormentilla* Stokes**

VN: Tormentil (E). Blutwurz; Tormentil (G). Potentille; Tormentille (F).

KE: Rhizome permitted for oral use. No CI, I. AE: Gastric complaints [BAnz nr.85 05.05.88].

SZ: Rhizome permitted as herbal tea. No CI, I. AE: GI-disturbances.

FR: Subterranean parts permitted for oral use (toxicological categories pd:2 ht/ae/wa:1 sa/ti:1).

SW: Classified as natural product.

***Primula veris* L. = *Primula officinalis* (L.) Hill.**

VN: Primrose (E). Primel; Schlüsselblume; Wiesen-Schlüsselblume (G). Primevère (officinale) (F).

KE: Flower permitted for oral use. CI: hypersensitivity. AE: GI-disturbances (occasionally). No I [BAnz nr.122 06.07.88].
Root permitted for oral use. No CI, I. AE: GI-disturbances (occasionally) [BAnz nr.122 06.07.88].

SZ: Flower permitted as herbal tea. No CI, AE, I, except for rare contact allergy.

FR: Flower permitted for oral use (toxicological categories pd:2 ht/ae/wa:1 sa/ti:1).
Root permitted for oral use (toxicological categories pd:2 ht/ae/wa:1 sa/ti:2).

BE: Root permitted as traditional cough remedy.

SW: Classified as natural product.

AS: *Primula elatior* (L.) Hill. [KE,SZ,FR].

***Prunus amygdalus* Stok. var. *dulcis* Koehne.**

VN: Sweet almond (E). Süße Mandel (G). Amande douce (F).

SW: Classified as natural product (seed classified as foodstuff).

***Prunus armeniaca* L.**

VN: Apricot (E). Aprikose (G). Abricot (F).

SW: Classified as natural product. The fruit is classified as a drug, which must normally be registered as pharmaceutical speciality.

***Prunus cerasus* L.**

VN: Sour cherry (E). Sauerkirsche (G). Cerisier griottier; Griottier (F).

FR: Fruit-stalk permitted for oral use (toxicological categories pd:2 ht/ae/wa:1 sa/ti:1).

SW: Classified as natural product and as a drug, which must normally be registered as pharmaceutical speciality.

AS: *Prunus avium* L. [FR].

***Prunus domestica* L.**

VN: Plum tree (E). Pflaumenbaum (G). Prunier (F).

FR: Fruit permitted as laxative.

SW: Classified as foodstuff.

***Prunus spinosa* L.**

VN: Blackthorn (E). Schlehdorn (G). Épine noire; Prunellier (F).

KE: Flower not permitted for therapeutic use. Usefulness is not documented adequately. No risks are known, however, and there is no objection to the use as an admixture to herbal teas [BAnz nr.101 01.06.90].

Fruit permitted for local use in mouth. No CI, AE, I [BAnz nr.101 01.06.90].

SW: Classified as natural product.

***Psidium guayava* L.**

VN: Guajava; Guava (E). Djamboe; Guayava (G). Goyavier (F).

SW: Fruit classified as natural product.

***Pterocarpus santalinus* L.**

VN: Red sandalwood; Red sanders (E). Roter Sandelbaum (G). Santal rouge (F).

KE: Wood not permitted for therapeutic use. Usefulness is not documented adequately. No risks are known, however [BAnz nr.193 15.10.87].

SZ: The addition of the wood to certain herbal tea mixtures is permitted.

Ptychopetalum olacoides **Benth. =** ***Acanthea virilis*** **L.**
VN: Muira-Puama (E). Muira-puama; Potenzbaum (G). Muira-puma (F).
KE: Wood not permitted for therapeutic use. Usefulness is not documented adequately. No risks are known, however [BAnz nr.193 15.10.87].
AS: *Ptychopetalum unicatum* Anselmino [KE].

Pulmonaria officinalis **L. =** ***Pulmonaria maculosa*** **(Liebl.) Gams**
VN: Dage of Jerusalem; Lungwort (E). (Echtes) Lungenkraut (G). Pulmonaire (F).
KE: Herb not permitted for therapeutic use. Usefulness is not documented adequately. No risks are known, however [BAnz nr.193 15.10.87].
SZ: The addition of the herb to certain herbal tea mixtures is permitted.

Pulsatilla pratensis **Mill. =** ***Anemone pratensis*** **L.**
VN: Meadow windflower (E). Nickende Küchenschelle; Wiesen-Kuhschelle (G). Pulsatilla des prés (F).
SW: Classified as natural product.

Pulsatilla vulgaris **Miller =** ***Anemone pulsatilla*** **L.**
VN: Meadow windflower (E). Küchenschelle (G). Anémone pulsatille (F).
KE: Herb not permitted for therapeutic use. Usefulness is not documented adequately. Higher doses may irritate the kidneys and urinary tract and pregnancy is an absolute CI [BAnz nr.223 30.11.85].
FR: Fresh flowering aerial parts permitted for oral use (toxicological categories pd:2 ht/ae/wa:1 sa/ti:1).

Pygeum africanum **Hook.f.**
SW: Classified as a drug, which must normally be registered as pharmaceutical speciality.

Pyrus malus **L. =** ***Malus sylvestris*** **(L.) Mill.**
VN: Apple tree (E). Apfelbaum (G). Pommier (F).
FR: Fruit permitted as laxative.

Quassia amara **L.**
VN: Bitter wood; Quassia wood (E). Bitterholz (G). Bois amer; Bois de quassia (F).
SW: Classified as natural product.
RM: Bitter wood is obtained not only from *Quassia amara* L. (= Surinam quassia), but also from *Picrasma excelsa* (Schwartz) Planch. (= Jamaica quassia) [34].

Quercus robur **L. =** ***Quercus pedunculata*** **Ehrh.**
VN: (English) Oak (E). Sommer-Eiche; Stiel-Eiche (G). Chêne (commun); Gravelier (F).

KE: Bark permitted for oral use. No CI for internal use. No AE. I: reduced absorption of alkaloids and other basic substances [BAnz nr.22a 01.02.90].
SZ: Bark permitted as herbal tea for non-internal purposes (mouthwash, gargle, foot-bath, hip-bath). No CI, AE, I.
SW: Classified as natural product.
AS: *Quercus petraea* (Matt.) Liebl. = *Quercus sessiliflora* Sal. [KE].

***Quillaja saponaria* Mol.**
VN: Quillaia; Quillaja (E). Seifenrindenbaum (G). Panama (F).
FR: Bark permitted for external use only (toxicological categories pd:-ht/ae/wa:1 sa/ti:1).
SW: Classified as natural product.
AS: *Quillaja smegmadermos* DC. [FR].

***Ranunculus ficaria* L. = *Ficaria ranunculoides* Moench.**
VN: Figwort; Pilewort (E). Feigwurz; Scharbockskraut (G). Ficaire (F).
FR: Root permitted for external use only (toxicological categories pd:-ht/ae/wa:1 sa/ti:1).

***Raphanus sativus* L. var. *niger* (Mill.) S. Kerner**
VN: Black radish (E). Schwarzer Rettich (G). Radis noir (F).
KE: Root permitted for oral use. CI: cholelithiasis. No AE, I [BAnz nr.177a 24.09.86].
FR: Root permitted for oral use (toxicological categories pd:2 ht/ae/wa:1 sa/ti:1).
Juice of fresh plant permitted without specifications.
SW: Classified as natural product.
AS: KE also permits ssp. *niger* (Miller) DC var. *albus* DC.

***Rauwolfia serpentina* (L.) Bentham ex Kurz**
VN: Rauwolfia; Snakewood (E). Rauwolfia; Schlangenholz (G). Arbre aux serpents; Rauwolfia (F).
KE: Root permitted for oral use. CI, AE and I of the toxic alkaloid reserpine [BAnz nr.173 18.09.86].
SW: *Rauwolfia* species are classified as drugs, which must normally be registered as pharmaceutical speciality.

***Rhamnus catharticus* L.**
VN: Buckthorn (E). Purgierdorn (G). Nerprun (F).
KE: Fruit permitted for oral use. CI, AE, I of anthranoid laxatives [BAnz nr.101 01.06.90].
SZ: Fruit permitted for short-term use as herbal tea. CI, AE, I of anthranoid laxatives.
FR: Fruit pulp permitted as laxative.

***Rhamnus frangula* L. = *Frangula alnus* Miller**

VN: Buckthorn (E). Faulbaum (G). Bourdaine; Frangule (F).
KE: Bark permitted for oral use. CI, AE, I of anthranoid laxatives [BAnz nr.228 05.12.84].
SZ: Bark permitted for short-term use as herbal tea. CI, AE, I of anthranoid laxatives.
FR: Bark permitted for short-term oral use (max. 8–10 days) as a laxative by adults and children of 12 years and older. CI, AE and I of anthranoid laxatives.
BE: Bark and dry extract permitted as traditional laxative. Max. 10 daily doses/package.
SW: Classified as a drug, which must normally be registered as pharmaceutical speciality.
RM: As the fresh drug contains anthrones and is strongly emetic, it should be stored for at least one year or be submitted to an artificial aging process [KE].

***Rhamnus purshianus* DC. = *Frangula purshiana* (DC.) A. Gray ex J.C. Cooper**

VN: Cascara sagrada (E). Amerikanischer Faulbaum; Cascara (G). Cascara (F).
KE: Bark permitted for oral use. CI, AE, I of anthranoid laxatives [BAnz nr.228 05.12.84].
SZ: Bark permitted for short-term use as herbal tea. CI, AE, I of anthranoid laxatives.
FR: Bark permitted for short-term oral use (max. 8–10 days) as a laxative by adults and children of 12 years and older. CI, AE and I of anthranoid laxatives.
BE: Bark and dry extract permitted as traditional laxative. Max. 10 daily doses/package.
SW: Classified as a drug, which must normally be registered as pharmaceutical speciality.
RM: As the fresh drug contains anthrones and is strongly emetic, it should be stored for at least one year or be submitted to an artificial aging process [KE].

***Rheum palmatum* L.**

VN: Rhubarb (E). Rhabarber (G). Rhubarbe (de Chine) (F).
KE: Root permitted for oral use. CI, AE, I of anthranoid laxatives [BAnz nr.228 05.12.84 and BAnz nr.80 27.04.89].
SZ: Root permitted for short-term use as herbal tea. CI, AE, I of anthranoid laxatives.
FR: Root permitted for external use (toxicological categories pd:1 ht/ae/wa:1 sa/ti:1).
Rhizome permitted for short-term oral use (max. 8–10 days) as a

laxative by adults and children of 12 years and older. CI, AE and I of anthranoid laxatives.
SW: Classified as natural product (with a dose limitation).
AS: *Rheum officinale* Baill. [FR].

Rheum rhaponticum **L.**
VN: Garden rhubarb (E). Rapontik (rhabarber) (G). Rhapontic; Rhubarbe de France (F).
FR: Rhizome permitted for short-term oral use (max. 8–10 days) as a laxative by adults and children of 12 years and older. CI, AE and I of anthranoid laxatives.
AS: Related species [FR].
RM: Is sometimes considered an adulterant of *Rheum palmatum*, as it contains less anthracene derivatives. Can be identified by presence of stilbene derivatives, in particular rhaponticosid (= rhaponticin) [34].

Rhododendron ferrugineum **L.**
VN: Rostrote Alpenrose (G).
KE: Leaf not permitted for therapeutic use. No AE have been reported for herbal tea, but toxic diterpenes may be present and chronic use might lead to hydroquinone poisoning (due to the presence of arbutin) [BAnz nr.164 01.09.90].

Rhus toxicodendron **L.**
VN: Poison oak; Upright sumac (E). (Echter) Gift-Sumach (G). Sumac vénéneux (F).
SW: Classified as a drug, which must normally be registered as pharmaceutical speciality.

Ribes nigrum **L.**
VN: Black currant (E). Schwarze Johannisbeere (G). Cassissier; Groseillier noir (F).
SZ: Leaf permitted as herbal tea. No CI, AE, I.
FR: Leaf permitted for oral use (toxicological categories pd:2 ht/ae/wa:1 sa/ti:1).
Fresh fruit permitted for oral use (toxicological categories pd:1 ht/ae/wa:1 sa/ti:1).
BE: Leaf permitted as traditional diuretic and as traditional antiarthritic agent.
SW: Leaf and fruit classified as foodstuff and as natural product.

Ricinus communis **L.**
VN: Castor-oil plant (E). Wunderbaum (G). Ricin commun (F).
SZ: Refined oil is permitted as such. CI: intestinal obstruction, unexplained stomach ache. AE: frequent use produces electrolyte losses

(I with cardiac glycosides); also gastric irritation, allergic skin reactions. Should not be used for prolonged period.
SW: Classified as a drug, which must normally be registered as pharmaceutical speciality.

Rosa canina **L.**
VN: Brier hip (E). Hundsrose (G). Églantier; Rosier sauvage (F).
KE: Pseudofruit ("Hagebuttenschalen"), fruit ("Hagebuttenkerne") and pseudofruit with fruits ("Hagebutten") are not permitted for therapeutic use. Usefulness is not documented adequately. No risks are known, however, and there is no objection to the use of the pseudofruit or the pseudofruit with fruits as an admixture to herbal teas [BAnz nr.164 01.09.90].
SZ: The addition of the pseudofruit to certain herbal remedies is permitted.
FR: Pseudofruit is permitted for oral use (toxicological categories pd:1 ht/ae/wa:1 sa/ti:1).
AS: Pharmacopoea Helvetica VII permits *Rosa pendulina* L. as source plant [34].

Rosa gallica **L.**
VN: French rose; Red rose (E). Französische Rose; Rote Rose (G). Rose rouge; Rosier (F).
KE: Petal permitted for local use in the mouth. No CI, AE, I [BAnz nr.164 01.09.90].
FR: Flower-bud and petal permitted for oral use (toxicological categories pd:1 ht/ae/wa:1 sa/ti:1).
AS: *R. centifolia* L. and *R. damascena* Mill. [8]. KE specifies *Rosa gallica* L., *R. centifolia* L. and their varieties.

Rosa multiflora **Thunb.**
SW: Classified as natural product.

Rosmarinus officinalis **L.**
VN: Rosemary (E). Rosmarin (G). Romarin (F).
KE: Leaf permitted for oral use. No CI, AE, I [BAnz nr.223 30.11.85].
SZ: Leaf permitted as herbal tea. CI: pregnancy. No AE, I.
FR: Leaf and flowering top permitted for oral use (toxicological categories pd:1 ht/ae/wa:1 sa/ti:1).

Rubia tinctorum **L.**
VN: Madder (E). Färberröte; Krapp (G). Garance (des teinturiers) (F).
KE: Root permitted for oral use. CI: pregnancy, lactation. AE: harmless red discoloration of the urine. No I [BAnz nr.173 18.09.86].
SW: Classified as natural product.

RM: KE has prepared a revised monograph, in which the therapeutic use of madder root will no longer be permitted because of its genotoxic risks.

***Rubus fruticosus* L.**

VN: Blackberry; Bramble (E). Brombeere (G). Ronce (noire) (F).

KE: Leaf permitted for oral use. No CI, AE, I [BAnz nr.22a 01.02.90]. Root not permitted for therapeutic use. Usefulness is not documented adequately. No risks are known, however [BAnz nr.22a 01.02.90].

SZ: Leaf and root permitted as herbal tea. No CI, AE, I.

FR: Leaf and root permitted for oral use (toxicological categories pd:2 ht/ae/wa:1 sa/ti:1).

SW: Classified as natural product.

AS: FR only speaks about "ronce" (*Rubus* sp.) in general.

***Rubus idaeus* L.**

VN: Raspberry (E). Himbeere (G). Framboisier (F).

KE: Leaf not permitted for therapeutic use. Usefulness is not documented adequately. No risks are known, however [BAnz nr.193 15.10.87].

SW: Classified as natural product.

***Ruscus aculeatus* L.**

VN: Butcher's broan (E). Mäusedorn; Stechender Mäusedorn (G). Fragon épineux; Petit houx (F).

KE: Rhizome permitted for oral use. No CI or I. AE: rarely gastric complaints, nausea [BAnz nr.127 12.07.91].

FR: Subterranean parts permitted for oral use (toxicological categories pd:2 ht/ae/wa:1 sa/ti:1).

***Ruta graveolens* L.**

VN: Rue (E). Gartenraute; Weinraute (G). Rue officinale (F).

KE: Leaf and herb not permitted for therapeutic use. Usefulness is not documented adequately. The essential oil is toxic and can produce contact dermatitis. Phototoxic reactions are possible (furocoumarins) [BAnz nr.43 02.03.89].

SW: Classified as a drug, which must normally be registered as pharmaceutical speciality.

AS: KE specifies ssp. *vulgaris* Willkomm.

***Saccharomyces cerevisiae* Meyen**

VN: Yeast (E). Bierhefe (G). Levure de bière (F).

KE: Cell (faex medicinalis) permitted for oral use. No CI. AE: headache; flatulence (from fermentable yeast). I: MAO-inhibitors (hypertensive reaction) [BAnz nr.85 05.05.88].

AS: *Candida utilis* (Henn.) Rodden et Kreyer Van Rey [KE].

***Salix alba* L.**

VN: (White) willow (E). Silber-Weide (G). Aubier (blanc); Saule (F).
KE: Bark permitted for oral use. CI, AE, I: on theoretical grounds similar to those of the salicylates. [BAnz nr.228 05.12.84].
SZ: The inclusion of the bark in certain herbal tea mixtures is permitted.
FR: Stem bark permitted for oral use (toxicological categories pd:2 ht/ae/wa:1 sa/ti:1).
BE: Bark permitted as traditional antiarthritic agent.
SW: Classified as natural product.
AS: *Salix purpurea* L., *Salix fragilis* L. and other equivalent spp.; at least 1% of total salicin should be present [KE].
Salix purpurea L., *Salix irminalis* L. [FR].
A German text book prefers 3 out of 8 considered spp. because their salicin content is sufficient: *Salix purpurea*, *Salix daphnoides* and *Salix fragilis* [34].
SW also classifies *Salix nigra* Marsh. as natural product.

***Salvia lavandulaefolia* Vahl. = *Salvia officinalis* L. ssp. *lavandulaefolia* (Vahl.) Gams.**

VN: Sauge d'Espagne (F).
FR: Leaf and flowering top permitted for oral use (toxicological categories pd:2 ht/ae/wa:1 sa/ti:2).

***Salvia officinalis* L.**

VN: Sage (E). Salbei (G). Sauge officinale (F).
KE: Leaf permitted for oral use. CI: pregnancy (essential oil/alcoholic extracts). AE: prolonged use of essential oil/alcoholic extracts may produce epileptiform cramps. No I [BAnz nr.228 05.12.84].
SZ: Leaf permitted as herbal tea. No CI, AE, I. Should not be used for prolonged period.
FR: Leaf and flowering top permitted for oral use (toxicological categories pd:2 ht/ae/wa:1 sa/ti:2). The level of active constituents has to be limited.
BE: Leaf permitted as traditional stomatological.
SW: Classified as natural product.
RM: A German text book specifies ssp. *minor* (Gmelin) Gams. and ssp. *major* (Garsault) Gams. but excludes ssp. *lavandulaefolia* (Vahl) Gams., because this is considered a separate species [34].

***Salvia sclarea* L.**

VN: Clary sage (E). Muskateller-Salbei (G). Sauge sclarée; Toute-bonne (F).
FR: Leaf and flowering top permitted for oral use (toxicological categories pd:2 ht/ae/wa:1 sa/ti:2).

***Sambucus nigra* L.**

VN: Black elder (E). (Schwarzer) Holunder (G). Sureau noir (F).
KE: Flower permitted for oral use. No CI, AE, I [BAnz nr.50 13.03.86].
SZ: Flower permitted as herbal tea. No CI, AE, I.
FR: Flower and fruit permitted for oral use (toxicological categories pd:1 ht/ae/wa:1 sa/ti:1).
Stem bark also permitted for oral use (toxicological categories pd:2 ht/ae/wa:1 sa/ti:2).
SW: Classified as natural product.
BE: Flower permitted as traditional diuretic.
AS: SW also classifies other *Sambucus* species as natural product.

***Sanguinaria canadensis* L.**

VN: Bloodroot (E). Kanadische Blutwurzel (G). Sanguinaire (F).
SW: Classified as natural product.

***Sanicula europaea* L.**

VN: Sanicle (E). Sanikel (G). Sanicle (commun) (F).
KE: Herb permitted for oral use. No CI, AE, I [BAnz nr.177a 24.09.86].

***Santalum album* L.**

VN: Weißes Sandelholz (G).
KE: Wood permitted for oral use. CI: diseases of renal parenchym. AE: nausea, skin itching. No I. Not to be used for more than 6 weeks without consulting physician [BAnz nr.43 02.03.89].
SW: Classified as natural product.

***Saponaria officinalis* L.**

VN: Soapwort (E). (Gemeines) Seifenkraut (G). Saponaire (officinale) (F).
KE: Herb not permitted for therapeutic use. Usefulness is not documented adequately. Contains irritating triterpene saponins [BAnz nr.80 27.04.89].
Root permitted for oral use. No CI, I. AE: gastric irritation (rarely) [BAnz nr.80 27.03.89].
SW: Classified as natural product.

***Saraca indica* L.**

SW: Classified as natural product.

***Sarothamnus scoparius* (L.) Wimm. ex Koch = *Cytisus scoparius* (L.) Link**

VN: (Scotch) Broom (E). (Gemeiner) Besenginster (G). Genêt à balai (F).
KE: Flower not permitted for therapeutic use. Usefulness is not documented adequately. Contains only low level of alkaloids (major alkaloid spartein) so that toxic alkaloidal effects should not be expected. CI: hypertension. I: MAO-inhibitors (the flower may

contain over 2% of tyramine). There is no objection to the use as an admixture in herbal teas in levels up to 1% [BAnz nr.11 17.01.91]. Herb permitted for oral use. No CI, AE. I: MAO-inhibitors (due to tyramine content) [BAnz nr.11 17.01.91].

SZ: Herb permitted as herbal tea. CI: Hypertension, pregnancy. No AE, I.

FR: Flower permitted for oral use (toxicological categories pd:2 ht/ae/wa:1 sa/ti:2).

RM: According to KE, hydroalcoholic preparations of the herb should contain max. 1 mg/ml of the alkaloid spartein.

***Sassafras albidum* (Nutt.) Nees**

VN: Sassafras (E). Sassafras (G). Sassafras (F).

SW: Classified as foodstuff.

RM: As sassafras wood contains 1–2% of essential oil consisting for about 80% of the toxic and hepatocarcinogenic compound safrole, prolonged use is generally discouraged [34].

***Satureja montana* L.**

VN: Winter Savory (E). Bergbohnenkraut (G). Sarriette des montagnes (F).

FR: Leaf and flowering top permitted for oral use (toxicological categories pd:1 ht/ae/wa:1 sa/ti:1).

Schisandra chinensis* (Turcz.) *Baill.

VN: Magnoliavine (E).

SW: Classified as natural product.

***Schizonepeta tenuifolia* (Bth.) Brig. = *Nepeta japonica* Maxim.**

SW: Classified as a drug, which must normally be registered as pharmaceutical speciality.

***Scopolia carniolica* Jacq.**

VN: Glockenbilsenkraut (G).

KE: Rhizome permitted for oral use. CI, AE, I of belladonna alkaloids [BAnz. nr.177a 24.09.86].

***Scrophularia nodosa* L.**

VN: Figwort (E). Knotige Braunwurz (G). Scrofulaire noueuse (F).

FR: Root and flowering top permitted for oral use (toxicological categories pd:2 ht/ae/wa:1 sa/ti:1).

AS: FR speaks about "scrofulaire" in general. In France, two different *Scrophularia* spp. are known under this vernacular name: *S. nodosa* L. (scrofulaire noueuse) and *S. umbrosa* Dumort. = *S. aquatica* L. (scrofulaire aquatique).

***Secale cereale* L.**

VN: Rye (E). Roggen (G). Seigle (F).
FR: Fruit permitted as laxative.

***Sedum telephium* L.**

VN: Livelong (E). Knolliges Steinkraut; Rote Fetthenne (G). Grand orphin (F).
SW: Classified as natural product.
AS: SW also classifies *Sedum roseum* Scop. as natural product.

***Selenicereus grandiflorus* (L.) Britton et Rose = *Cereus grandiflorus* (L.) Mill.**

VN: Night-blooming cereus (E). Königin der Nacht (G). Ciege à grandes fleurs (F).
KE: Flower and herb not permitted for therapeutic use. Usefulness is not documented adequately. No risks are known, however [BAnz nr.22a 01.02.90].
SW: Classified as natural product.

***Senecio nemorensis* L. ssp. *fuchsii* (Gmel.) Celak**

VN: (Fuchs)kreuzkraut (G).
KE: Herb not permitted for therapeutic use. Usefulness is not documented adequately. Contains hepatotoxic and carcinogenic pyrrolizidine alkaloids. The use in diabetes mellitus may keep from therapy with proven effectiveness [BAnz nr.138 27.07.90].

***Serenoa repens* (Bartr.) Small = *Sabal serrulata* (Michx.) Nutall ex Schultes**

VN: Saw palmetto (E). Zwergpalme (G). Palmier de l'Amérique du Nord (F).
KE: Fruit permitted for oral use. No CI, I. AE: gastric complaints (rarely). As improvement is symptomatic without eliminating prostatic hypertrophy, a physician should be consulted regularly [BAnz nr.43 02.03.89].
SW: Classified as natural product.

***Silybum marianum* (L.) Gaertn. = *Carduus marianus* L.**

VN: St. Mary's thistle (E). Mariendistel (G). Chardon-Marie (F).
KE: Fruit permitted for oral use. No CI, I. AE: occasionally slight laxative effect [BAnz nr.50 13.03.86].
Herb not permitted for therapeutic use. Usefulness is not documented adequately. No risks are known, however [BAnz nr.49 11.03.92].
SZ: Fruit permitted as herbal tea. No CI, I, AE.
FR: Fruit permitted for oral use (toxicological categories pd:1 ht/ae/wa:1 sa/ti:1).
SW: Classified as foodstuff and as natural product.

***Sinapis alba* L. = *Brassica alba* Boiss.**
VN: White mustard (E). Weißer Senf (G). Moutarde blanche (F).
KE: Seed permitted for external use only. CI: children younger than 6 years; renal disease (mustard oil is absorbed through skin). AE: skin and nervous damage (prolonged use). Should not be used for more than 2 weeks [BAnz nr.22a 01.02.90].
SW: *Sinapis* species are classified as foodstuff.

***Smilax regelii* Kill et C.V. Morton = *Smilax utilis* Hemsley**
VN: Sarsaparilla (E). Sarsaparilla (G). Salsepareille (F).
KE: Root not permitted for therapeutic use. Usefulness is not documented adequately. Gastric and renal toxicity as well as drug interactions are possible [BAnz nr.164 01.09.90].
SW: SW classifies "sarsaparille" as natural product.
AS: *Smilax aristolochiaefolia* Miller and *Smilax febrifuga* Kunth. [KE].

***Solanum dulcamara* L.**
VN: Dogwood; Sweet bitter (E). Bittersüß (G). Douce-amère (F).
KE: Stalk permitted for oral use. No CI, AE, I [BAnz nr.101 01.06.90].
RM: According to a Dutch textbook, excessive use of stalk preparations has been associated with serious poisoning [44].

***Solidago serotina* Ait. = *Solidago gigantea* Ait.**
VN: Riesengoldrute (G).
KE: Herb permitted for oral use. No CI, AE, I [BAnz nr.193 15.10.87].
SZ: Herb permitted as herbal tea. CI: patients with chronic renal disease should first consult a physician. No AE, I.
AS: KE specifies *Solidago serotina* Ait. = *S. gigantea* Ait. and S. *canadensis* L. and their hybrids.

***Solidago virgaurea* L.**
VN: Golden rod (E). (Echte) Goldrute (G). Solidage; Verge d'or (F).
KE: Herb permitted for oral use. No CI, AE, I [BAnz nr.193 15.10.87].
SZ: Herb permitted as herbal tea. CI: patients with chronic renal disease should first consult a physician. No AE, I.
FR: Flowering top permitted for oral use (toxicological categories pd:2 ht/ae/wa:1 sa/ti:1).
BE: Flowering top permitted as traditional diuretic.
SW: Classified as natural product.
AS: *Solidago virgaurea* is no longer generally available. More common source plants of trade products are *Solidago gigantea* Ait. and *Solidago canadensis* L. [34].

***Sophora japonica* L.**
SW: Classified as natural product.

***Sorbus aucuparia* L.**

VN: Mountain-ash; Quickbeam (E). Eberesche; Vogelbeerbaum (G). Sabier des oiseleurs; Sorbier (F).

KE: Fruit not permitted for therapeutic use. Usefulness is not documented adequately. No risks are known, however [BAnz nr.122 06.07.88].

SW: Classified as foodstuff and as natural product.

***Spinacia oleracea* L.**

VN: Spinach (E). Spinat (G). Épinards (F).

KE: Leaf not permitted for therapeutic use. Usefulness is not documented adequately. No risks are known, however [BAnz nr.85 05.05.88].

***Stachys officinalis* (L.) Trévisan = *Betonica officinalis* L.**

VN: Betony (E). Betonie; Heilziest (G). Bétoine (F).

FR: Leaf permitted for oral use (toxicological categories pd:2 ht/ae/wa:1 sa/ti:1).

***Stellaria media* (L.) Vill. = *Alsine media* L.**

VN: Chickweed (E). Vogelmiere. (G). Morsgeline; Mouron des oiseaux (F).

SW: Classified as natural product.

***Sterculia tomentosa* Guill. et Perr.**

VN: Karaya (E). Karaya (G). Karaya; Sterculia (F).

FR: Gum permitted as laxative.

AS: *Sterculia urens* Roxb. [FR].

***Stevia rebaudiana* (Bert.) Hemsley = *Eupatorium rebaudianum* Bert.**

SW: Classified as natural product.

***Strophanthus kombe* Oliv.**

VN: Strophantus (E). Strophantus (G). Strophantus (F).

SW: Classified as a drug, which must normally be registered as pharmaceutical speciality.

AS: SW also classifies *Strophanthus gratus* Baill. as a drug, which must normally be registered as pharmaceutical speciality.

***Strychnos nux-vomica* L.**

VN: Nux vomica (E). Brechnußbaum (G). Vomiquier (F).

KE: Seed not permitted for therapeutic use. Usefulness is not documented adequately for most advocated uses. Contains the toxic alkaloid strychnine [BAnz nr.173 18.09.86].

SW: Classified as a natural product (with a dose limitation) and as a drug, which must normally be registered as pharmaceutical speciality.

***Styrax tonkinensis* (Pierre) Craib. et Hartw. = *Anthostyrax tonkinensis* Pierre**
SW: The balsamic resin (= Siam benzoin) is classified as natural product.

***Swertia chirata* Buch. Ham.**
SW: Classified as natural product.

***Symphytum officinale* L. = *Symphytum consolida* Gueldenst. ex Ledeb.**
VN: (Common) comfrey (E). Beinwell (G). Consoude (grande) (F).
KE: Herb, leaf, root permitted for external use only. No CI, AE, I. Skin should be intact and pregnant user should first consult physician. External dosage of pyrrolizidine alkaloids max. 100 μg/day for max. 4–6 weeks/year [BAnz nr.138 27.07.90].
FR: Root permitted for external use only (toxicological categories pd:-ht/ae/wa:1 sa/ti:1).
SW: Classified as a drug, which must normally be registered as pharmaceutical speciality.

***Syzygium aromaticum* (L.) Merr. et L.M. Perry = *Caryophyllus aromaticus* L. = *Eugenia caryophyllata* Thunb.**
VN: Clove (E). Gewürznelkenbaum (G). Giroflier (F).
KE: Flower-bud permitted for local use in the mouth. No CI, AE, I [BAnz nr.223 30.11.85].
FR: Flower-bud permitted for oral use (toxicological categories pd:1 ht/ae/wa:1 sa/ti:1).
BE: Flower-bud permitted as traditional stomatological.
SW: Classified as natural product.

***Syzygium cumini* (L.) Skeels = *Syzygium jambolana* (Lam.) DC.**
VN: Java plum (E). Jambolanapflaume (G). Jambolanier (F).
KE: Bark permitted for oral use. No CI, AE, I [BAnz nr.76 23.04.87]. Seed not permitted for therapeutic use. Usefulness is not documented adequately. Should not be used instead of antidiabetic therapy with proven effectiveness [BAnz nr.76 23.04.87].

***Tabebuia* species**
VN: Ipe roxo; Pau d'arco; Taheebo (E).
SW: Bark classified as a drug, which must normally be registered as pharmaceutical speciality.

***Tamarindus indica* L.**
VN: Tamarind (E). Tamarindenbaum (G). Tamarinier (de l'Inde) (F).
FR: Fruit pulp permitted as laxative.
BE: Pulp permitted as traditional laxative.
SW: Classified as natural product.

***Tanacetum parthenium* (L.) Schultz Bip. = *Chrysanthemum parthenium* (L.) Bernh.**

VN: Feverfew (E). Mutterkraut (G). Camomille grande (F).
FR: Aerial parts permitted for oral use (toxicological categories pd:2 ht/ae/wa:1 sa/ti:2).
SW: Classified as natural product.

***Taraxacum officinale* G.H. Weber ex Wigger s.l. = *Taraxacum dens-leonis* Desf.**

VN: Dandelion (E). Löwenzahn (G). Dent de lion; Pissenlit (F).
KE: Root with herb permitted for oral use. CI: biliary obstruction, empyema of gall-bladder, ileus. AE: Gastric complaints. No I [BAnz nr.228 05.12.84 and BAnz nr.164 01.09.90].
SZ: Root with herb permitted as herbal tea. CI: biliary inflammation or obstruction; intestinal obstruction. No AE, I.
FR: Leaf and root permitted for oral use (toxicological categories pd:1 ht/ae/wa:1 sa/ti:1).
SW: Classified as natural product.
AS: Related species [FR].

***Terminalia chebula* Retz. = *Myrobalanus chebula* Gaertn.**

VN: Myrobalan (E).
SW: Classified as natural product.
AS: SW also classifies *Terminalia bellirica* (Gaertn.) Roxb. as natural product.

***Tetragonolobus maritimus* (L.) Roth.**

SW: Classified as natural product.

***Teucrium chamaedrys* L.**

VN: Common germander (E). Edler Gamander (G). Germandrée petit-chêne (F).
FR: Flowering aerial parts permitted for oral use (toxicological categories pd:2 ht/ae/wa:1 sa/ti:1).[1]

***Teucrium marum* L.**

VN: Cat thyme (E). Amberkraut; Katzenkraut (G). Germandrée maritime; Thym de chat (F).
FR: Flowering top permitted for oral use (toxicological categories pd:2 ht/ae/wa:1 sa/ti:1).

***Teucrium polium* L.**

VN: Germandrée tomenteuse (F).

---

[1] See the note added in proof on p. 317

FR: Aerial parts permitted for oral use (toxicological categories pd:2 ht/ae/wa:1 sa/ti:1).

***Theobroma cacao* L.**

VN: Cacao (E). Cacao (G). Cacao (F).

KE: Seed and seed-shell not permitted for therapeutic use. Usefulness is not documented adequately. There is no objection, however, to the use of the seed as an admixture. CI: hypersensitivity. AE: allergic reactions with skin manifestations and migraine [BAnz nr.40 27.02.91].

***Thuja occidentalis* L.**

VN: American arbor vitae (E). Abendländischer Lebensbaum (G). Thuya (du Canada) (F).

SW: Classified as a drug, which must normally be registered as pharmaceutical speciality.

***Thymus serpyllum* L.**

VN: Mother of thyme; Wild thyme (E). Quendel; Wilder Thymian (G). Serpolet; Thym sauvage (F).

KE: Herb permitted for oral use. No CI, AE, I [BAnz nr.193 15.10.87].

SZ: The addition of the herb to certain herbal tea mixtures is permitted.

FR: Leaf and flowering top permitted for oral use (toxicological categories pd:1 ht/ae/wa:1 sa/ti:1).

BE: Herb permitted as traditional cough remedy and as traditional digestive aid.

SW: Classified as natural product.

***Thymus vulgaris* L.**

VN: Common thyme; Garden thyme (E). Echter Thymian; Römischer Quendel (G). Thym (commun); Thym vrai (F).

KE: Herb permitted for oral use. No CI, AE, I [BAnz nr.228 05.12.84].

SZ: Herb permitted as herbal tea. No CI, AE, I.

FR: Leaf and flowering top permitted for oral use (toxicological categories pd:1 ht/ae/wa:1 sa/ti:1).

BE: Herb permitted as traditional cough remedy and as traditional digestive aid.

AS: *Thymus zygis* L. [FR].

***Tilia cordata* Mill. = *Tilia sylvestris* Desf.**

VN: Lime tree (E). Linde; Winterlinde (G). Tilleul (sauvage) (F).

KE: Inflorescence permitted for oral use. No CI, AE, I [BAnz nr.164 01.09.90].

Leaf not permitted for therapeutic use. Usefulness is not documented adequately. No risks are known, however, and there is no objection to use as admixture to herbal teas [BAnz nr.164 01.09.90].

Wood and charcoal not permitted for therapeutic use. Usefulness is

not documented adequately. No risks are known, however [BAnz nr.164 01.09.90].
SZ: Inflorescence permitted as herbal tea. No CI, AE, I.
FR: Inflorescence permitted for oral use (toxicological categories pd:1 ht/ae/wa:1 sa/ti:1).
Sap-wood permitted for oral use (toxicological categories pd:2 ht/ae/wa:1 sa/ti:1).
BE: Inflorescence, powder and extract permitted as traditional tranquillizer.
SW: Classified as natural product.
AS: *Tilia platyphyllos* Scop. = *T. grandifolia* Ehrh. as alternative source for the inflorescence [KE,SZ,FR], the sap-wood [FR], the leaf, the wood and the charcoal [KE].

***Tilia tomentosa* Moench = *Tilia argentea* Desf.**
VN: Silberlinde (G).
KE: Flower not permitted for therapeutic use. Usefulness is not documented adequately. No risks are known, however, and there is no objection to use as an admixture to herbal teas [BAnz nr.164 01.09.90].

***Trifolium pratense* L.**
VN: Red clover; Wild clover (E). Wiesenklee (G). Trèfle des prés (F).
SW: Classified as natural product.

***Trigonella foenum-graecum* L.**
VN: Fenugreek (E). Bockshornklee (G). Fénugrec (F).
KE: Seed permitted for oral use. No CI, I. AE: skin reactions to repeated external use [BAnz nr.22a 01.02.90].
FR: Seed permitted for oral use (toxicological categories pd:1 ht/ae/wa:1 sa/ti:-).
SW: Classified as foodstuff and as natural product.

***Triticum aestivum* L. = *Triticum vulgare* Vill. = *Triticum sativum* Lamk.**
VN: Common wheat (E). Weizen (G). Blé (F).
FR: Bran permitted as laxative.

***Tropaeolum majus* L.**
VN: (Common) nasturtium (E). Kapuzinerkresse (G). Capucine (F).
FR: Fresh leaf permitted for oral use (toxicological categories pd:1 ht/ae/wa:- sa/ti:1).

***Turnera diffusa* Willd.**
VN: Damiana (E). Damiana (G). Damiana (F).
KE: Leaf and herb not permitted for therapeutic use. Usefulness is not documented adequately. No risks are known, however [BAnz nr.43 02.03.89].
SW: Classified as natural product.

***Tussilago farfara* L.**

VN: Coltsfoot (E). (Gemeiner) Huflattich (G). Pas d'âne; Tussilage (F).

KE: Flower, herb, root not permitted for therapeutic use. Usefulness is not documented adequately. Contains hepatotoxic pyrrolizidine alkaloids (PA) in all plant parts [BAnz nr.138 27.07.90].
Leaf is permitted for oral use. CI: pregnancy, lactation. No AE, I. Dosage max. 10 μg PA/day (herbal tea) or max. 1 μg PA/day (extracts, expressed sap) for max. 4–6 weeks per year [BAnz nr.138 27.07.90].

SZ: Leaf is permitted as herbal tea. No CI, AE, I.

SW: Classified as a drug, which must normally be registered as pharmaceutical speciality. Not accepted.

***Urginea maritima* (L.) Baker = *Scilla maritima* L.**

VN: Sea-onion; Squill (E). Meerzwiebel (G). Scille (F).

KE: Bulb permitted for oral use. CI, AE and I of cardiac glycosides [BAnz nr.154 21.08.85].

SW: Classified as a drug, which must normally be registered as pharmaceutical speciality.

***Urtica dioica* L.**

VN: (Common) nettle (E). Große Brennessel (G). Ortie dioique (F).

KE: Herb and leaf permitted for oral use. No CI, AE, I [BAnz nr.76 23.04.87].
Root permitted for oral use. No CI, I [BAnz nr.173 18.09.86]. AE: mild GI-complaints (occasionally) [BAnz nr.43 02.03.89].

SZ: Herb permitted as herbal tea. No CI, AE, I.

FR: Aerial parts permitted for oral use (toxicological categories pd:1 ht/ae/wa:1 sa/ti:1).
Root permitted for oral use (toxicological categories pd:2 ht/ae/wa:1 sa/ti:1).

SW: Classified as natural product.

AS: KE specifies *Urtica dioica* L., *Urtica urens* L. and/or their hybrids as source plants for the herb, leaf, and root.

***Usnea barbata* (L.) Wiggers emend. Mot.**

VN: Bartflechte (G).

KE: Thallus permitted for local use in mouth. No CI, AE, I [BAnz nr.80 27.04.89].

AS: Other *Usnea* spp., in particular *U. florida* (L.) Fries, *U. hirta* (L.) Hoffmann and *U. plicata* (L.) Fries [KE].

***Vaccinium myrtillus* L.**

VN: Bilberry (E). Blaubeere; Heidelbeere (G). Airelle (myrtille); Myrtille (F).

KE: Fruit permitted for oral use. No CI, AE, I [BAnz nr.76 23.04.87]. Leaf not permitted for therapeutic use. Usefulness is not documented adequately. Higher doses or prolonged use can produce chronic poisoning; chronic administration of 1.5 g/kg/day is lethal in animals [BAnz nr.76 23.04.87].

FR: Fruit permitted for oral use (toxicological categories pd:1 ht/ae/wa:1 sa/ti:1).
Leaf permitted for oral use (toxicological categories pd:2 ht/ae/wa:1 sa/ti:1).

BE: Leaf permitted as traditional stomatological.

SW: Classified as foodstuff and as natural product.

AS: SW also classifies *Vaccinium oxycoccus* L. and *Vaccinium vitis-idaea* L. as foodstuff and natural product.

***Valeriana officinalis* L.**

VN: Valerian (E). (Echter) Baldrian (G). Herbe aux chats; Valériane (officinale) (F).

KE: Root permitted for oral use. No CI, AE, I [BAnz nr.90 15.05.88].

SZ: Root permitted as herbal tea and as tincture. No CI, AE or I, except for an effect of the tincture on driving ability.

FR: Subterranean parts permitted for oral use (toxicological categories pd:2 ht/ae/wa:1 sa/ti:2). The level of active constituents has to be limited.

BE: Subterranean parts, powder, extract, tincture permitted as traditional tranquillizer.

SW: Classified as natural product and as a drug, which must normally be registered as pharmaceutical speciality.

AS: Cultivated varieties [FR].

RM: Preparations with a standardised valepotriate content are mostly prepared from *Valeriana edulis* Nutt. ssp. *procera* (Mexican valerian) and *Valeriana wallichii* DC. (Indian valerian) [34].

***Veratrum album* L.**

VN: False helleborine; White hellebore (E). Weißer Germer; Weiße Nieswurz (G). Hellebore blanc; Vératre blanc (F).

SW: *Veratrum* species, such as *Veratrum album*, are classified as drugs, which must normally be registered as pharmaceutical speciality.

***Verbascum densiflorum* Bertol.**

VN: Mullein (E). Großblumige Königskerze (G). Bouillon blanc (F).

KE: Flower permitted for oral use. No CI, AE, I [BAnz nr.22a 01.02.90].

FR: Peeled flower permitted for oral use (toxicological categories pd:- ht/ae/wa:1 sa/ti:-).

AS: *Verbascum phlomoides* L. [KE,FR] and *Verbascum thapsus* L. [FR].

Verbena officinalis **L.**

VN: European vervain (E). (Echtes) Eisenkraut (G). Verveine officinale (F).
KE: Herb not permitted for therapeutic use. Usefulness is not documented adequately. No risks are known, however, and the addition to herbal preparations is not excluded categorically [BAnz nr.22a 01.02.90].
FR: Aerial parts permitted for oral use (toxicological categories pd:2 ht/ae/wa:1 sa/ti:1).
SW: Classified as natural product.

Veronica officinalis **L.**

VN: Speedwell (E). Ehrenpreis (G). Thé d'Europe; Véronique officinale (F).
KE: Herb not permitted for therapeutic use. Usefulness is not documented adequately. No risks are known, however [BAnz nr.43 02.03.89].
SW: Classified as natural product.

Viburnum prunifolium **L.**

VN: Black haw; (Sweet) viburnum (E). (Amerikanischer) Schneeballbaum; Viburnum (G). Viburnum; Viorne (américain) (F).
FR: Stem bark permitted for oral use (toxicological categories pd:2 ht/ae/wa:1 sa/ti:1).

Vinca minor **L.**

VN: Evergreen; Wintergreen (E). Kleine Immergrün; Wintergrün (G). Petite pervenche (F).
KE: Herb not permitted for therapeutic use. Usefulness is not documented adequately. Hematological changes (leucocytopenia, lymphocytopenia, reduced globulin levels) have been observed in animals [BAnz nr.173 18.09.86].
SW: Classified as a drug, which must normally be registered as pharmaceutical speciality.

Viola odorata **L.**

VN: Common violet; Garden violet (E). Märzveilchen; Veilchen (G). Violette de mars; Violette odorante (F).
FR: Flower permitted for oral use (toxicological categories pd:1 ht/ae/wa:1 sa/ti:1).
SW: Classified as natural product.
AS: *Viola calcarata* L. and *Viola lutea* Huds. [FR].

Viola tricolor **L.**

VN: Heartsease; (Wild) pansy (E). Ackerstiefmütterchen; Ackerveilchen (G). Pensée sauvage; Violette tricolore (F).
KE: Herb permitted for external use only. No CI, AE, I [BAnz nr.50 13.03.86].

SZ: Herb permitted as herbal tea for external use only. No CI, AE, I.
FR: Flowering aerial parts permitted for oral use (toxicological categories pd:2 ht/ae/wa:1 sa/ti:1).
SW: Classified as natural product.
AS: KE and FR specify ssp. *vulgaris* (Koch) Oborny and ssp. *arvensis* (Murray) Gaud. as principal source plants.

***Viscum album* L.**
VN: (European) mistletoe (E). Mistel (G). Gui (F).
KE: Herb permitted only for parenteral injection. CI: hypersensitivity to proteins, chronic progressive infections (e.g., tuberculosis). AE: allergic and other reactions. No I [BAnz nr.228 05.12.84].
SW: Classified as natural product (with a dose limitation) and as a drug, which must normally be registered as pharmaceutical speciality.
RM: The viscotoxins are not absorbed orally and may have necrotising effects in higher doses [34].

***Vitex agnus-castus* L.**
VN: Chaste tree (E). Keuschbaum (G). Agneau chaste; Gatillier (F).
KE: Fruit permitted for oral use. No CI, I. AE: skin reactions [BAnz nr.90 15.05.85].
SW: Classified as a drug, which must normally be registered as pharmaceutical speciality.

***Vitis vinifera* L.**
VN: Vine (E). Weinrebe; Weinstock (G). Vigne rouge; Vigne vinifère (F).
FR: Leaf permitted for oral use (toxicological categories pd:2 ht/ae/wa:1 sa/ti:1).
SW: Classified as foodstuff and as natural product.

Xanthomonas campestris
SW: Xanthan gum (produced by fermentation of a carbohydrate with *Xanthomonas campestris*) is classified as foodstuff (with a dose limitation) and as natural product.

***Xysmalobium undulatum* (L.) R. Brown**
VN: Uzara (G).
KE: Root permitted for oral use. CI: Use of cardioactive glycosides. No AE, I. Consult physician, when diarrhoea lasts for more than 3–4 days [BAnz nr.164 01.09.90].
RM: Contains cardelonide glycosides and has digitalis-like cardiac activity in higher doses [KE].

***Zanthoxylum clava-herculis* Lour.**
SW: Classified as natural product.

***Zea mays* L.**
VN: Indian corn; Maize (E). Mais (G). Maïs (F).
FR: Style permitted for oral use (toxicological categories pd:2 ht/ae/wa:1 sa/ti:1).
BE: Style permitted as traditional diuretic.

***Zingiber officinale* Roscoe**
VN: Ginger (E). Ingwer (G). Gingembre (F).
KE: Rhizome permitted for oral use. No CI, AE, I. Should not be used for vomiting in pregnancy [BAnz nr.85 05.05.88 and BAnz nr.164 01.09.90].
BE: Rhizome permitted as traditional digestive aid.

***Zizyphus jujuba* Miller = *Z. sativa* Gaertn. = *Z. vulgaris* Lamk. = *Rhamnus zizyphus* L.**
VN: Jujubier (F).
FR: Fruit (deprived of seed) permitted for external use (toxicological categories pd:- ht/ae/wa:1 sa/ti:1).

Unspecified
KE: Pollen permitted for oral use. CI: Hypersensitivity to pollen. AE: GI-complaints (rarely). No I [BAnz nr.11 17.01.91].

Acknowledgements

I am very much obliged to the following persons for their provision of valuable data on national legislations: Konstantin Keller (Berlin, Germany); Agnes Artiges and Marie-Hélène Loulergue (Paris, France); Pat Adamo (Rockville, United States); Brenley Milsom (Canberra, Australia); and Inger Näsman (Uppsala, Sweden).

References

1. Battaglino G (1987) EEC Directives and Recommendations in the Pharmaceuticl Field. Milano, Organizzazione Editoriale Medico Farmaceutica, pp 391–392
2. Anonymous (1989) Quality of herbal remedies. In: The rules governing medicinal products in the European Community. Volume III. Guidelines on the quality, safety and efficacy of medicinal products for human use. Luxembourg: Office for Official Publications of the European Communities, pp 31–37
3. De Smet PAGM (1992) Toxicological outlook on the quality assurance of herbal remedies. In: De Smet PAGM, Keller K, Hänsel R, Chandler RF, red. Adverse Effects of Herbal Drugs. Volume 1. Heidelberg: Springer-Verlag pp 1–72
4. Keller K (1991) Legal requirements for the use of phytopharmaceutical drugs in the Federal Republic of Germany. J Ethnopharmacol 32:225–229
5. Anonymous (1992) Bekanntmachung über die Zulassung und Registrierung von Arzneimitteln. Bundesanzeiger (herausgegeben von Bundesminister der Justiz) 3.1.1984 (nr.1); 5.12.1984 (nr.228); 15.5.1985 (nr.90); 21.8.1985 (nr.154); 30.11.1985

(nr.223); 13.3.1986 (nr.50); 18.9.1986 (nr.173); 24.9.1986 (nr.177a); 23.4.1987 (nr.76); 15.10.1987 (nr.193a); 5.5.1988 (nr.85); 6.7.1988 (nr.122); 2.3.1989 (nr.43); 27.4.1989 (nr.80); 1.2.1990 (nr.22a); 13.3.90 (nr.50); 1.6.1990 (nr.101); 27.7.1990 (nr.138); 1.9.1990 (nr.164); 17.1.1991 (nr.11); 27.2.1991 (nr.40); 18.3.1991 (nr.54); 19.4.1991 (nr.74); 12.7.1991 (nr.127); 21.9.1991 (nr.178); 11.3.1992 (nr.49).

6. Braun R, red (1991) Standardzulassungen für Fertigarzneimittel. Text und Kommentar. Stand: März 1991. Stuttgart: Deutscher Apotheker Verlag
7. Artiges A (1991) What are the legal requirements for the use of phytopharmaceutical drugs in France? J Ethnopharmacol 32:231–234
8. Anonymous (1986) Avis aux fabricants concernant les demandes d'autorisation de mise sur le marché de specialités pharmaceutiques à base de plantes. Fascicule spécial no. 86/20 bis. Paris: Direction de la Pharmacie et du Médicament, Ministère des Affaires Sociales et de l'Emploi
9. Anonymous (1987) Avis aux fabricants sur les specialités pharmaceutiques à base de drogues végétales à visée laxative. Paris: Direction de la Pharmacie et du Médicament, Ministère des Affaires Sociales et de l'Emploi
10. Anonymous (1990) Avis aux fabricants concernant les demandes d'autorisation de mise sur le marché des médicaments à base de plantes. Fascicule spécial no. 90/22 bis. Paris: Direction de la Pharmacie et du Médicament, Ministère des Affaires Sociales et de la Solidarité
11. Anonymous (1989–1991) Omzendbrief nr.367 aan de vergunninghouders en de industrie-apothekers. Brussel: Algemene Farmaceutische Inspectie, Ministerie van Volksgezondheid en Leefmilieu, september 1989, mei 1990, januari 1991 en juli 1991
12. Bradley PR (1990) European monographs – a way to harmonization. Lecture presented at the first international symposium of the European Scientific Cooperative for Phytotherapy (ESCOP). Brussels: October 22, 1990
13. Anonymous (1990) Gamolenic acid in atopic eczema: Epogam. Drug Ther Bull 28:69–70
14. Buhagiar C (1991) Efamast. Int Pharm J 5:58–60
15. Nightingale SL (1987) Regulation of food, drugs and medical devices in the USA. World Health Forum 8:461–468
16. Adamo PT (1992) Division of Regulatory Guidance Center for Food Safety and Applied Nutrition, Food and Drug Administration, Washington DC. Personal communication
17. Tyler VE (1987) Herbal medicine in America. Planta Med pp 1–4
18. Tyler VE (1987) The New Honest Herbal. A sensible guide to herbs and related remedies. 2nd edn. George F. Stickley Company, Philadelphia
19. Der Marderosian A, Liberti LE (1988) Natural product medicine. A scientific guide to foods, drugs, cosmetics. George F. Stickley Company, Philadelphia pp 93–110
20. Anonymous (1990) FDA proposes banning 258 nonprescription drug ingredients. Clin Pharm 9:598
21. Department of Health and Human Services (1991) Weight control products for over-the-counter human use; certain active ingredients. Fed Reg 56:37792–37799
22. Anonymous (1991) US herbal product market studied. Marketletter 18 (November 18):25
23. Anonymous (1975) Safe and unsafe herbs in herbal teas. Department of Health Education, and Welfare. Public Health Service. Food and Drug Administration, Washington DC
24. Anonymous (1991) Food and Drug Administration Code of Federal Regulations. 4-1-91 Edition. Washington: Department of Health & Human Services, §172.510 and §182.10–20
25. Hausen BM (1985) Lorbeer-Allergie. Ursache, Wirkung und Folgen der äußerlichen Anwendung eines sogenannten Naturheilmittels. Dtsch Med Wschr 110:634–638
26. Czygan F-C. Senfsamen, Schwarze. In: Wichtl M, red (1989) Teedrogen. Ein Handbuch für die Praxis auf wissenschaftlicher Grundlage. 2. Auflage. Stuttgart: Wissenschaftliche Verlagsgesellschaft pp 449–451

27. Michaels E (1986) Canada lags in acceptance, regulation of herbal remedies. Can Med Ass J 135:547–548
28. Moulds RFW, McNeil JJ (1988) Herbal preparations – to regulate or not to regulate? Med J Aust 149:572–574
29. Anonymous (1988) Guidelines for importers of therapeutic substances into Australia. Department of Community Services and Health, Canberra
30. Anonymous (undated) Regulations for natural products in Sweden. Uppsala: Medical Products Agency
31. Anonymous (1991) Risk evaluation of health-food products. Report of a nordic project group. Stockholm, Nordic Council
32. Hoppe HA (1975) Drogenkunde. Band 1. Angiospermen. 8. Auflage. Berlin: Walter de Gruyter
33. Penso G (1983) Index Plantarum Medicinalium Totius Mundi Eorumque Synonymorum. Milano: Organizzazione Editoriale Medico Farmaceutica
34. Wichtl M, red. (1989) Teedrogen. Ein Handbuch für die Praxis auf wissenschaftlicher Grundlage. 2. Auflage. Stuttgart: Wissenschaftliche Verlagsgesellschaft
35. Der Marderosian A, Liberti LE (1988) Natural product medicine. A scientific guide to foods, drugs, cosmetics. Philadelphia: George F. Stickley Company
36. Duke JA (1985) Handbook of medicinal herbs. Boca Raton: CRC Press
37. Launert E (1981) Hamlyn Guide to Edible and Medicinal Plants of Britain and Northern Europe. London: Hamlyn
38. Lust JB (1974) The Herb Book. New York: Bantam Books
39. Madaus G (1979) Lehrbuch der biologischen Heilmittel. Band I–III. Hildesheim: Georg Olms Verlag
40. Millspaugh CF (1974) American Medicinal Plants. New York: Dover Publications
41. Osol A, Farrar GE (1955) The Dispensatory of the United States of America. 25th edn. Philadelphia: J.B. Lippincott Company
42. Reynolds JEF, red (1989) Martindale The Extra Pharmacopoeia. 29th edn. London: The Pharmaceutical Press
43. Spoerke Jr DG (1980) Herbal Medications. Santa Barbara: Woodbridge Press Publishing Co
44. Van Hellemont J (1988) Fytotherapeutisch compendium. Tweede druk. Utrecht: Bohn, Scheltema & Holkema
45. Vogel VJ (1970) American Indian medicine. Norman: University of Oklahoma Press
46. Anonymous (1989) Drogues a usage medicamenteux. Unpublished working document. Paris: Direction de la Pharmacie et du Médicament, Ministère des Affaires Sociales et de la Solidarité
47. Schilcher H (1988) Pflanzliche Diuretika. In: Reuter HD, Deininger R, Schulz V, red. Phytotherapie. Grundlagen – Klinik – Praxis. Stuttgart: Hippokrates Verlag, pp 223–233

Abies, *Picea* and *Pinus* Species

D. Corrigan

Botany

The family Pinaceae, one of the major conifer taxa, is divided into several genera of which *Abies*, *Picea* and *Pinus* are among the largest. *Abies*, commonly known as fir, consists of 50 species, *Picea* usually known as spruce, also contains about 50 species, while *Pinus* or pine numbers between 70 and 100 species. These three genera, found mainly in the northern hemisphere, contain many commercially important forest trees. Among the most important species are *Abies alba* (L.) Karst (silver fir), *Abies balsamea* (L.) Mill. (balsam fir), *Abies sibirica* Ledebe (Siberian fir), *Picea abies* (L.) Karst (Norway spruce), *Picea mariana* (Mill.) B.S.P., *Pinus mugo* Turra (dwarf or pumilio pine), *Pinus palustris* Mill. (longleaf pine), *Pinus strobus* (white pine) and *Pinus sylvestris* L. (scots pine) [1].

Chemistry

Many of these coniferous species are commercially important, and for this reason they have been extensively investigated chemically. A diversity of compounds has been isolated from the needles, bark, oleoresin and wood of the various species [2]. Typically the essential oils contain significant quantities of α- and β-pinene, d-limonene, Δ^3-carene, α-terpineol and β-phellandrene as well as many other monoterpenes. The proportions of each component are subject to a considerable degree of variation not only between the individual genera and species but also within species [3,4]. Norin [2] has extensively reviewed the chemistry of the different genera. He noted the presence in *Pinus* species of stilbenes and dihydrostilbenes, flavanones and flavones, resin acids such as abietic and pimaric acid, macrocyclic diterpenes, labdane diterpenes, serratane triterpenes, caffeic and related acids, lignans and norditerpenoids. Colophony resin (rosin) and turpentine are obtained from the oleoresin produced by *Pinus* species [5]. The exact species used depends on the geographical source. Turpentine or oil of turpentine is the essential oil obtained by steam distillation of the crude oleoresin. The remaining solid resin constitutes colophony which

Adverse Effects of Herbal Drugs, Vol. 2
(ed. by P.A.G.M. De Smet, K. Keller, R. Hänsel, R.F. Chandler)

consists of diterpene resin acids such as abietic acid. Both products can also be produced by solvent extraction of the chipped wood from pine stumps or as by-products of the paper pulping industry. There is wide variation in chemical composition due to the differences in species used and their geographical location. All turpentine oils contain α-pinene and may also contain β-pinene. The Δ^3-carene content varies depending on the source. "Sulphate" oils produced as a by-product of the paper industry tend to be high in Δ^3-carene, while oils from the oleoresin obtained by "tapping" the trees directly, have low or negligible amounts of this compound [6]. Mirov [7] has studied the oleoresin products (gum turpentine) and has reported that some pines, e.g., *P. jeffreyi*, produce significant amounts of hydrocarbons such as *n*-heptane and undecane.

The chemical composition of the *Abies* species, e.g., *Abies alba*, is essentially similar to that of *Pinus* with α-pinene and l-limonene being the main components of the needle oil [8]. Abietic acid and related resin acids have been identified. Abienol, a diterpene of the labdane type, is one of the major constituents of Canada balsam (derived from *A. balsamea*). Sesquiterpene acids such as juvabione have also been found in this genus. Flavonoids and lanostane-type triterpenes have been isolated from the bark of a number of *Abies* species [2].

Monoterpenes and diterpenoid resin acids are typical constituents of *Picea* species as are simple lignin-related phenols, e.g., vanillin, lignans, flavonoids and stilbenes [2,9].

A variety of coniferous essential oils available commercially including pine oil [CAS-8002-09-3] obtained, according to Martindale [10], by extraction and fractionation or by steam distillation of the wood of *Pinus palustris* and other species of *Pinus*. The main constituent is α-terpineol. Pumilio pine oil [CAS-8000-26-8] is obtained by distillation of the fresh needles of *Pinus mugo* var *pumilio* [10]. Leung [11] refers to this oil as dwarf pine needle oil and refers to the oil from *P. sylvestris* as scotch pine needle oil. Martindale [10] refers to this latter oil as *Oleum Pini sylvestris* observing that the oil now sold under this name is often a distillate from the leaves and twigs of various conifers. Opdyke [8,12] has produced separate monographs on oils from the cones of *Abies alba* and from the needles of the same species. However, Martindale [10] does not include entries on these oils referring only to Siberian fir oil [Oleum Abietis] [CAS-8002-09-3], which it states is distilled from the fresh leaves of *Abies sibirica* and has similar properties to pumilio pine oil. Norway spruce needle oil and extract from *Picea abies* are also listed as being used commercially [13].

Pharmacology and Uses

A range of products obtained from plants of all three genera are used medicinally. The needles (particularly *Pinus sylvestris*) and the bark (*Pinus strobus*) are used commercially. Both spruce and pine needles are reportedly used in the form of teas for bronchial conditions, as is a syrup made from white pine bark (*Pinus strobus*) [11,14]. The oils are used for a variety of purposes. Pine oil for instance is used as a disinfectant and in the form of an inhalation for respiratory tract conditions [10]. Pumilio pine oil is also used for this purpose. Some oils are used as flavourings (Siberian fir oil), while many embrocations, salves, ointments, etc. for rheumatism, sprains, fibrositis and related conditions contain these oils. They are particularly popular for use in medicinal baths.

According to Weiss [15], pine baths are the most widely used and most thoroughly investigated of the herbal baths. The scots pine (*Pinus sylvestris*) is used along with the Norway spruce (*Picea abies* or *P. excelsa*) as well as the common silver fir (*Abies alba*). The extract used is a combination of the essential oil produced by distillation added to the inspissated (partially concentrated under vacuum) aqueous extract. This extract can be obtained from the needles and young shoots and can contain 15% of tannic acid as well as the volatile oil. Both extracts can also be produced from the bark giving a tannin content of 26–28%. Weiss [15] comments that the irritant effect is correspondingly greater and notes that this product is used to treat persistent rheumatic conditions. A bath extract containing smaller amounts of volatile oil and prepared from the wood can also be used. The pine baths are used for nervous diseases, rheumatic and neuralgic conditions. The physiological effects of these baths was investigated by Von Spindler [16] in 1913, who reported that extracts from pine needles contained only 1–1.5% of essential oil and that the tannin content was the major source of activity. He found that pine needle baths stimulated metabolism and circulation, as shown by a decrease in uric acid and an increase of urea. Inhalation of the volatile oil was said to add to the effect.

Turpentine is used externally as a rubefacient liniment for rheumatic conditions [13]. Earlier editions of Martindale [10,17] contained details of a preparation called Dutch or Haarlem drops containing 15 parts of turpentine, 1 part of sulphur and 4 parts of linseed oil. A dose of 0.3 to 2 ml was used for lumbago and rheumatism. The 29th edition of Martindale [18] contains details of proprietary ear drops containing 10% turpentine oil. This oil is also included in a number of salve formulations. Terebene, prepared from turpentine by the addition of cold sulphuric acid which converts the pinene into limonene, is preferred to turpentine for inhalation purposes [10].

Colophony is mainly used pharmaceutically as an ingredient of some collodions and plaster-masses. Pine or Stockholm tar is obtained by the destructive distillation of the stems and roots of various *Pinus* species. Consisting of a mixture of hydrocarbons and phenols [19], it is mainly used as an ingredient of bath additives, shampoos, ointments and creams used for the treatment of eczema and psoriasis [13].

Boyd and Pearson [20] found that oil of turpentine markedly increased the output of respiratory tract fluid (R.T.F.) when administered by gastric tube to guinea pigs. They further reported that "Oil of pine in the form of *Oleum abietis* BP (oil of Siberian fir)" augmented the output of R.T.F. but not to the same extent as turpentine.

High levels of vitamin C have been reported in pine needle concentrates and in *Picea excelsa* by a number of Russian workers [21,22]. These products were used to successfully treat scurvy in laboratory animals [23] and in humans. Verkhratskii [24] claimed that this effect was due to the polyphenols of the spruce needles used which, when added to liver homogenates of rabbits on a scurvy producing diet, enhanced the reduction of dehydroascorbic acid to ascorbic acid.

The essential oils from *Picea abies* and *Pinus sylvestris* show some antibacterial activity against *E. coli* and *S. aureus*. This activity increases as the oil ages and is also dependent on the chemotype chosen for distillation [4].

Other biological activities reported for these species include inhibition of PAF (platelet-activating factor) activity by a lipid fraction from pine pollen [25] and the 52% inhibition of human plasma cholinesterase by a methanolic extract of *Picea jezoensis* bark [26]. The authors postulated that this effect was possibly due to proanthocyanidins. Interestingly, Bastide and co-workers [27] have reported that the proanthocyanoside extract from *Pinus maritimus* inhibited elastase [E.C.34.21.11] and that it had an angioprotective effect in rats, although it was less effective than extracts from *Vitis vinifera*.

Sakagami et al. [28] reported that the hot water extract of the cones of *Pinus parviflora* Sieb et Zucc. has a folk reputation in Japan as a treatment for gastric cancer. They found that some fractions of the hot water and NaOH extracts from the cones of this species have immunopotentiating activity as well as displaying antitumour, antimicrobial and antiviral (*Herpes simplex* and influenza) activities. One fraction known as PC6 causes *in vitro* inhibition of HIV virus by binding to HIV-1 reverse transcriptase. These actions have been tentatively ascribed to a complex of lignin-like polyphenolic skeleton with a molecular matrix of unknown components.

Pharmacokinetics

Tobin et al. [29] reported that α-terpineol found in a pine oil disinfectant had an apparent half-life of about 12 minutes after i.v. injection of 0.033 ml/kg of pine oil into a horse. α-Terpineol was no longer detectable in plasma after 2 hours. According to work by Rommelt et al., cited by Opdyke [30], α- and β-pinene and limonene were detected in the exhaled air of young pigs and one human subject when they had been immersed in baths containing 150 ml of a proprietary pine-oil mixture in 450 litres of water. The terpenes were detected within 20 minutes, reaching maximum levels 50–75 minutes after the start of the bath and remaining detectable after 1 day.

Adverse Reaction Profile

The oils from *Abies alba* needles [8], from *Pinus mugo* [30] and *Pinus sylvestris* [31] were all granted GRAS (Generally Recognised As Safe) status by the Flavouring Extract Manufacturers' Association (FEMA) in 1965. The Council of Europe includes *Abies alba* cone oil and needle oil and *Pinus mugo* in its list of substances, spices and seasonings deemed admissible for use with a possible limitation of the active principle in the final product. In the case of *Pinus sylvestris* oil the Council temporarily permitted its use as flavouring agent because toxicological and technological data were insufficient [31]. In the U.K. the GSL (General Sales List) limits the maximum strength of this oil to 9 mg in inhalant capsules; to 6 mg in lozenges and throat tablets and to 0.05 mg/5 ml in cough syrups [32]. The Food and Drug Administration in the U.S. has approved the above three oils and turpentine oil for food use, while colophony and white pine bark have only been approved for use in alcoholic beverages [5,11].

In France an infusion of *Pinus sylvestris* shoots is accepted for product registration purposes as being "traditionally used during benign acute bronchial disorders" and for local use as a mouthwash and gargle for oral hygiene, and as such no toxicological study is required. However, when the whole powder is supplied then a reduced toxicological study is required [33].

The sale of medicinal products containing sulphurated turpentine oil (e.g., Haarlem Drops) is prohibited in the Netherlands and in Germany [34,35].

General Animal Data

Reported LD_{50} values for the conifer oils are relatively high; for example, Von Skramlik [36] reported the acute oral LD_{50} values in rats for *Pinus mugo* oil to be 10.64 gms/kg body weight. The corresponding value for *Pinus sylvestris* was 6.88 g/kg and for turpentine 5.76 g/kg. According to sources quoted by Opdyke [8,12,30,31] the acute oral LD_{50} in rats and the acute dermal LD_{50} in rabbits exceeded 5 g/kg body weight for *Abies alba* oils as well as the two pine oils.

Tobin et al. [29] investigated a case of suspected acute intoxication in a thoroughbred horse by injection of a commercial pine oil disinfectant. After intravenous injection of 0.1 ml/kg, death due to massive pulmonary oedema occurred within minutes, with observed blood and tissue levels of α-terpineol of between 150 and 300 ppm. Other horses survived doses of 0.033 ml/kg of oil although marked histopathological changes were seen in the lungs of those animals which survived the initial injection period. These changes included intraseptal oedema in the ventral portions of the lungs, interstitial pneumonia, alveolar congestion and oedema with fibrin formation. The alveolar macrophages were pleomorphic and proliferating in large patchy areas.

Okanishi [37] states that pine needle oil is more toxic to mice than sandalwood or vetivert oils. On the other hand, Primavori [38] injected *Pinus pumilio* (*P. mugo*) oil solubilised in sorbitol monostearate intravenously into animals without toxic effect. Inhalation toxicity for pine essential oils was determined by Kachanov [39], using mice. The LD_{50} was reported to be 7.3 mg/litre of air while the tolerated dose was 2 mg/litre of air. Timajeev et al. [40] reported that single administration of rosin and pine oil had no profound toxic effects but that repeated administration resulted in morphological and functional changes in liver cells, and the exocrine pancreas. This group found that rosin (colophony) decreased the rate of protein metabolism while DNA formation was markedly inhibited by pine oil.

General Human Data

Craig [41] has reviewed a number of studies of poisoning in childhood involving volatile oils. He noted that of 54 deaths in British children between 1931 and 1951 caused by volatile oils, turpentine was involved in 2 of the cases, but of 74 cases of accidental poisoning seen in the Scottish cities of Edinburgh and Aberdeen in the same period, 25 involved turpentine. He reported that turpentine produces a wide range of toxic effects including vomiting, stupor, convulsions, irritation of the urinary tract, choking sensation, pyrexia, ataxia, shock, tachycardia, sweating and leucocytosis. Craig [41] concluded from a review of 26 cases that turpentine poisoning is mild relative to that of the other volatile oils although he gave details of a case from the literature where an 11-month-old girl was given two teaspoonfuls of spirits of turpentine as an anthelmintic. Convulsions occurred a few hours later and the child became comatose, with cyanosis, hyperpyrexia and marked tachypnoea and tachycardia. She died a few hours after the convulsions without regaining consciousness. Martindale [10] states that a dose of 140 ml (15 ml in children) may be fatal but Craig [41] also notes that a woman of 46 who had gastric lavage within 15 minutes of taking 300 mls of turpentine in a suicide attempt developed no symptoms. Craig compared his findings with those recorded by Rubin et al. in a general survey of poisonings in Washington in 1949. In their 11 cases Rubin et al. found coma or drowsiness in six, fever in four, vomiting in four and pneumonia in one.

Hill et al. [42] report a case of recurrent pine oil poisoning in an infant who required six admissions in a period of six months for episodes consisting of coughing, respiratory depression, hematemesis, coma, dehydration and mouth lesions. Electroencephalograms were interpreted as compatible with metabolic or toxic encephalopathy.

Martindale [17] includes details of two reports of toxicity to turpentine. The first deals with workers in a factory manufacturing a shoe-cream containing turpentine. The toxicity was considered to be due to inhalation and absorption through the skin and the use of high α-pinene concentrations. In addition to symptoms of giddiness, burning of the face, throat and anus, and frequent painful micturition, three workers had bladder ulcers, two had rectal inflammation, one had leucocytosis and one had renal inflammation. The second report concerns two boys, one who drank an unknown volume of turpentine and the other who was exposed to turpentine vapour at home. Both developed profuse petechiae on their bodies and in the mouth. The thrombocyte count was lowered and bleeding time prolonged. The bone marrow became normoblastic and there was abundant erythropoiesis.

In contrast, Komarov [23] has reported that 52 cases of scurvy were successfully treated for up to twenty days with pine needle concentrate with no harmful effects even in cases of kidney disorders.

Cardiovascular Reactions

A digitalis-like action on the isolated toad heart was reported by Primavori [38] when solubilised *Pinus pumilio* oil was injected, but there was no change in blood pressure even with high doses. Jaeger et al. [43] reported that rabbits injected i.v. with turpentine showed elevated heart and respiration patterns.

Central Nervous System Reactions

Inhalation or subcutaneous injection of the oil from *P. mughus* (sic) and *P. pumilio* produces in frogs and white mice after a short time, excitations, depression, paralysis and death [44]. Sazonova [45] reports that a laboratory worker exposed for long unspecified periods to pine oil vapour experienced drowsiness and headache but also concluded that pine oil was acceptable as a pediculicide. Rats treated orally with 5 ml of pine oil showed no specific brain lesions [43]. Rabbits treated i.v. with turpentine showed no CNS lesions upon necropsy 6 hours post intoxication [43]. Gornel and Goldman [46] cite references which show that the toxicity of pine oil distillates commonly shows up as CNS excitement followed by depression, resulting in symptoms such as transient excitement, giddiness, headache and a sensation of drunkenness. More severe toxic effects lead to ataxia, delirium, progressive stupor, coma and death.

Dermatological Reactions

Opdyke [8,12,30] concludes that the oils from *Abies alba* and *Pinus sylvestris* are generally non-irritating, non-sensitising and non-phototoxic in both animal tests and in some patch tests with human volunteers. *Pinus pumilio*

(*P. mugo*) oil was reported to be irritating to human skin and in patch tests with 21 patients with essential oil dermatoses. Both it and *Pinus sylvestris* oil gave positive reactions due to the presence of Δ^3-carene [30,31].

Mitchell and Rook [47] include a number of reports of dermatitis and contact sensitivity to the wood, needles and balsams (resins) of a variety of *Abies*, *Picea* and *Pinus* species. It is suggested that stilbenes and hydroxy-stilbenes, e.g., pinosylvin and its derivatives, may be involved in the sensitivity but it is also strongly suggested that Δ^3-carene from the essential oil is the major eczematogenic factor in the oils and particularly in certain turpentines. Jadassohn [48] reports on the exacerbation of turpentine dermatitis in a painter after he had eaten sweets made from pine or spruce buds. A review of turpentine by Pirila [6] cited extensively in Mitchell and Rook [47] noted that the incidence of turpentine dermatoses had declined in countries where turpentine had been replaced by hydrocarbon solvents. Both colophony and wood tar are also reported to have irritant and sensitising effects. Colophony is well known as a sensitising agent, with Mitchell and Rook recording numerous cases from the literature documenting contact dermatitis due to colophony used in adhesive plasters, physiotherapy wax, fabrics and hair lacquers.

Karlberg et al. [49] studied the allergenic potential of abietic acid, colophony and a pine resin concentrate in 563 patients with contact dermatitis. Fourteen showed an isolated sensitivity to colophony and two to the pine-resin. Six patients reacted to both. Guinea pig tests showed that the pure resin concentrate was a grade I allergen [least likely to induce contact allergy] while abietic acid was a grade III and colophony a grade IV allergen. They concluded that the risk of becoming sensitised to the resin acids in pine oil products was low but that patients already sensitised to colophony might get a recurrence after contact with products containing pine oil.

Foussereau et al. [50] reported different allergologic profiles among 13 persons allergic to colophony. Some reacted only to abietylic alcohol while others did not react to abietic acid. They further noted that methyl abietate used as a plasticiser in some "hypoallergic" sticking plasters had an allergising effect in 6 out of 12 cases.

Hematological Reactions

Okanishi [37] reported that pine oils produced leucocytosis in the mouse. Kachanov [39] noted that cats exposed to pine oil vapours for 24 hours showed no change in erythrocyte count when investigated at the end of the inhalation period, two hours later and after twenty-two hours. However, seven out of ten animals had a transitory increase in leucocytes of 24–47%. Two cats had leukopenia. Removal of the carotid sinus prevented the leukopenic response but removal of the spleen had no effect. Kachanov [39] suggested that the decrease in eosinophils indicated adrenal involvement.

Gastrointestinal Reactions

Thesen [35] refers to reports that sulphurated turpentine oils can produce diarrhoea when taken in large amounts.

Metabolic Reactions

Eisyment [51] reported that lactating cows given *Picea* bark, which had been included in the silage, had total blood lipids 17% greater than controls.

Neurological Reactions

Gornel and Goldman [46], reporting on a case of an abortion induced by pine oil-based disinfectant, stated that their patient developed a peripheral neuropathy about four weeks after instilling up to 180 mls of a 1 in 2 dilution of the oil product in water into her uterus. This neuropathy progressed to involve feet, legs, knees, hands, elbows and shoulders and then gradually subsided so that the patient had no further disability.

Renal Reactions

Dysuria, hematuria, glycosuria and proteinuria have been noted as toxic effects of pine and turpentine oils according to Gornel and Goldman [46]. Their patient who had induced an abortion with pine oil and soap, developed renal failure within 24 hours. Renal biopsy after 6 weeks indicated focal fibrosis and tubular atrophy. Thesen [35] records that the consumption of large amounts of sulphurated turpentine oils can result in the irritation of the urinary tract with pain and hematuria. Mancini [44] has stated that rabbits have tolerated daily doses of 0.3–1 g of *P. mugo* oil per kg for several weeks without renal lesions and that almost the entire oil was eliminated in the urine as glucuronates. Weiss [52] states that extended use of pine wood tar as a keratoplastic and antiseptic may cause renal irritation due to absorption and may be detected through the presence of phenols from the tar which cause urine to blacken when left standing in air.

Respiratory Tract Reactions

Quander and Moseley [53] described a case of pulmonary oedema in a woman who induced an abortion by intrauterine injection of turpentine and water.

Following the injection of 0.1 ml/kg of pine oil into the jugular vein of a horse, the lungs became very hemorrhagic, congested and oedematous but did not collapse. Similar histopathological changes were noted in an animal given 0.033 ml/kg [29].

Rats treated orally with 5 ml pine oil and rabbits injected i.v. with turpentine both showed pulmonary oedema and hemorrhage upon post-mortem examination [43].

Drug Interactions

Jori et al. [54] reported that a dose of pumilio pine oil of 500 mg/kg had no effect on the *in vivo* metabolism and pharmacological activity of pentobarbitone (25 mg/kg) in rats or *in vitro* on the metabolism of aminopyrine, p-nitroanisole and aniline by rat liver.

Fertility, Pregnancy and Lactation

There are reports that a decoction of the branch tips of long leaf pine [*Pinus palustris* Mill.] is used for menstrual cramps in southeastern South Carolina [55] and that Indian women from northwestern United States took water extracts of pine needles to induce abortion [56]. A number of reports have appeared linking pine needle consumption with abortion and pregnancy complications in cattle [56]. This has been linked by Wagner and Jackson [57] to the presence of phytoestrogens in ponderosa pine (*Pinus ponderosa*). Paul et al. [58] have reported that ovarian steroidogenesis in rats was reduced after treatment with *Pinus lambertiana* with a reduction in ovarian and uterine weights.

Murphy et al. [56] report that abortion in cows may occur within 48 hours after ingestion of pine needles. Weak calves which later died and retained placentas are also frequent occurrences after pine needle consumption, according to references cited by Murphy et al. This group administered 1 g/kg/day of an aqueous extract of either *Pinus palustris* Mill. or *Pinus taeda* L. needles orally to female Sprague/Dawley rats four days prior to mating and continued through to the twentieth day of gestation. The average number of resorptions and fetal deaths was significantly larger and the average number of implantations lower in the group dosed with *P. palustris* extract compared to dams dosed with distilled water. There were no significant differences between the litters dosed with *P. taeda* extract and those of the control group. No toxic effects were noted in the dams in any of the treatment groups. In addition pregnant rats were dosed [1 g/kg/day] on days 6–15 of gestation. No teratogenic or abortive effects of the extracts were noted leading to the conclusion that the effect on implantation is significant in the early stages of pregnancy in rats.

More recently Jensen et al. [59] have evaluated histopathological and physiological changes in cows having premature births after eating *P.*

ponderosa needles. Premature calving of weak or dead calves accompanied by retained placentas was induced in eight of nine pregnant cows fed a 9 kg/head/day mixture of ponderosa pine needles and alfalfa at 7.5 months of gestation. Serum progesterone levels in the treated cows decreased progressively and were 0.4 to 1.5 ng/ml at the time of calving. The number of binucleate trophoblastic giant cells in placentomes was less than normal and the number of necrotic luteal cells in corpora lutea was greater than normal. The authors noted that the substance(s) within pine needles which cause these histological changes remain to be characterised.

Quander and Moseley [53] cite a number of reports of attempts at abortion using either pine oil disinfectant or turpentine, in addition to their own case report of abortion induced by a 20-year-old woman who injected a mixture of turpentine and water into her uterus. In one of the cases cited the patient recovered rapidly without abortion and eventually delivered a normal term child. In their own case Quander and Moseley record that the patient's ability to conceive remained unimpaired but noted that in a third case the patient's condition required laparotomy and bilateral salpingo-oophorectomy before recovery. Gornel and Goldman [46] reported the case of a 31-year-old woman who induced an abortion by instilling into her uterus about 75–150 ml of a 1 in 2 mixture of pine oil [70%] and neutral soap [14%] in water, resulting in uremia, acute pyelonephritis, anemia, peripheral neuropathy and renal damage as already noted.

Mutagenicity and Carcinogenicity

Roe and Field [60] stated that turpentine oil and α-pinene were weak promoters of tumour formation by 9,10-dimethyl-12-benzanthracene in mice, although earlier references cited by these authors indicate that turpentine was more or less ineffective in the mouse, in contrast to a report in 1941 that it promoted skin tumour development in rabbit skin. These different results were ascribed to differences in the composition of the oil. Nagao et al. [61] reported that the flavone tectochrysin from "*Pinus pumila*" (*P. pumilio*?) showed no mutagenic activity when tested with *Salmonella typhimurium* strains TA98 and TA100 in the presence of rat liver S-9 mix.

References

1. Dallimore W, Jackson AB (1966) A Handbook of Coniferae and Gingkoaceae. 4th edn. (revised by Harrison SG). London: Edward Arnold
2. Norin T (1972) Some aspects of the chemistry of the order Pinales. Phytochemistry 11:1231–1242
3. Roberts DR (1970) Within tree variation of monoterpene hydrocarbon composition of slash pine oleoresin. Phytochemistry 9:809–815

4. Chalchat JC, Garry RPh, Michet A, Bastide P, Mahuret R (1987) Correlation composition chimique/activité antimicrobienne. III Influence du vieillessement naturel et provoque sur l'activité de trois huiles essentielles de resineux vis-a-vis d'Escherichia coli. Plantes Med Phytother 21:218–235
5. Leung AY (1980) Encyclopedia of common natural ingredients used in food, drugs and cosmetics. New York: Wiley-Interscience, pp 314–316
6. Pirila V (1968) Pattern of sensitivity to different terpenes. Contact Dermatitis Newsletter London 3:48 [cited in Mitchell J, Rook A (1979) Botanical Dermatology. Vancouver: Greengrass, pp 520–521]
7. Mirov NT (1961) Composition of gum turpentines of pines. U.S. Dept. Agric. Forest Service Techn Bull No. 1239
8. Opdyke DLJ (1974) Abies Alba oil from needles. Fd Cosmet Toxicol 12 (Suppl): 811
9. V. Schantz M (1965) Über die zusammensetzung der ätherischen Öle bei verschiedenen Picea arten. Planta Med. 13:369–381
10. Reynolds JEF (ed) (1982) Martindale. The Extra Pharmacopoeia 28th Edn. London: The Pharmaceutical Press, pp 682–685
11. Leung AY (1980) Encyclopedia of common natural ingredients used in food, drugs and cosmetics. New York: Wiley-Interscience, pp 266–269
12. Opdyke DLJ (1974) Abies Alba oil from cones. Fd Cosmet Toxicol 12 (Suppl): 809–810
13. Arzneiburo der Bundesvereinigung Deutscher Apothekerverbande Pharmazeutische Stoffliste (1990) 7 Auflage. Frankfurt am Main: Werbe – und Vertriebsgesellschaft Deutscher Apotheker
14. Williamson EM, Evans FJ (1988) Potters new cyclopaedia of botanical drugs and preparations by Wren RC. Saffron Walden: The C.W. Daniel Company Ltd, pp 216–217
15. Weiss RF (1988) Herbal Medicine. Gothenburg and Beaconsfield: AB Arcanum and Beaconsfield Publishers, p 347
16. V. Spindler O (1913) The physiological effect of pine needle baths. Schweiz Wchschr 51:338–340 [per Chem Abstr 1913; 7:3795]
17. Wade A (ed) (1977) Martindale The Extra Pharmacopoeia 27th edn. London: The Pharmaceutical Press, pp 1027–1028
18. Reynolds JEF (ed) (1989) Martindale The Extra Pharmacopoeia 29th edn. London: The Pharmaceutical Press, p 1067
19. Morton JF (1977) Major medicinal plants. Springfield: Thomas, pp 13–21
20. Boyd EM, Pearson GL (1946) On the expectorant action of volatile oils. Am J Med Sci 211:602–610
21. Tul'chinskaya KZ (1935) Antiscorbutic vitamin concentrates obtained from some products of no food value. Proc Inst Sci Research Food Ind (USSR) 3:131–144 [per Chem Abstr 1936; 30:3481]
22. Gakh JV (1936) The antiscorbutic properties of the scotch pine (*Pinus sylvestris*) and the spruce (*Picea excelsa*). Arch Sci Biol (USSR) 42:145–146
23. Komarov SN (1936) The curative action of anti-scorbutic pine needle concentrate. Proc Sci Inst Vitamin Research USSR 1:127–30 [per Chem Abstr 1937; 31:1853]
24. Verkhrats'kii NS (1957) Biological activity of polyphenols of spruce needles. Ukrain Biokhim Zhur 29:479–484 [per Chem Abstr 1958; 52:8306]
25. Siafaka-Kapadai A, Demopoulos CA, Andrikopoulos NK (1986) Biological activity of lipids of pine pollen on platelet aggregation in correlation with PAF. Biochem Int 12:33–41
26. Katoh Y et al. (1986) Inhibition of human plasma cholinesterase *in vitro* by extracts of plants in Hokkaido. Hokkaidoritsu Eisei Kenkyushoho 36:63–65 [per Chem Abstr 1987; 106:1916–20]
27. Jonadet M, Meumer MT, Bastide P (1983) Anthocyanosides extraits de *Vitis vinifera*, de *Vaccinium myrtillus* et de *Pinus maritimus*. I. Activités inhibitrices vis-a-vis de l'elastase *in vitro*. II. Activités angioprotectrices comparées *in vivo*. J Pharm Belg 38:41–46

28. Sakagami H, Oh-hara T, Kaiya T et al. (1989) Molecular species of the antitumor and antiviral fraction from Pine cone extract. Anticancer Res 9:1593–1598
29. Tobin T, Swerczek TW, Blake JW (1976) Pine oil toxicity in the horse: drug detection, residues and pathological changes. Res Commun Chem Path Pharmac 15:291–301
30. Opdyke DLJ (1976) Pinus pumilio oil. Fd Cosmet Toxicol 14:843–844
31. Opdyke DLJ (1976) Pinus sylvestris oil. Fd Cosmet Toxicol 14:845–846
32. D.H.S.S. (U.K.) (1984) The Medicines (Products other than Veterinary Drugs) (General Sale List) Order SI No. 769
33. Ministère des Affaires Sociales de France (1990) Avis aux Fabricants concernant les demandes d'autorisation de mise sur le marché de medicaments à base de plantes. Bulletin Officiel No. 90/22 bis
34. Anonymous (1987) Kroonberoep Haarlemmerolie ongegrond. Pharm Weekbl 122:949
35. Thesen R (1988) BGA-Warnung vor Piperazin und Terpentinöl. Pharm Ztg 133(50):29
36. Von Skramlik E (1959) Über die giftigkeit und Verträglichkeit von ätherischen Ölen. Pharmazie 14:435–445
37. Okanishi T (1928) Some pharmacological actions of sandalwood oil, vetivert oil and pine needle oil. Fol. Pharmacol Jap 7:77–85 [per Chem Abst 1930; 24:658]
38. Primavori GG (1960) Pharmacological researches on action of the essential oil from *P. pumilio*. Atti Soc Toscana Sci Nat Pisa Processi Verbali e mem Ser B 67:6–23 [per Chem Abstr 1962; 56:1960]
39. Kachanov AD (1961) Pharmacological characterisation of essential oils from pine. TR. Leningr-Khim Farmatsevt Inst 210–214 [per Chem Abstr 1963; 58:14617]
40. Timajeev VP, Agranovskii MZ, Samarin AA, Polyakova TI (1981) Biological effects of rosin, pine oil and adhesives and their probable mechanism of action. TRLSGMI 65–69 [per Chem Abstr 1983; 98:210999]
41. Craig JO (1953) Poisoning by the volatile oils in childhood. Arch Dis Child 28:475–483
42. Hill RM, Barer J, Leighton Hill L, Butler CM, Harvey DJ, Horning MG (1975) An investigation of recurrent pine oil poisoning in an infant by the use of gas chromatography–mass spectrometric methods. J Pediatrics 87:115–118
43. Jaeger RW, De Castro F, Blair J, Whittler M (1978) The brain in hydrocarbon intoxication. Vet Hum Toxicol 20:103
44. Mancini A (1925) Pharmacological study of the oil of knee pine. Boll Chim Farm 64:449–459
45. Sazonova NA (1945) Toxicity of pine oil. Farmakol i Toksikol 8:50 [per Chem Abstr 1946; 40:5845]
46. Gornel DL, Goldman R (1968) Acute renal failure following hexol-induced abortion. J Am Med Assoc 203:168–170
47. Mitchell J, Rook A (1979) Botanical Dermatology. Vancouver: Greengrass, pp 514–523
48. Jadassohn W (1960) Étude sur l'eczema du a des substances chimiquement connues. Acta Allergologica 15 (Suppl VII):185–190
49. Karlberg A-T, Boman A, Wahlberg JE (1980) Allergenic potential of abietic acid, colophony and pine resin – HA. Clinical and experimental studies. Contact Dermatitis 6:481–487
50. Foussereau J, Schlewer G, Chabeau G, Reimeringer A (1980) Étude allergologique d'intolerances a la colophone. Dermatosen 28:14–15
51. Eisyment TA (1983) Lipid composition of bovine blood in relation to the inclusion of tree bark in the diet. Fiziol Biokhim OSN Povysh Prod S-Kh Zhivotn Bashkirov BA Ed. 108–112 [per Chem Abstr 1985; 102:184156]
52. Weiss RF (1988) Herbal Medicine. Gothenburg and Beaconsfield: AB Arcanum and Beaconsfield Publishers, p 329
53. Quander MF, Moseley JE (1964) Abortion, chemical peritonitis and pulmonary edema following intrauterine injection of turpentine. Obstet Gynecol 24:572–574

54. Jori A, Bianchetti A, Prestini PE (1969) Effect of essential oils on drug metabolism. Biochem Pharmacol 18:2081–2085
55. Morton JF (1973) Plant products and occupational materials ingested by esophageal cancer victims in South Carolina. Quart J Crude Drug Res 13:2005–2022
56. Murphy JC, Craig JC, Pace HB, El-Sohly M, Watson ES (1977) Evaluation of an aqueous extract of pine needles utilising the rat reproductive system. Quart J Crude Drug Res 15:193–197
57. Wagner WD, Jackson LL (1977) Phytoestrogen from *P. ponderosa* assayed by competitive binding with 17 β-estradiol to mouse uterine cytosol. Theriogenology 19:507–516
58. Paul B, Deb C, Banik S (1980) Ovarian steroidogenesis in rats after treatment with *P. lambertiana*. Indian J Exp Biol 18:26–28
59. Jensen R, Pier AC, Kaltenbach CC, Murdoch WJ, Becerra VM, Mills KW, Robinson JL (1989) Evaluation of histopathologic and physiologic changes in cows having premature births after consuming ponderosa pine needles. Am J Vet Res 50:285–289
60. Roe FJC, Field WEH (1965) Chronic toxicity of essential oils and certain other products of natural origin. Fd Cosmet Toxicol 3:311–324
61. Nagao M, Morita N, Yahagi Y et al (1981) Mutagenicities of 61 flavonoids and 11 related compounds. Environ Mut 3:401–419

Anthranoid Derivatives – General Discussion

J. Westendorf

Botany

The chemical class of naturally occurring anthranoids comprises some hundreds of structurally related compounds, present in many species of the plant families: Liliaceae (*Aloe*, *Hawertia*, *Eremus*), Hypericaceae (*Hypericum*), Polygonaceae (*Rheum*, *Rumex*, *Polygonum*, *Fagopyrum*, *Oxygonum*), Rhamnaceae (*Rhamnus*), Rubiaceae (*Galium*, *Rubia*, *Morinda*), Caesalpiniaceae (*Cassia*, *Gleditschia*), Fabaceae (*Andira*), Verbenaceae (*Tectona*), and Scrophulariaceae (*Digitalis*). Anthranoids are also present in Ascomycetes, such as *Penicillium* and *Aspergillus* species.

Of primary pharmaceutical interest are mainly anthranoid-containing plants with laxative or cathartic action, such as *Aloe*, *Cassia*, *Rhamnus* and *Rheum*. In addition, *Rubia tinctorum* L. is used in the treatment of kidney and bladder stones [1].

Chemistry

Naturally occurrally anthranoids are oxo-, hydroxy-, and hydroxy-oxo-derivatives of anthracene. Most of these compounds are derivatives of 9,10-anthraquinone (= AQ). Reduction of the anthraquinones (= AQs) leads to anthrones and their tautomeric anthranols, which are also present as dimers. The aromatic hydrogens may be substituted by functional groups, such as methoxy, hydroxymethyl, and carboxy groups. Many AQs are present in plants as glycosides. A comprehensive review of the naturally occurring anthranoids is given by Thomson [2].

AQ-containing plants are mainly used medicinally for their laxative or cathartic action. The presence of hydroxy groups in positions 1 and 8 of the AQ nucleus is essential for the laxative action of these compounds. Although the composition of herbal AQ preparations is very complex, only a few AQs and their glycosides are responsible for the cathartic action. An overview is given in Table 1.

Adverse Effects of Herbal Drugs, Vol. 2
(ed. by P.A.G.M. De Smet, K. Keller, R. Hänsel, R.F. Chandler)

Table 1. Occurrence of laxative anthranoid derivatives in medicinal plants

Anthranoid derivative	Occurrence
Aglycones	
Chrysophanol	*Aloe, Cassia, Rhamnus, Rheum, Rumex*
Aloe-emodin	*Aloe, Cassia, Rhamnus, Rheum*
Rhein	*Cassia, Rheum, Rumex*
Danthron	*Cinchona*
Emodin	*Rhamnus, Rheum, Rumex*
Physcion	*Cassia, Haronga, Rhamnus, Rheum*
Glycosides	
Sennosides	*Cassia, Rheum*
Aloins	*Aloe, Cassia*
Frangulosides	*Rhamnus*
Glucofrangulines	*Rhamnus*
Cascarosides	*Rhamnus*

Table 2. Occurrence of non-laxative anthranoid derivatives in some plants belonging to the *Rubiaceae*

Anthranoid derivative	Occurrence
Alizarin	*Rubia tinctorum, Cinchona*
Lucidin	*Rubia tinctorum*
Rubiadin	*Rubia tinctorum, Galium, Cinchona*
Purpuroxanthin	*Rubia tinctorum*
Purpurin	*Rubia tinctorum, Cinchona*

Rubia tinctorum contains primarily AQs which are substituted in one aromatic ring only. These compounds are without laxative action. The most important AQs of this plant are listed in Table 2. Most of the AQs in *Rubia tinctorum* and other species of Rubiaceae also occur as glycosides, such as glucosides and primverosides [2].

Numerous qualitative and quantitative procedures for the determination of AQs in drugs and plant material have been reported in the literature [3–8]. The methods include extraction of the material with different organic solvents, such as chloroform, acetone, ethanol, ethylacetate and separation of the AQs by TLC, HPLC and GC (after silylation).

Pharmacology and Uses

Most of the AQ-containing drugs are used as laxatives. Depending on the dose and the type of drug used, a soft or fluid stool is produced. Although intensive research has been performed, the mechanism of action is still unclear. However, there is no doubt that the AQs exert their action on the colonic mucosa. The higher the concentration of these compounds in the colon, the more vigorous their laxative action. AQ-glycosides, which are transported to the colon without prior absorption are more potent than AQ-aglycones, which are partially absorbed in the stomach and duodenum. The presence of the intestinal flora is essential for the laxative action of the glycosides and, possibly, also for the effect of the aglycones [9].

It is believed that AQs act by disturbing the equilibrium between the absorption of water from the intestinal lumen via an active sodium transport [10] and the secretion of water into the lumen by the hydrostatic blood pressure or a prostaglandin-dependent chloride secretion [11,12]. Anthrones, formed from AQs or their glycosides via reduction by the intestinal flora are most likely the active metabolites [13]. These anthrones are highly reactive and about 100-fold more cytotoxic than their parent AQs [14]. The laxative action could, therefore, also be the result of a cytotoxic effect of the anthrones on the intestinal mucosa. It should be noted that diarrhoea is a common side effect in cancer patients treated with cytotoxic drugs. It is also interesting in this context that anthrones are used, together with other cytostatic drugs and potent glucocorticoids, for the treatment of psoriasis, a hyperproliferative disease of the skin [15].

A comparison of the laxative potency of a variety of anthranoids in mice showed the following sequence of increasing activity: chrysophanol = aloe-emodin = aloe-emodin anthrone $<$ aloe-emodin dianthrone = aloe-emodin diglucoside $<$ rhein $\ll$ sennidin $<$ sennoside A $<$ crude glycoside concentrate prepared from senna pod (as sennosides A & B) = senna pod standard (as sennosides A & B). Danthron and emodin were inactive in the assay [16]. However, it should be considered that the laxative action of anthranoids is mediated by the intestinal flora, which is rather different between man and rodents. Moreover, the relative inactivity of the anthrones does not reflect their intrinsic activity on the colonic mucosa but the fact that these compounds do not reach this place in sufficiently large quantities due to prior absorption or metabolic transformation to less active compounds.

There is only limited information available about a possible litholytic activity of the AQs present in *Rubia tinctorum* (alizarin, purpurin, lucidin) [1] and it remains doubtful, whether they exert a disintegrating effect on the surface of calcium-containing kidney and bladder stones.

Pharmacokinetics

Most of the herbal anthranoid-containing preparations contain complex mixtures, consisting of AQ-aglycones as well as AQ-glycosides. As the fate of both groups in the organism is very different, they will be treated separately.

Table 3. Excretion of anthranoid aglycones following oral administration to laboratory animals

Compound	animal	Excretion (%) urine	faeces	total	Ref.
Rhein	rat	17.2	1.7	18.9	17
Danthron	rat	15.8	0.9	16.7	18
Danthron	rat	26.5	7.0	33.5	19
Alizarin	rat	10.4	ND		20
^{14}C-Emodin	rat	22.0	68	90.0	21
Rhein	mouse	2–5	2–6	4–11	22
Aloe-Emodin	mouse	3–9	16–31	19–40	22
Chrysophanol	mouse	2–3	34–45	36–48	22

AQ-Aglycones

Animal pharmacokinetic studies have been performed with rhein, aloe-emodin, emodin, alizarin, chrysophanol and lucidin. All of these AQs showed a considerable renal excretion after administration by oral gavage, which demonstrates their intestinal absorption. An overview is given in Table 3.

Qualitatively, glucuronide and sulfate conjugates of AQs were detected in the urine as well as in the faeces. This suggests that the AQs enter the faeces via biliary excretion. The fact that there is a loss of more than 50%, when the detection is performed by a spectrophotometric method, indicates a considerable breakdown of the AQ-chromophore, possibly the result of bacterial metabolism in the colon. This has been demonstrated by incubation of danthron with *Streptomyces aureofaciens* [23].

A rapid absorption has been demonstrated after oral application of ^{14}C-rhein to rats [24]. There was also evidence of a considerable enterohepatic circulation in these experiments. Even after direct application of rhein to the colon, the absorption was quite efficient. This indicates that rhein, which can be liberated from sennosides in the colon by the glucosidases of the intestinal flora, is systemically available. The distribution of rhein was normal, with relatively high concentrations in the parenchymatous organs. There was a remarkable retention of radioactivity in the kidneys which could not be extracted by organic solvents. Similar observations have been made with ^{14}C-emodin [20] and with ^{14}C-lucidin (own unpublished results). It seems likely, therefore, that a special metabolism of AQs takes place in the kidney, which leads to a covalent binding to macromolecules. This observation may be of pathological importance.

Pharmacokinetic data in man are only available for alizarin [25]. After oral administration of 210 mg alizarin, the renal excretion was 18–36%, whereas 21–33% were excreted via the faeces. No alizarin could be detected in the bile of one patient treated with this compound. This is in contrast to the animal experiments with ^{14}C-rhein [24], ^{14}C-emodin [21], and ^{14}C-lucidin (own unpublished results).

No phase one-metabolites of rhein and alizarin have been detected after oral administration to rats. Emodin was partially oxidized to emodic acid [21]. A similar observation was made by us after application of ^{14}C-chrysophanol to rats. The compound was oxidized to aloe-emodin and rhein (own unpublished results). The hydroxymethyl-AQ lucidin, however, was partially reduced in the rat to rubiadin [26].

AQ-Glycosides

AQ-glycosides are much more hydrophilic than their corresponding aglycones. Substantial absorption through the intestinal wall is therefore unlikely. After ingestion of AQ-glycosides, most of the compounds will be directly transported to the colon (a small amount may be cleaved by glycosidases of the intestinal wall). The AQ-glycosides are then metabolized by the intestinal flora. If the compounds contain a 1,8-dihydroxy-structure in their AQ-nucleus, highly reactive anthrones will be formed, which are responsible for the laxative action. This happens, for instance, to the sennosides, the metabolism of which has been reviewed by Lemli [27].

If the glycosides do not have this structure, no anthrones are formed and no laxative action is observed. This latter group of glycosides includes ruberythric acid (alizarin primeveroside) and lucidin primeveroside, which are both present in *Rubia tinctorum*. We observed that after oral administration the former compound is metabolized by rats to alizarin and 1-hydroxyanthraquinone [28]. The latter compound was carcinogenic in rats after chronic treatment [29]. Lucidin primeveroside is transformed by rats to lucidin and rubiadin [26]. Both compounds are highly genotoxic in a battery of short-term tests [30,31].

Adverse Reaction Profile

General Animal Data

Only limited investigations are available that deal with the toxicity of anthranoid derivatives in laboratory animals. Most of these studies have been performed with senna extracts (see also the separate monograph about *Cassia* spp. elsewhere in this volume). The acute toxicity of sennosides A & B was investigated in mice [32]. The LD_{50} for i.v. injection was 4100 mg/kg and >5000 mg/kg for the oral route of administration. In contrast, the toxicity of a partially purified senna extract (20% Ca-sennosides) was considerably higher, namely 172 mg/kg i.v. and 2500 mg/kg p.o. This difference is believed to be due to the presence of free aglycones in the extract. However, for the i.v. route the effect of non-physiological high calcium concentrations may also account for the toxicity.

General Human Data

According to Cooke [33], 20–30% of people above age 60 take laxatives at least once a week. Most of these drugs contain AQs as their active principles. A study of 700 patients with pathological symptoms caused by laxative abuse showed that about 80% were taking senna and related AQ-drugs [34]. The reasons for the excessive use of such laxatives are manifold and include psychiatric abnormalities, such as depression, personality disorders and anorexia nervosa [35]. Laxative abuse may also occur as a variant of bulimia [36]. The typical patient (in 90% of the cases a female) complains of chronic constipation, has a gross misconception of what constitutes normal bowel habits, and/or has an abnormal desire for weight loss or removal of body wastes. The laxative abuse syndrome (LAS) includes symptoms of massive loss of electrolytes with many secondary consequences, as well as pathological changes of the colonic mucosa [33–35,37–41], which will be discussed in special sections below.

A harmless side effect of the use of AQ-containing drugs is a discolouration of the urine and faeces, which may interfere with certain diagnostic tests [42].

AQ-containing laxatives should not be used (a) by children younger than 12 years (b) in inflammatory intestinal diseases (colitis ulcerosa, Crohn's disease), ileus or subileus, and painful syndromes of unknown origin (c) for more than 8–10 days [43]. However, as most of these drugs are not prescribed by physicians, it is difficult to control that all consumers pay sufficient attention to these contra-indications. Many symptoms outlined above and in the following subheadings are summarized in the literature as "laxative abuse". The frequency of their occurrence makes it questionable, whether herbal AQ-containing laxatives should be available without prescription.

Gastro-Intestinal Reactions

Chronic consumption of AQ-containing laxatives leads to a characteristic pigmentation of the colonic and rectal mucosa. This phenomenon is called "melanosis coli" [38–40]. It is caused by a deposition of insoluble condensation products, which occur spontaneously by condensation of highly reactive intermediates of anthranoid derivatives, such as anthrones, in the colon. These black particles are taken up by macrophages superficially within the lamina propria. After cessation of drug intake the pigmentation is reversible within 4–12 months [33]. Melanosis coli is a valuable diagnostic parameter for the detection of chronic abuse of AQ-containing laxatives, but it is without pathological impact. More critical are morphological alterations of the anus and rectum, caused by excessive use of cathartic agents, such as AQ-containing drugs. Fissures, cryptitides and stenoses of the anus have been observed in 11–25% of 700 patients with chronic abuse of laxatives [34]. These symptoms were not always reversible and often required surgical operations. In 7–12% of the patients perianal thromboses and haemorrhoidal prolapses have been observed. It seems possible, however, that a haemorrhoidal history in these patients was the reason for taking laxatives.

Other pathological alterations caused by laxatives can be found in the colon. These are characterized by damage of the smooth muscles and myenteric plexi, which result in decreased peristalsis and possible paralysis of the muscular activity. In progressive stages a considerable loss of cell regeneration is also observed, together with inflammatory processes, which may be indistinguishable from other inflammatory bowel diseases, such as colitis ulcerosa [41]. It is likely that these symptoms are due to the very aggressive nature of the anthrones, formed from AQs by bacterial metabolism in the large bowel. We showed that anthrones are 100-fold more cytotoxic than their corresponding AQs [44]. It should be considered that intestinal damage is a common phenomenon during treatment of cancer patients with cytotoxic drugs.

Hepatic Reactions

A case of toxic hepatitis has been reported after the excessive use of senna by a young female patient [45]. It should be noted that hepatic damage has also been observed in animal studies after the feeding of danthron to rats [46] or mice [47]. As the anthraquinones form highly reactive anthrones in the colon, it is likely that, after absorption and transportation to the liver, these compounds are able to induce liver damage. It seems possible that further cases of liver damage caused by AQs have not been associated with the uptake of these drugs, because the physicians treating these patients did not even know that they were taking AQ-containing laxatives.

Metabolic Reactions

AQ-containing laxatives cause increased losses of water and electrolytes. The potassium depletion of the body may be up to 25–50% [33]. The loss of potassium is partly due to direct excretion via the faeces and partly caused by the loss of sodium as a result of secondary hyperaldosteronism. The loss of potassium is responsible for symptoms, such as renal tubular nephropathy, a decrease of overall muscular activity and cardiac complications, such as arrythmia and bradycardia. Patients receiving cardiac glycosides are especially sensitive.

Some patients with laxative abuse may also have a history of misusing drugs made from ipecacuanha root. However, the hypokalemic form of muscular weakness caused by anthranoid laxatives can be differentiated from emetine-induced myopathy by muscle biopsy [36].

Osteopathic Reactions

Chronic purgative abuse has been associated with a painless deforming artropathy mainly effecting the hands. Clubbing of the fingers with or without hypertrophic osteopathy has also been attributed to the chronic use of purgatives in excessive doses [48–52].

Renal Reactions

Renal malfunction may occur as a consequence of the massive loss of electrolytes during the abuse of laxatives. As experiments with radioactive anthraquinones have shown that anthraquinones accumulate in the kidneys [21,24,26], it seems possible that these compounds are able to cause histopathological damage in these organs. However, no reports are available to support this hypothesis.

Drug Interactions

AQ-containing laxatives might potentially decrease the transit time of concomitantly administered oral drugs and thereby decrease their absorption [53]. Due to an excessive loss of potassium caused by laxative abuse the toxicity of cardiac glycosides may be increased. The drugs may also interfere with the potassium-retaining effects of potassium-sparing diuretics [35]. It has been speculated that senna preparations play a potentiating role in the development of analgesic nephropathy [54]. This speculation is in keeping with the general notation that dehydration may be an aggrevating risk factor in analgesic nephropathy [55].

Fertility, Pregnancy and Lactation

There is no evidence from the literature that AQs are teratogenic or embryotoxic. Swedish [56] and Australian [57] categorization systems on drug use in pregnancy allocate sennosides into the category of drugs which may be assumed to have been used by a large number of pregnant women without any definite disturbance in the reproductive process having been noted so far. Investigations with sennosides in rats and rabbits have not yielded evidence of reproductive toxicological effects [58]. It should be noted, however, that investigations made with sennosides may not be transferable to other AQs. Because some AQs are mutagenic and carcinogenic in rodents, adverse effects on the fetus can not be completely excluded, when these compounds are ingested by the mother. High doses of AQ-containing cathartics might also stimulate endometrial activity and provoke abortion [59].

AQs are partly excreted into the mother's milk. A cathartic effect in the infant seems, therefore, possible [60,61]. However, a study in 20 women with a post partum intake of a standardized senna preparation showed that only minimal amounts of rhein were observable in the milk, and the risk for the infant to develop diarrhoea was claimed to be minimal [62]. The WHO Working Group on Drugs and Human Lactation reached the conclusion that the risk of inducing diarrhoea in a suckling infant by administering senna glycosides to its mother appears to be negligible and that breast feeding should be regarded as safe [63]. The French health authorities exclude senna from their general rule that herbal anthranoid laxatives should not be used during lactation [43].

Most AQ-containing herbal medicines contain genotoxic anthraquinones, such as lucidin (*Rubia tinctorum*), aloe-emodin (*Aloe*, *Rheum*, *Rhamnus*) or emodin (*Rheum*, *Rhamnus*). Even senna contains small amounts of aloe-emodin (sennosides C and D). The excretion of these AQs into breast milk has not been investigated, but it is likely that these compounds are excreted at least at the same rate as rhein. As the conjugated fraction of rhein in the study of Faber and Strenge-Hesse [62] has not been measured, the total amount of AQ excreted may be higher. Due to these suggestions a risk to the infant can not be completely excluded. Therefore, the use of all AQ-containing drugs by breast-feeding mothers remains questionable.

Mutagenicity and Carcinogenicity

Extensive information is available from the literature about the genotoxicity of AQs in *in vitro* short-term tests, but very few experiments have been performed *in vivo*. The spectrum of AQs detected in medicinal plants is very complex and it is not possible to discuss all of these compounds in this chapter. Instead the main focus will be on major AQ-constituents only.

A great variety of AQs have been investigated for possible mutagenicity in the *Salmonella*/microsome assay [64–67]. Positive results have been obtained with danthron, chrysophanol, aloe-emodin and emodin (in the group of laxative AQs) but not with rhein. Of the AQs present in *Rubia tinctorum*, lucidin, purpurin and purpuroxanthin were mutagenic, whereas alizarin was inactive [67]. The anthrones, anthralin and chrysarobin, have also been tested for possible mutagenicity in *Salmonella* [44]. Mutagenicity was achieved with chrysarobin but not with anthralin. The latter compound was very toxic to the bacteria and it seems possible that this toxicity overcomes possible mutagenic effects.

In V79 Chinese hamster fibroblasts, the AQs emodin, aloe-emodin, lucidin, purpurin and purpuroxanthin have been demonstrated to induce mutations in the HGPRT-gene locus [67]. Emodin has also been reported by another author [68] to be non-mutagenic in this assay, but the compound was mutagenic in the mouse carcinoma cell line FM3A [69]. The AQs danthron, chrysophanol, rhein and alizarin were not mutagenic in V79 cells [67]. The anthrones of danthron (anthralin), aloe-emodin and chrysophanol (chrysarobin) were also non-mutagenic, but these compounds were highly cytotoxic (in the range of 1 μg/ml) [44].

Various AQs have been tested for the induction of DNA repair in primary rat hepatocytes. Emodin, aloe-emodin, purpuroxanthin, purpurin, and lucidin were active in this assay, alizarin was weakly active and rhein and chrysophanol were inactive [67]. The same result was obtained in the *in vitro* transformation assay with mouse C3H/M2 fibroblasts [70].

Only two AQs have been investigated for possible tumor induction in rodents. After feeding danthron to rats (1% of the diet, for 16 months), 7/12 animals developed tumors of the large bowel. Four of these tumors were adenocarcinomas. No tumor was observed in the control animals [46]. Danthron was also tested for possible tumor induction in mice [47]. The animals received a diet supplemented with 0.2% danthron for a period of 500 days. All treated mice which survived 500 days developed adenomatous hyperplasia of the cecum and colon. No such tumor was observed in the control group. Hepatocellular carcinomas were also observed in danthron-treated mice (4/17) but not in the control group (0/19). 5/19 Adenomas were observed in the liver of control animals, in contrast to 9/17 adenomas in the treated animals.

1-Hydroxyanthraquinone, which is not a laxative, has also been investigated for possible tumor induction in rats [29]. It has been detected as a metabolite of alizarin primeveroside in rats, the latter compound being one of the main AQ-constituents of *Rubia tinctorum* [71]. Thirty animals received a diet containing 1% of 1-hydroxyanthraquinone over a period of 480 days. The following tumors were observed: 10 adenomas and 5 adenocarcinomas of the cecum; 12 adenomas and 11 adenocarcinomas of the colon; 12 hyperplastic nodules and 4 hepatocellular carcinomas of the liver; 4 papillomas and 1 glandular adenoma of the forestomach. No tumor was observed in 30 control animals.

Comparison of the *in vitro* genotoxicity results obtained with danthron and 1-hydroxyanthraquinone with that of other AQs does not imply a special risk for these two compounds. Both are weak mutagens in *Salmonella* and induce unscheduled DNA synthesis (UDS) in primary rat hepatocytes [28,71]. These effects are also produced by various other AQs, such as lucidin, emodin and aloe-emodin. It has to be suspected, therefore, that these latter AQs may be carcinogenic as well.

One case has been published where the chronic application of danthron in a young female was held responsible for the occurrence of a leiomyosarcoma of the small intestine [72]. A recent epidemiological study, performed at Lübeck, Germany, has demonstrated a threefold increase of the incidence of colon carcinoma in patients with a history of chronic abuse of anthranoid laxatives [73]. The "Melbourne colorectal study" clearly demonstrates that colon cancer is not related to obstipation itself [74]. The data from Siegers [73] are yet preliminary and have to be corroborated by further studies. However, it has to be taken into consideration from these investigations and from the animal and *in vitro* experiments that AQ-containing laxatives may be carcinogenic in man.

The AQ danthron has been withdrawn from the market in European and some non-European countries because of its carcinogenic action in rodents. As a consequence, more people now use AQ-containing laxatives made from plants, which have not been restricted. From the chemical and biological point of view, however, there is no rationale for different regulations for danthron and the genotoxic AQs that are present in herbal remedies.

References

1. Gebhardt M (1979) Erste vorläufige Ergebnisse einer Studie über die litholytische Wirksamkeit von Urol auf Calciumoxalatsteine. Fortschr Urol Nephrol 14 (Suppl): 34–40
2. Thomson RH (1987) Naturally occurring quinones III: Recent advances. London: Chapman and Hall, pp 347–606
3. Berg W, Herrmann M, Kraft R (1974) Zur Strukturaufklärung von neuen Anthrachinon-Derivaten aus Rubia tinctorum L. 1. Mitteilung. Pharmazie 29:478–482
4. Berg W, Hesse A, Herrmann M, Kraft R (1975) Zur Strukturaufklärung von neuen Anthrachinonderivaten aus Rubia tinctorum L. 2. Mitteilung. Pharmazie 30:330–334
5. Auterhoff H (1951) Die chemische Wertbestimmung des Rhabarbers. Dtsch Apoth Ztg 23:415–417
6. Stahl E, Meußen HG, Jahr H (1985) Über den Gehalt der verschiedenen Hydroxyanthracenderivate in Rhabarberwurzeln und -zubereitungen. Dtsch Apoth Ztg 125:1478–1480
7. Chao Yung Su S, Ferguson NM (1973) Extraction and separation of anthraquinone glycosides. J Pharm Sci 62:899–901
8. Reynolds T (1985) The compounds in aloe leaf exudates: A review. Bot J Linn Soc 90:157–177
9. Dreessen M, Eyssen H, Lemli J (1981) The metabolism of sennosides A and B by the intestinal microflora. J Pharm Pharmacol 33:679–681
10. Wanitschke R, Karbach U (1988) Influence of rhein on rat colonic Na^+, K^+-ATP-ase and permeability *in vitro*. Pharmacology 36 (Suppl 1):98–103
11. Beubler E, Kollar G (1988) Prostaglandin-mediated action of sennosides. Pharmacology 36 (Suppl 1):85–91
12. Clauss W, Domkos G, Leng-Peschlow E (1988) Effect of rhein on electrogenic chloride secretion in rabbit distal colon. Pharmacology 36 (Suppl 1):104–110
13. Van Os FHL (1976) Some aspects of the pharmacology of anthraquinone drugs. Pharmacology 14 (Suppl 1):18–29
14. Dominiak M, Marquardt H (1990) Anthrones in comparison to their corresponding anthraquinones are severely cytotoxic but not genotoxic. Naunyn Schmiedebergs Arch Pharmacol 341 (Suppl):106

15. Wiegrebe W, Gerber A, Kappler J, Bayerl Ch (1979) Untersuchungen zum Stoffwechsel antipsoriatisch wirksamer Anthronderivate. Arzneim Forsch 29: 1083–1088
16. Fairbairn JW, Moss JR (1970) The relative purgative activities of 1,8-dihydroxyanthracene derivatives. J Pharm Pharmacol 22:584–593
17. Lemmers L (1979) Absorption, metabolism and excretion of sennoside A and B in the rat. Pharm Weekbl Sci Ed 1:1–9
18. Lemmers L (1978) Metabolisme en werkingsmechanisme van laxerende antraceenderivaten. Thesis, Leuven
19. Breimer DP, Baars RJ (1976) Pharmacokinetics and metabolism of anthraquinone laxatives. Pharmacology 14 (Suppl 1):30–47
20. Mähner B, Dulce HJ (1968) Ausscheidungsprodukte von Hydroxyanthrachinonen im Harn von Ratten. Z Klin Chem 6:99–102
21. Bachmann M, Schlatter CV (1981) Metabolism of ^{14}C-emodin in the rat. Xenobiotica 11:217–225
22. Moss MJR (1969) Thesis, University of London
23. Cudlin J, Steinerova N, Semera P, Vokoun J (1978) Microbial analogy of Bayer-Villiger reaction with anthraquinone derivative. Collect Czech Chem Comm 43: 1808–1810
24. Lang W (1988) Pharmacokinetics of ^{14}C-labelled rhein in rats. Parmacology 36 (Suppl 1):158–171
25. Lorenz D, Lücker PW, Krumbiegel G, Memmicke WH, Wetzelsberger N (1985) Pharmacokinetic studies of alizarin in man. Meth Find Exp Clin Pharmacol 7: 637–643
26. Poginsky B, Blömeke B, Westendorf J, Marquardt H (1990) Metabolism and DNA interaction of hydroxyanthraquinones present in Rubia tinctorum. Naunyn Schmiedebergs Arch Exp Pharm (Suppl) 341:106
27. Lemli J (1988) Metabolism of sennosides- An overview. Pharmacology 36 (Suppl 1):126–128
28. Blömeke B, Poginsky B, Schmutte Ch, Marquardt H, Westendorf J (1992) Formation of genotoxic metabolites from anthraquinone glycosides, present in Rubia tinctorum L. Mutat Res 265:263–272
29. Mori H, Yoshimi N, Iwata H, Mori Y, Hara A, Tanaka T, Kawai K (1990) Carcinogenicity of naturally occurring 1-hydroxyanthraquinone in rats: induction of large bowel, liver and stomach neoplasms. Carcinogenesis 11:799–802
30. Westendorf J, Poginsky B, Marquardt H, Groth G, Marquardt H (1988) The genotoxicity of lucidin, a natural component of Rubia tinct. L., and lucidinethylether, a component of ethanolic Rubia extracts. Cell Biol Toxicol 4:225–239
31. Poginsky B, Hewer H, Blömeke B, Westendorf J, Marquardt H, Phillips DH (1991) Evaluation of DNA-binding activity of hydroxyanthraquinones occurring in Rubia tinctorum L. Carcinogenesis 12:1265–1271
32. Marvola M, Koponen A, Hiltunen R, Hieltala P (1981) The effect of raw material purity on the acute toxicity and laxative effect of sennosides. J Pharm Pharmacol 33:108–109
33. Cooke, TW (1981) Laxative abuse. Acta Gastro Ent Belg 44:448–458
34. May H (1982) Mißbrauch von Abführmitteln, nachweisbare Schäden an Kolon, Anus und Stoffwechsel. Ärtztezeitschr Naturheilverf 7:365–371
35. Oster JR, Materson BJ, Rogers AI (1980) Laxative abuse syndrome. Amer J Gastroenterol 74:451–458
36. De Smet PAGM, Vulto AG (1987) Drugs used in non-orthodox medicine. In: Dukes MNG, red. Side effects of drugs – Annual 11. Amsterdam: Elsevier pp 422–431
37. Pietrusco RG (1977) Use and abuse of laxatives. Am J Hosp Pharm 34:291–300
38. Virchow R (1847) Die pathologischen Pigmente. Virchows Arch Path Anat 1:379
39. Bockus HL, Willard JH, Bank J (1933) Melanosis coli: the etiologic significane of the anthracene laxatives: a report of 41 cases. J Am Med Assoc 101:1–6

40. Wittoesch JHR, Jackman RJ, Mc Donald JR (1958) Melanosis coli: general review and study of 887 cases. Dis Colon Rect 1:172–180
41. Smith B (1973) Pathologic changes in the colon produced by anthraquinone purgatives. Dis Colon Rect 16:455
42. Reynolds JEF, red (1989) Matindale The Extra Pharmacopoeia. 29th edn. London: The Pharmaceutical Press, p 1106
43. Anonymous (1989) Leitfaden für Hersteller von Phytopharmaka mit abführender Wirkung, die Gegenstand eines vereinfachten Zulassungsverfahrens sein können. Pharm Ind 51:858–863
44. Westendorf J, Poginsky B, Dominiak M, Blömeke B, Marquardt H (1990) DNA-interaction and mutagenicity of hydroxyanthraquinones and their corresponding anthrones. Proc Am Assoc Cancer Res 31:565
45. Beuers U, Spengler U, Pape GR (1991) Hepatitis after chronic abuse of senna. Lancet 337:372–373
46. Mori H, Sugie S, Niwa K, Takahashi M, Kawai K (1985) Induction of intestinal tumours in rats by chrysazin. Brit J Cancer 52:781–783
47. Mori H, Sugie S, Niwa K, Yoshimi N, Tanaka T, Hirono I (1986) Carcinogenicity of chrysazin in large intestine and liver of mice. Jpn J Cancer Res 77:871–876
48. Prior J, White I (1978) Tetany and clubbing in a patient who ingested large quantities of senna. Lancet 2:947
49. Frier BM, Scott RDM (1977) Osteomalacia and arthropathy associated with prolonged abuse of purgatives. Br J Clin Pract 31:17
50. Silk DBA, Gibson JA, Murray CRH (1975) Reversible finger clubbing in a case of purgative abuse. Gastroenterology 68:790
51. Malmquist J, Ericsson B, Hulten-Nosslin MB, Jepson JO, Ljungberg O (1980) Finger clubbing and aspartylglucosamin excretion in a laxative-abusing patient. Postgrad Med 56:862
52. Armstrong RD, Crisp AJ, Graham R, Woolf DL (1981) Hypertophic osteoartropathy and purgative abuse. Br Med J 282:1836
53. McEvoy GK, Litvak K, red (1990) AHFS Drug Information 90. Bethesda: American Society of Hospital Pharmacists
54. Wainscoat JS, Finn R (1974) Possible role of laxatives in analgesic nephropathy. Br Med J 4:697–698
55. Dukes MG (1988) Antipyretic analgesics. In: Dukes MNG, red. Side effects of drugs. 11th edn. Amsterdam: Elsevier pp 156–169
56. Berglund F, Flodh H, Lundborg P, Prame B, Sannerstedt R (1984) Drug use during pregnancy and breast feeding. A classification system for drug information. Acta Obstet Gynecol Scand 1984; Suppl. 126:1–55
57. Australian Drug Evaluation Comittee (1989) Medicines in pregnancy. An Australian categorization of risk. Canberra: Australian Government Service
58. Mengs U (1986) Reproductive toxicological investigations with sennosides. Arzneim Forsch 36:1355–1358
59. Maiwald L (1986) Klinische Relevanz anthrachinonhaltiger Drogen. Z Phytother 7:153–156
60. Greenhalf JO, Leonard HS (1973) Laxatives in the treatment of constipation in pregnant and breast feeding mothers. Practitioner 210:259–263
61. Knowles JA (1973) Effects on the infant of drug therapy in nursing mothers. Drug Ther 3:57–65
62. Faber P, Strenge-Hesse A (1988) Relevance of rhein excretion into breast milk. Pharmacololgy 36 (Suppl 1):212–220
63. Bennett PN, red (1988) Drugs and human lactation. Amsterdam: Elsevier, pp 88–89
64. Brown J, Brown R (1976) Mutagenesis by 9,10-anthraquinone derivatives and related compounds in Salmonella typhimurium. Mutat Res 40:203–224
65. Brown J, Dietrich P (1979) Mutagenicity of anthraquinone and benzanthrone derivatives in the Salmonella/microsome test: activation of anthraquinone glycosides by enzymic extracts of rat cecal bacteria. Mutat Res 66:9–24

66. Tikkanen L, Matsushima T, Natori S (1983) mutagenicity of anthraquinones in the Salmonella preincubation test. Mutat Res 116:297–304
67. Westendorf J, Marquardt H, Poginsky B, Dominiak M, Schmidt J, Marquardt H (1990) Genotoxicity of naturally occurring hydroxyanthraquinones. Mutat Res 240: 1–12
68. Bruggeman IM, Van Der Hoeven JCM (1984) Lack of activity of the bacterial mutagen emodin in HGPRT and SCE assay with V79 chinese hamster cells. Mutat Res 138:219–224
69. Morita H, Umeda M, Masuda T, Ueno Y (1988) Cytotoxic and mutagenic effects of emodin on cultured mouse carcinoma FM3A cells. Mutat Res 97:81–102
70. Wölfle D, Schmutte Ch, Westendorf J, Marquardt H (1991) Hydroxyanthraquinones as tumor promoters: Enhancement of malignant transformation of C3H mouse fibroblasts and growth stimulation of primary rat hepatocytes. Cancer Res 50: 6540–6544
71. Kawai K, Mori H, Sugie S, Yoshimi N, Inoue T, Nakamura T, Nozawa Y, Matsushima T (1986) Genotoxicity in the hepatocyte/DNA repair test and toxicity to liver mitochondria of 1-hydroxyanthraquinone and several dihydroxyanthraquinones. Cell Biol Toxicol 4:457–467
72. Patel PM, Selby PJ, Deacon J, Chilvers C, McElwain TJ (1989) Anthraquinone laxatives and human cancer: an association in one case. Postgrad Med J 65:216–217
73. Siegers CP (1992) Anthranoid laxatives and colorectal cancer. TIPS 13:229–231
74. Kune GA, Kune S, Watson LF (1988) The role of chronic constipation, diarrhea, and laxative use in the etiology of large-bowel cancer. Dis Colon Rectum 31:507–512

Anthranoid Derivatives – *Aloe* Species

J. Westendorf

Botany

The genus *Aloe*, which belongs to the family of Asphodelaceae (formerly Liliaceae), comprises about 300 species. Of principal pharmaceutical interest are *Aloe ferox* Mill. and *Aloe barbadensis* Mill. The latter species is also known as *Aloe vera* L. or *Aloe vulgaris* Lamk. [1]. The dried leaf exudates of *Aloe ferox* and its hybrids and of *Aloe barbadensis* are used medicinally under the names of Cape Aloe and Curaçao Aloe, respectively.

Chemistry

Leaf exudates of *Aloe* species contain a variety of anthranoid derivatives. 9,10-Anthraquinones in the free aglycone form are only present at low levels. Among these are aloe-emodin, chrysophanol, aloe-saponarin I, aloe-saponarin II, laccaic-acid-D-methyl-ester, deoxyerythrolaccain, helminthosporin, and isoxanthorin [2].

The aloes usually contain high concentrations (e.g., 19–21%) of the C-glycosides aloin A and aloin B (stereoisomers of 10-glucosyl-aloe-emodinanthrone), together with aloinoside A and aloinoside B (aloin-11-O-α-L-rhamnoside). Curaçao aloe but not Cape aloe also contains 7-hydroxyaloins. Natal aloe, which is often used to adulterate medicinal aloes, contains the C-glucoside of 1-methoxy-2,8-dihydroxy-6-methylanthrone instead of aloin [4,5].

Besides anthranoid derivatives, aloe contains so-called resin substances [6]. Aloeresin A is a C-glycoside of 4-chromone esterified at C2 with *p*-coumaric acid [7]. Aloenin, the 6′-O-glucoside of 4-methoxy-6-(1-methyl-3,6-dihydroxyphenyl)-pyran-2-one has been identified in the leaves of *Aloe arborescens* Mill. [8] and isoeleutherol-5-O-glucoside has been isolated from the stems of *Aloe saponaria* Haw. [9].

Adverse Effects of Herbal Drugs, Vol. 2
(ed. by P.A.G.M. De Smet, K. Keller, R. Hänsel, R.F. Chandler)

Pharmacology and Uses

Two distinct components of aloe are used medicinally: the leaf exudate is used as a purgative, and the mucilaginous gel from the leaf parenchyma is used as a remedy against a variety of skin disorders [10].

The cathartic action of aloe leaf exudates is well documented. A soft stool is excreted after oral treatment with 50–200 mg aloe extract [1]. Higher doses produce diarrhoea with intestinal spasms and abdominal pain. Man is the most sensitive species. For instance, the effective dose for rats is about a hundred-fold higher [11]. The cathartic action is due to the presence of anthranoid derivatives (mainly aloin) which are metabolized by the intestinal flora to reactive anthrones. It has been demonstrated that, in contrast to rats, certain human intestinal bacteria are capable of cleaving aloin [12]. A more detailed description of the mechanisms involved in the cathartic action is presented in a general discussion on anthranoids elsewhere in this volume. Other reported pharmacological actions of aloe leaf exudates include anti-diabetic activity [13], cardiac stimulatory activity [14], and anti-bradykinin activity [15].

The mucilagenous pulp of the leaf parenchyma is used widely in cosmetics [16] and in remedies against various skin disorders [17], such as burns [18], radiation burns [19], and skin ulcers [20]. The pulp has also been used internally to treat peptic ulcers [21].

Pharmacokinetics

See the general discussion on anthranoid derivatives elsewhere in this volume.

Adverse Reaction Profile

A general discussion of adverse reactions of herbal medicines containing anthranoids is presented elsewhere in this volume.

General Animal Data

Systematic toxicity studies of aloe extracts in experimental animals are not available from the literature. A study of mice receiving 50 mg/kg/day of a dry aloe extract for a period of 12 weeks did not show severe pathological symptoms, nor any changes in electrolyte concentrations [22]. A two-fold increase of the sorbitol-dehydrogenase level in the treated animals was considered as a symptom of liver damage. A slight inflammatory reaction was also observed in the colonic mucosa of the treated animals.

General Human Data

The adverse effects of anthranoid-containing laxatives are reviewed in a general discussion elsewhere in this volume.

Allergic Reactions

Hypersensitivity to aloe has been rarely reported. Morrow et al. [23] describe a man, who had used *Aloe vera* gel orally for three years and topically for about one year. He developed pruritic eczematous dermatitis, and showed a positive skin patch test to the gel. Hogan [24] observed an erythematous, scaly, papular eruption in an elderly woman, after she had started treatment with jelly from an *Aloe vera* plant. Patch testing of the patient with various agents gave strong reactions to *Aloe vera* jelly, formaldehyde, and quarternium 15. Japanese authors have described four cases of allergic contact dermatitis to *Aloe arborescens* Mill. The leaf jelly of this species has been used in Japan to treat gastrointestinal disorders and topically for various skin diseases [25,26]. Another case of an allergic reaction to aloe leaves has been reported in the Russian literature [27].

Dermatological Reactions[1]

See the section on allergic reactions.

Fertility, Pregnancy and Lactation

A general discussion of the effects of herbal medicines containing anthranoids, when used during pregnancy or lactation, is presented elsewhere in this volume. It is often stated that aloe may not be used during pregnancy because of an abortive action. However, there are no animal data in the literature to support this statement.

Mutagenicity and Carcinogenicity

A general discussion of the mutagenic and carcinogenic properties of herbal medicines containing anthranoids is presented elsewhere in this volume. We investigated the mutagenicity of an aloe extract in *Salmonella typhimurium* and V79 cells and observed no activity. The extract was also inactive in the DNA-repair induction assay in primary rat hepatocytes (own unpublished

---

[1] See the note added in proof on p. 315

results). These negative results are due to the inability of the used systems to liberate mutagenic anthraquinone aglycones from the C-glycosides present in aloe extracts. However, it has to be taken into consideration that the mutagenic compound, aloe-emodin, is absorbed after cleavage of aloin by the intestinal flora and oxidation of the liberated aloe-emodin anthrone.

References

1. Steinegger E, Hänsel R (1988) Lehrbuch der Pharmakognosie auf phytochemischer Grundlage. Berlin: Springer Verlag, pp 165–166
2. Mathis C (1966) Comparative biochemistry of hydroxyquinones. In Swain T (Ed.) Comparative Phytochemistry. London: Academic Press, pp 245–270
3. Thomson RH (1971) Naturally occurring quinones. 2nd edition. New York: Academic Press
4. Wagner H (1985) Pharmazeutische Biologie: Drogen und ihre Inhaltsstoffe. 3rd edition. Stuttgart: Gustav Fischer Verlag, pp 221–222
5. Schneider G (1990) Arzneidrogen, Mannheim: Wissenschaftsverlag, pp 111–112
6. Böhme H, Kreutzig L (1964) Über die quantitative Ermittlung von Aloe mittels Papier- und Dünnschichtchromatographie. Arch Pharmazie 297:681–689
7. Gramatica P, Monti D, Speranza G, Manitto P (1982) Aloe revisited. The structure of aloeresin A. Tetrah Lett 23:2433–2424
8. Hirata T, Kushi Y, Suga T, Christensen A (1976) Structural studies of aloenin; the crystal structure of its aglycone. Chem Lett pp 393–396
9. Yagi A, Makino K, Nishioka I (1977) Studies on the constituents of Aloe saponaria Haw. III. The structures of phenol glucosides. Chem Pharm Bull 25:1771–1776
10. Reynolds T (1985) The compounds in aloe leaf exudates: a review. Bot J Linn Soc 90:157–177
11. Van Os FHL (1976) Some aspects of the pharmacology of anthraquinone drugs. Pharmacology 14 (Suppl 1):18–29
12. Che QM, Akao T, Hattori M, Kobashi K, Namba T (1991) Isolation of a human intestinal bacterium capable of transforming barbaloin to aloe-emodin anthrone. Planta Med 57:15–19
13. Ghannam N, Kingston M, Al-Meshaal IA, Tariq M, Parman N, Woodhouse N (1986) The antidiabetic activity of aloes: Preliminary clinical and experimental observations. Hormone Res 24:288–294
14. Yagi A, Shibata S, Nishioka I, Iwadare S, Ishida Y (1982) Cardiac stimulant action of constituents of Aloe saponaria. J Pharm Sci 71:739–741
15. Yagi A, Harada N, Yamada H, Iwadare S, Nishioka I (1982) Antibradykinin active material in Aloe saponaria. J Pharm Sci 71:1172–1174
16. Hoffenberg P (1979) Aloe vera. Eine alte Heilpflanze neu für die Kosmetik. Seifen-Öle-Fette-Wachse 105:499–502
17. Morton J (1961) Folk uses and commercial exploitation of aloe leaf pulp. Econ Bot 15:311–319
18. Cheney RH (1970) Aloe drug in human therapy. Quart J Crude Drug Res 10:1523–1530
19. Rowe TD, Lovell BK, Parks L (1941) Further observation on the use of Aloe vera leaf in the treatment of third degree x-ray reactions. J Am Pharm Assoc 30:266–269
20. Zawahry ME, Hegazy MR, Helal M (1973) Use of aloe in treating leg ulcers and dermatoses. Int J Dermatol 12:68–73
21. Blitz JJ, Smith JW, Gerard JR (1963) Aloe vera gel in peptic ulcer therapy: Preliminary report. J Am Osteopath Assoc 62:731–735
22. Siegers CP, Younes M, Herbst EW (1986) Toxikologische Bewertung anthrachinonhaltiger Laxanzien. Z Phytother 7:157–159

23. Morrow DM, Rapoport MJ, Strick RA (1980) Hypersensitivity to aloe. Arch Dermatol 116:1064–1065
24. Hogan DJ, (1988) Widespread dermatitis after topical treatment of chronic leg ulcers and stasis dermatitis. Can Med Assoc J 138:336–338
25. Shoji A (1982) Contact dermatitis to Aloe aborescens. Contact Dermatitis 8:164–167
26. Nakamura T, Kotajima S (1984) Contact dermatitis from Aloe aborescens. Contact Dermatitis 11:51
27. Sauchak UI (1977) Acute bullous allergic dermatitis due to local application of aloe leaves. Vestn Dermatol Venerol 12:44–45

Anthranoid Derivatives – *Cassia* Species

J. Westendorf

Botany

Two species of *Cassia* (family Caesalpiniaceae, formerly Leguminosae) are used as herbal medicines: *Cassia senna* L. = *Cassia acutifolia* Del. (yields Alexandrian senna) and *Cassia angustifolia* Vahl (yields Tinnevelly senna). The plant parts used medicinally are the dry leaves (Sennae Folium) and the mature pods (Sennae Fructus Acutifoliae, Sennae Fructus Angustifoliae).

Chemistry

Sennae Folium and Sennae Fructus contain mainly dianthrone glycosides (sennosides) as active components. Sennae Folium contains about 3% of anthra-glycosides, whereas Sennae Fructus contains about 5%. The sennosides A and B are the mesomeric forms of rhein dianthrone-8,8′-diglucoside, and sennosides C and D are the corresponding pair of rhein-aloe-emodin dianthrone-8,8′-diglucoside. Mono- and diglucosides of rhein and aloe-emodin and of the corresponding anthrones as well as free anthraquinones and dimeric anthrones (sennidines) are also present [1]. The genuine compounds are the glucosides of rhein anthrone and aloe-emodin anthrone, which form the sennosides by dimerisation during drying [2,3].

Pharmacology and Uses

Sennae Folium and Sennae Fructus are most popular remedies against constipation and they are present in numerous herbal laxative preparations sold throughout the world [1,2]. The laxative dose is 0.5–2 g [4]. Although the anthra-glycoside content of Sennae Fructus is higher than that of Sennae Folium the latter drug is more active at equal dosage. This is probably due to the higher content of aloe-emodin anthrone in the leaves. This is the most active compound of the laxative anthranoid derivatives [1,5].

Adverse Effects of Herbal Drugs, Vol. 2
(ed. by P.A.G.M. De Smet, K. Keller, R. Hänsel, R.F. Chandler)

The pharmacologic action of herbal anthranoid laxatives is presented in a general discussion elsewhere in this volume.

Pharmacokinetics

See the general discussion on anthranoid derivatives elsewhere in this volume.

Adverse Reaction Profile

The adverse reaction profile of herbal remedies containing anthranoid derivatives is presented in a general discussion elsewhere in this volume.

General Animal Data

The acute toxic dose of a senna extract was investigated in mice. The LD50 was 171 mg/kg after i.v. injection and 2500 mg/kg after oral administration. The LD50 for pure sennosides given orally to mice was about 4000 mg/kg. This difference has been explained by the presence of free anthra-aglycones in the plant extract [6,7]. Rats treated for a total of 11 weeks with a daily dose of 10 mg/kg of senna powder, virtually free of aglycones, did not show alterations of the intestinal mucosa, as examined by light and electron microscopy [8]. The administration of senna powder to cattle and horses produced damage of myofibrils [9,10].

It should be taken into consideration that toxicity data on anthranoid-containing laxatives obtained in experimental animals cannot be extrapolated to humans. There is a large difference in sensitivity between man and rodents, the latter being about a hundred-fold less sensitive [5].

General Human Data

Numerous cases of toxic symptoms following chronic consumption of senna preparations have been reported. Most of these are primary or secondary to the loss of electrolytes. These effects are produced also by other laxative drugs and are reviewed in a general disscussion about anthranoid-containing herbal remedies.

Hepatic Reactions

Beuers et al. [11] recently reported a rare case of hepatitis in a 26-year-old woman, who had been taking high doses of senna laxatives. One month before the first signs developed, the patient had supplemented her usual intake of 10 g senna leaves (in the form of a herbal tea) twice a week with an extract of senna fruit corresponding to a daily dose of 100 mg sennoside B (resulting in a tenfold excess of the recommended dose). There was no evidence of a viral, autoimmune, or metabolic cause, and histological examination suggested toxic damage. There was moderate portal and lobular infiltration by lymphocytes and histocytes with extensive cell necrosis around the central veins. Liver function improved within one week after stopping the senna treatment, and rapidly deteriorated again upon a rechallenge.

Osteopathic Reactions

Armstrong et al. [12] reported a case of a 21-year-old woman, who developed clubbing of digits and hypertrophic osteoarthropathy after taking at least 3 senna tablets daily for 3 years to control her weight. The patient also admitted to a period of secondary amenorrhoea of several months duration a year before. When the intake of senna was stopped, the patient's weight increased and within 6 months the clubbing had disappeared, though the periungual erythema persisted. The patient's rheumatic symptoms were less severe and controlled by non-steroidal anti-inflammatory drugs, though there was no regression of the radiological bone abnormalities. It was concluded that the presentation of clubbing with hypertrophic osteoarthropathy and purgative abuse was more than coincidental: there was no evidence of any other disease and, significantly, the patient's clubbing regressed and symptoms improved after stopping senna consumption.

Malmquist et al. [13] saw severe finger clubbing developed in a 35-year-old female patient with a previous history of anorexia nervosa during a period of senna laxative abuse. Pathological findings included urinary excretion of aspartylglucosamine and abnormal cytoplasmic inclusions in phagocytic cells on liver biopsy [13].

Further cases of osteoarthropathy have been reported [14–16].

Fertility, Pregnancy and Lactation

A general discussion of the effects of herbal medicines containing anthranoid derivatives, when used during pregnancy or lactation, is presented elsewhere in this volume. It has been stated that the use of senna preparations during pregnancy and lactation is safe [17–19]. However, as the drug contains the sennosides C and D, with the genotoxic aloe-emodin as aglycone, one should consider a risk for the infant, even if this compound crosses the placenta or enters the mother's milk in very small amounts (See the general discussion on anthranoid derivatives elsewhere in this volume).

Mutagenicity and Carcinogenicity

A general discussion of the mutagenic and carcinogenic properties of herbal medicines containing anthranoid derivatives is presented elsewhere in this volume.

References

1. Hänsel R, Haas H (1983) Therapie mit Phytopharmaka. Berlin: Springer Verlag, pp 162–163
2. Atzorn R, Weiler EW, Zenk H (1981) Formation and distribution of sennosides in Cassia angustifolia, as determined by a sensitive and specific radioimmunoassay. Planta Med 41:1–14
3. Miething H, Boventer W, Hänsel R (1986) Densitometrische Gehaltsbestimmung von Aloe-emodinglycosiden in Sennesfrüchten und Blättern und der wäßrigen Zubereitungen. Pharm Ztg 131:747–749
4. Wagner H (1985) Pharmazeutische Biologie: Drogen und ihre Inhaltsstoffe. 3rd edition. Stuttgart: Gustav Fischer Verlag, pp 223–224
5. Van Os FHL (1976) Some aspects of the pharmacology of anthraquinone drugs. Pharmacology 14 (Suppl 1):18–29
6. Marvola M, Koponen A, Hiltunen R, Hieltala P (1981) The effect of raw material purity on the acute toxicity and laxative effect of sennosides. J Pharm Pharmacol 33:108–109
7. Hieltala P, Marvola M, Parviainen T, Lainonen H (1987) Laxative potency and acute toxicity of some anthraquinone derivatives, senna extracts and fractions of senna extracts. Pharmacol Toxicol (Copenhagen) 61:153–156
8. Dufour P, Gendre P, Meunier JM, Cannelas J (1983) tolerance of mouse intestinal mucosa to a chronic ingestion of senna powder. Ann Pharm Franç 41:571–578
9. Schmitz DG, Denton JH (1977) Senna bean toxicity in cattle. Southwest Vet 30:165–170
10. Martin BW, Terry MK, Bridges CH, Bailey EM (1981) Toxicity of Cassia occidentalis in the horse. Vet Hum Toxicol 23:416–417
11. Beuers U, Spengler U, Pape GR (1991) Hepatitis after chronic abuse of senna. Lancet 337:372–373
12. Armstrong RD, Crisp AJ, Grahame R, Woolf DL (1981) Hyperthrophic osteoarthropathy and purgative abuse. Br Med J 282:1836
13. Malmquist J, Hulten-Nosslin M, Ericsson B, Jeppsson J, Ljungberg O (1980) Finger clubbing and aspartylglucosamine excretion in a laxative abusing patient. Postgrad Med J 56:862–864
14. Prior J, White I (1978) Tetany and clubbing in a patient who ingested large quantities of senna. Lancet 2:947
15. Frier BM, Scott RDM (1977) Osteomalacia and arthropathy associated with prolonged abuse of purgatives. Br J Clin Pract 31:17
16. Silk DBA, Gibson JA, Murray CRH (1975) Reversible finger clubbing in a case of purgative abuse. Gastroenterology 68:790
17. Grospietsch G (1991) Agiolax in Schwangerschaft und Stillzeit unbedenklich? Med Mo Pharm 14:184–185
18. Faber P, Strenge-Hesse A (1988) Relevance of rhein excretion into breast milk. Pharmacology 36 (Suppl 1):212–220
19. Köhlen ML, De Smet PAGM, Helling EAM, Merkus FWHM (1990) Het gebruik van geneesmiddelen tijdens de lactatie. In: De Smet PAGM, Van Loenen AC, Offerhaus L, Van der Does E, red. Medicatiebegeleiding. De medisch-farmaceutische achtergronden van verantwoord geneesmiddelengebruik. Houten: Bohn Stafleu Van Loghum, pp 195–223

Anthranoid Derivatives – *Rhamnus* Species

J. Westendorf

Botany

Three species of the genus *Rhamnus* (Rhamnaceae) are used for medicinal purposes: *Rhamnus frangula* L. (syn. *Frangula alnus* Mill.), *Rhamnus purshianus* DC (syn. *Frangula purshiana* (DC) J.G. Cooper), and *Rhamnus catharticus* L. Vernacular names are:

- *Rhamnus frangula*: breaking buckthorn (English); Faulbaum (German); bourgene (French).
- *Rhamnus purshianus*: Amerikanischer Faulbaum (German).
- *Rhamnus catharticus*: buckthorn (English), Kreuzdorn (German), nerprun (French).

The following plant parts are used as laxatives:

- Rhamni Frangulae Cortex (dry bark of branches and stems from *Rhamnus frangula* L.
- Rhamni Purshiani Cortex, syn. Cascara Sagrada (dry bark of *Rhamnus purshianus* DC).
- Rhamni Cathartici Fructus (ripe berries of *Rhamnus catharticus* L.).

Chemistry

Rhamni Frangulae cortex contains at least 6.0% anthranoid derivatives, mainly as glycosides. Most important are glucofrangulin A (6-O-(α-L-rhamnosyl)-8-O-(β-D-glucosyl)-emodin, and glucofrangulin B (6-O-(α-D-apiosyl)-8-O-(β-D-glucosyl)-emodin. Beside these diglycosides the cortex also contains the monoglycosides frangulin A (6-O-(α-L-rhamnosyl)-emodin) and frangulin B (6-O-(α-D-apiosyl)-emodin). Further anthranoid derivatives present in the drug are emodin anthrone-6-O-rhamnoside (franguloside) and the corresponding glycosides of physcion and chrysophanol. In the fresh bark the anthranoid derivatives are mainly present in the reduced (anthrone) form. Because anthrones are irritant to the gastric mucosa, the

Adverse Effects of Herbal Drugs, Vol. 2
(ed. by P.A.G.M. De Smet, K. Keller, R. Hänsel, R.F. Chandler)

material has to undergo oxidation prior to medicinal use. This is achieved by storage for a period of at least one year or heating to 100°C for some hours. The latter procedure is especially responsible for a partial or total degradation of the glycosides. Therefore, the drug can also contain the aglycones emodin, physcion and chrysophanol [1–3]. A variety of naphthaline glycosides have also been detected [4].

Rhamni purshiani cortex has a quite different composition, even though *Rhamnus purshianus* is botanically related to *Rhamnus frangula*. In contrast to *R. frangula*, which contains only O-glycosides, *R. purshianus* mainly contains mixed O,C-glycosides, which account for about 80% of the anthranoid derivatives. Most important are the cascarosides A and B, which are 8-β-O-glucosides of aloin A and B, and the cascarosides C and D, which contain chrysophanol instead of aloe-emodin. The pure C-glycosides aloin A and B and desoxyaloin A and B and the 8-β-O-glucosides of aloe-emodin, emodin and chrysophanol are also present. The total amount of anthranoid derivatives is about 6%. Like Rhamni Frangulae Cortex, the bark of *R. purshianus* has to undergo oxidation prior to medicinal use [1–3].

Rhamni cathartici fructus contains 2% of anthranoid derivatives, mainly glucofrangulines and frangulines. Other compounds present are flavonol glycosides [1].

Pharmacology and Uses

Rhamni Frangulae Cortex and Rhamni Purshiani Cortex are widely used as laxatives. The action of the latter drug is more drastic than that of the former and it is comparable to that of aloe [3]. The effective dose in man is 100–300 mg p.o. Rats require 300 mg/kg to achieve a laxative effect [5]. The anthra-glycosides are active in the colon after glycosidic cleavage and reduction to the anthrones. A detailed description is presented in a general discussion on anthranoids elsewhere in this volume.

Adverse Reaction Profile

A general discussion of the adverse reactions of herbal medicines containing anthranoid derivatives is presented elswhere in this volume.

General Animal Data

No information is available about the toxicity of preparations from *Rhamnus* species in experimental animals.

General Human Data

See the general discussion on anthranoid derivatives elsewhere in this volume.

Fertility, Pregnancy and Lactation

A general discussion of the effects of herbal medicines containing anthranoid derivatives, when used during pregnancy and lactation, is presented elsewhere in this volume.

Mutagenicity and Carcinogenicity

A general discussion of the mutagenic and carcinogenic effects of herbal medicines containing anthranoid derivatives is presented elsewhere in this volume. We investigated an extract of Rhamni Frangulae Cortex in the *Salmonella* microsome assay with strain TA 1537 and in the DNA repair induction assay with primary rat hepatocytes and observed positive effects in both systems (unpublished results). The effects are most probably due to the presence of emodin in the extract.

References

1. Wagner H (1985) Pharmazeutische Biologie. Stuttgart: Gustav Fischer Verlag, pp 219–221
2. Schneider G (1990) Arzneidrogen. Mannheim: Wissenschaftsverlag, pp 112–113
3. Hänsel R, Haas H (1983) Therapie mit Phytopharmaka. Berlin: Springer Verlag, pp 164–165
4. Rosca M, Cucu V (1975) Naphthaline glycosides from the bark of *Rhamnus frangula*. Planta Med 28:178–181
5. Van Os FHL (1976) Some aspects of the pharmacology of anthraquinone drugs. Pharmacology 14 (Suppl 1):18–29

Anthranoid Derivatives – *Rheum* Species

J. Westendorf

Botany

The genus *Rheum* belongs to the family of the Polygonaceae and contains about 40 species, which are difficult to distinguish. The two species of major medicinal interest are *Rheum palmatum* L. and *Rheum officinale* Baill. Vernacular names are Chinese rhubarb (English), chinesischer Rhabarber (German), rhubarbe de Chine (French). The plant part used medicinally is the root (Rhei Radix). The French health authorities not only allow laxative preparations from *Rheum palmatum* or *Rheum officinale* but also consider *R. rhaponticum* L. (Rhubarbe de France) as an acceptable source plant of laxative products [1]. The stalks of *Rheum undulatum* L. (= *R. rharbarbarum* L.) are a popular vegetable in many parts of Europe and North America.

Chemistry

Rhei Radix contains about 3–4% of anthranoid derivatives. Most of these are 1- or 8-O-mono- and diglycosides of the anthraquinones rhein, emodin, aloe-emodin, chrysophanol and physcion. A number of homo- and heterodianthrones and their glycosides (sennosides A, B, C and D) are also present [2–4]. Other phenolic components are tannic acids and hydroxycinnamic acids. All *Rheum* species contain relatively large amounts of oxalic acid.

Stilbene derivatives with an estrogen-like action, such as rhaponticin, are present in *Rheum rhaponticum* and *Rheum undulatum*, but not in *Rheum palmatum* [5,6]. The presence of rhaponticin is, therefore, an important chemotaxonomic marker for testing adulteration of medicinal rhubarb (*R. palmatum*) with *R. rhaponticum* or *R. undulatum* [7].

Recently, Kubo et al. [8] described the isolation of two stilbene glycosides, 4′-*O*-methylpiceid and rhapontin, from the dried root of *Rheum palmatum*. The actually studied material was a crude drug purchased at a local Indonesian marketplace, however, and the report does not make clear how the correct botanical origin of this sample was secured.

Adverse Effects of Herbal Drugs, Vol. 2
(ed. by P.A.G.M. De Smet, K. Keller, R. Hänsel, R.F. Chandler)

Pharmacology and Uses

The roots of Chinese rhubarb are mainly used as a laxative. The action is mediated by anthraquinones and anthraquinone glycosides, which are reduced to anthrones by the intestinal flora. The latter compounds exert an anti-absorptive and hydragogue action on the colonic mucosa. The purgative action of the anthranoids is partly reduced by the presence of tannins. In small doses of 0.05–0.2 g, the laxative action may even turn into constipation [2].

In Chinese medicine, rhubarb root is also used for many other medicinal purposes. One of these is the treatment of patients with bleeding from gastric and duodenal ulcer with alcoholic rhubarb extracts. It has been reported that about 90% of 312 cases have been cured (the stool occult blood changing from positive to negative within two days) [9]. Other reasons for the use of rhubarb in Chinese medicine are acute jaundice, acute appendicitis, incomplete intestinal obstruction, amenorrhoea, hematemesis, hypercholesterolemia, burns, carbuncles and furuncles [10].

Pharmacokinetics

See the general discussion on anthranoid derivatives elsewhere in this volume.

Adverse Reaction Profile

A general discussion of adverse reactions of herbal medicines containing anthranoid derivatives is presented elsewhere in this volume.

General Animal Data

No information is available about the toxicity of extracts from *Rhei radix* in experimental animals.

General Human Data

Some cases of severe poisoning with death have been reported after the ingestion of **leaves** from *Rheum rhaponticum* [11–13]. The most critical symptom was acute renal failure, and the suggested cause was the precipitation of the constituent oxalic acid by the formation of calcium oxalate in the renal tubules.

Two non-fatal cases of renal failure and icterus occurred after the ingestion of rhubarb **leaves** by two children aged 4 and 6 years respectively

[14]. The calculated amount of oxalic acid ingested (0.2–0.8 g) was too small to account for the symptoms observed. The authors, therefore, suspected that anthranoids might have been responsible for the poisoning of the children. However, no analysis was presented to support this hypothesis.

Like other anthranoid laxatives, Rhei Radix may cause severe damage to the large intestine and a substantial loss of electrolytes, if the drug is used chronically. A description of these adverse effects is given in a general discussion on anthranoid derivatives elswhere in this volume.

Allergic Reactions

Diffey et al. [15] describe a home wine maker, who developed a severe dermatitis in light-exposed areas, a week after he had produced rhubarb wine (mainly exposing his right hand), using cherry rhubarb, normal rhubarb, wine yeast compound (sugar, dried yeast, diammonium phosphate, ammonium sulphate), and yeast nutrient. The patient had been sitting in the sun four days after the production of the wine. Coupling of this history with the dermatological findings (vesicobullous hand dermatitis with edema and scaling of the face, neck and lips) suggested photoallergic contact dermatitis to the rhubarb wine. Routine patch test to cherry rhubarb and normal rhubarb were negative, but photopatch testing with the rhubarb wine showed reduction of the minimal erythema doses to UVA radiation.

Dermatological Reactions

See the section on allergic reactions.

Hepatic Reactions

See the section on general human data.

Renal Reactions

See the section on general human data.

Fertility, Pregnancy and Lactation

A general discussion of the effects of herbal medicines containing anthranoid derivatives, when used during pregnancy or lactation, is presented elsewhere in this volume.

Mutagenicity and Carcinogenicity

A general discussion of the mutagenic and carcinogenic properties of herbal medicines containing anthranoid derivatives is presented elsewhere in this volume.

Methanolic and aqueous extracts of *Rheum rhabarbarum* were reported to be mutagenic in *Salmonella typhimurium* strain TA 98 [16].

References

1. Anonymous (1990) Avis aux fabricants concernant les demandes d'autorisation de mise sur le marché des médicaments à base de plantes. Bulletin Officiel no. 90/22 bis. Paris: Ministère des Affairs Sociales et de la Solidarité
2. Steinegger E, Hänsel R (1988) Lehrbuch der Pharmakognosie auf phytochemischer Grundlage. Berlin: Springer, pp 153–156
3. Stahl E, Menßen HG, Jahn H (1985) Über den Gehalt der verschiedenen Hydroxyanthracenderivate in Rhabarberwurzeln und – zubereitungen. Dtsch Apoth Ztg 125:1478–1480
4. Oshima Y, Ohno Y, Kajiyama K, Takahashi K (1986) High-performance liquid chromatographic separation of rhubarb constituents. J Chromatogr 360:303–306
5. Csupor L (1971) Spektralphotometrische Bestimmung des Rhaponticins und des Desoxy-rhaponticins in Rhizoma Rhei rhapontici (L.). Arch Pharm Ber Dtsch Pharm Ges 304:32–35
6. Kashiwada Y, Nonaka GI, Nishioka I (1984) Rhubarb Rhei rhizoma 6. Isolation and characterization of stilbenes. Chem Pharm Bull (Tokyo) 32:3501–3517
7. Engelshowe R (1985) Rhabarber-Eine alte Droge-noch immer aktuell. Pharmazie in unserer Zeit 14:40–49
8. Kubo I, Murai Y, Soediro I, Soetarno S, Sastrodihardjo S (1991) Efficient isolation of glycosidase inhibitory stilbene glycosides from *Rheum palmatum*. J Nat Prod 54:1115–1118
9. Zhou H, Jiao D (1990) 312 cases of gastric and duodenal ulcer bleeding treated with three kinds of alcoholic extract rhubarb tablets. Chung Hsi I Chieh Ho Tsa Chih 10:131–132, 150–151
10. Peigen X, Liyi H, Liwei W (1984) Ethnopharmacologic study of chinese rhubarb. J Ethnopharmacol 10:275–293
11. Robb HF (1919) Death from rhubarb leaves due to oxalic acid poisoning. J Am Med Assoc 73:627–628
12. Jacobciner H, Raybin HW (1962) Rhubarb poisoning. NY State J Med 62:1676–1678
13. Anonymous (1917) Poisoning from rhubarb leaves. J Am Med Assoc 68:1954
14. Streicher E (1964) Akutes Nierenversagen und Ikterus nach einer Vergiftung mit Rhabarber Blättern. Dtsch Med Wschr 89:2379–2381
15. Diffey BL, Lawlor EF, Hindson TC (1984) Photoallergic contact dermatitis to rhubarb wine. Photodermatology 1:43–44
16. Van der Hoeven J, Hogenkamp-Kalisvaart M, Fennis J, Alink GM, Voragen A, Koeman JH (1981) Natural mutagens in lettuce (*Lactuca sativa*) and rhubarb (*Rheum rhabarbarum*). Mutat Res 85:305–306

Anthranoid Derivatives – *Rubia* Species

J. Westendorf

Botany

The genus *Rubia* (Rubiaceae) contains a variety of plants that are used for medicinal purposes. The most important species is *Rubia tinctorum* L. Vernacular names include madder (English); Färberröte, Krapp (German); garance (French); and robbia (Italian). The plant part used medicinally is the root (Rubiae Radix). Other *Rubia* species of medicinal interest are: *Rubia cordifolia* L., *Rubia sikkimensis* Kurz., *Rubia peregrina* L., *Rubia iberica* C. Koch, and *Rubia petiolaris* DC.

Chemistry

Madder root contains a variety of hydroxyanthraquinones, mainly as glycosides. Among these are alizarin, alizarin-2-β-primeveroside (ruberythric acid), lucidin, lucidin-3-β-primeveroside, rubiadin, rubiadin-3-β-primeveroside, 2,4-dihydroxyanthraquinone-3-carboxylic acid (munjistin), purpurin, purpurin-3-carboxylic acid (pseudopurpurin), pseudopurpurin-3-β-primeveroside (galiosin), anthragallol, and purpuroxanthin. Traces of further anthraquinones have also been detected [1]. Asperuloside and chlorogenic acid have been detected in all parts of *Rubia tinctorum* [2]. Other *Rubia* species contain a similar spectrum of hydroxyanthraquinones. An interesting group of cyclic hexapeptides with antitumor properties has been observed in *Rubia cordifolia*, but not in *Rubia tinctorum* [3].

Pharmacology and Uses

Root extracts of *Rubia tinctorum* L. are used for the treatment of kidney and bladder stones [4]. It is hypothesized that the anthraquinones present in these extracts are the active principles [3]. After absorption and excretion in the urine, these compounds are said to exert a disintegrating effect on the surface of calcium-containing stones in the urinary tract. To our knowledge

Adverse Effects of Herbal Drugs, Vol. 2
(ed. by P.A.G.M. De Smet, K. Keller, R. Hänsel, R.F. Chandler)

no direct evidence is given by animal or human studies to support this hypothesis.

Pharmacokinetics

It has been demonstrated that lucidin primeveroside and alizarin primeveroside, the two main anthranoid derivatives present in Rubiae Radix, are metabolized and excreted in the urine after oral gavage to rats and that alizarin primeveroside is metabolized to 1-hydroxyanthraquinone [5]. The latter compound has been shown to have carcinogenic activity in rats [6].

See also the general discussion on anthranoid derivatives elsewhere in this volume.

Adverse Reaction Profile

A general discussion of adverse reactions of herbal medicines containing anthranoid derivatives is presented elsewhere in this volume.

General Animal Data

No information is available about the toxicity of extracts of Radix Rubiae Tinctorum in experimental animals.

General Human Data

See the general discussion on anthranoid derivatives elsewhere in this volume.

Fertility, Pregnancy and Lactation

A general discussion of the effects of herbal medicines containing anthranoid derivatives, when used during pregnancy and lactation, is presented elsewhere in this volume.

Mutagenicity and Carcinogenicity

A general discussion of the mutagenic and carcinogenic properties of herbal medicines containing anthranoid derivatives is presented elsewhere in this volume.

Extracts of Radix Rubiae Tinctorum were demonstrated to induce mutations in *Salmonella typhimurium*, strains TA 98 and TA 100. The induction of DNA repair in primary rat hepatocytes by the same extracts has also been demonstrated [7]. Additionally, the formation of DNA-adducts has been observed by the ^{32}P-postlabeling method after treatment of mice with extracts of Radix Rubiae Tinctorum [8]. This DNA-damage was due to the presence of the anthraquinone lucidin in these extracts. The latter compound has been demonstrated to be highly genotoxic in a variety of short term assays [9,10].

Due to these data, the German Federal Health department has now prepared a negative short communication about *Rubia tinctorum*, and it is expected that the drug will disappear from the market.

References

1. Wijnsma R, Verpoorte R (1986) Anthraquinones in the Rubiaceae. Progr Chem Org Nat Prod 49:79–149
2. Schneider G (1990) Arzneidrogen. Mannheim: Wissenschaftsverlag, p 117
3. Itokawa H, Takeya K, Mori N, Kidokoro S, Yamamoto H (1984) Studies on antitumour cyclic hexapeptides RA obtained from Rubiae radix, Rubiaceae (IV): Quantitative determination of RA-VII and RA-V in commercial Rubiae radix and collected plants. Planta Med 50:313–316
4. Schilcher H (1984) Pflanzliche Urologika. Dtsch Apoth Ztg 124:2431
5. Blömeke B, Poginsky B, Schmutte Ch, Marquardt H, Westendorf J (1992) Formation of genotoxic metabolites from anthraquinone glycosides, present in *Rubia tinctorum* L. Mutat Res 265:263–272
6. Mori H, Yoshimi N, Iwata H, Mori Y, Hara A, Tanaka T, Kawai K (1990) Carcinogenicity of naturally occurring 1-hydroxyanthraquinone in rats: induction of large bowel, liver and stomach neoplasms. Carcinogenesis 11:799–802
7. Poginsky B (1989) Vorkommen und Genotòxizität von Anthracenderivaten in Rubia tinctorum L. Dissertation, Hamburg
8. Poginsky B, Westendorf J, Blömeke B, Marquardt H, Hewer A, Grower PL, Phillips DH (1991) Evaluation of DNA-binding activity of hydroxyanthraquinones occurring in Rubia tinctorum L. Carcinogenesis 12:1265–1271
9. Westendorf J, Marquardt H, Poginsky B, Dominiak M, Schmidt J, Marquardt H (1990) Genotoxicity of naturally occurring hydroxyanthraquinones. Mutat Res 240:1–12
10. Westendorf J, Poginsky B, Marquardt H, Groth G, Marquardt H (1988) The genotoxicity of lucidin, a natural component of Rubia tinctorum L., and lucidinethylether, a component of ethanolic *Rubia* extracts. Cell Biol Toxicol 4:225–239

Arctium Species

P.A.G.M. De Smet

Botany

Burdock root (E.), Klettenwurzel (G.) or racine de bardane (F.) is obtained from several species of the genus *Arctium* (Asteraceae). The most common source plants are [1–7]:

- *Arctium lappa* L. = *A. majus* Bernh. = *Lappa major* Gaertn. (Große Klette in German);
- *Arctium minus* (Hill) Bernh. = *Lappa minor* Hill (Kleine Klette in German);
- *Arctium tomentosum* Mill. = *Lappa tomentosa* (Spinnwebklette or Filzklette in German);
- *Arctium nemorosum* Lej. et Court. (Hausklette in German).

In addition to the root, the herb and fruits of burdock may also be used medicinally. According to a German text book, however, the trade in these plant parts is relatively small [3].

Chemistry

Burdock **roots** contain large amounts of carbohydrate in the form of inulin (up to 45% in *A. lappa*, up to 27% in *A. minus*, and up to 19% in *A. tomentosum*). The root of *A. lappa* also yields 0.06–0.18% of volatile oil, tannin, sitosterol, stigmasterol, resin, mucilage, 0.4–0.8% of fatty oil, sugar, and acids [3,4].

Washino et al. [8] reported numerous different components of the essential oil of burdock root, including phenylacetaldehyde, benzaldehyde, 2-alkyl-(C_3-C_5)-3-methoxypyrazines and 2-methoxy-3-pyrazine, costic acid, dehydrocostuslactone and dehydrodihydrocostuslactone. Schulte et al. [2] identified 14 polyacetylenes in fresh root samples of different burdock source plants with tridecadiene-(1,11)-tetrayne-(3,5,7,9) (up to 1.5 mg%), tridecene-(1)-pentayne-(3,5,7,9,11) (up to 1.1 mg%) and tridecatriene-

Adverse Effects of Herbal Drugs, Vol. 2
(ed. by P.A.G.M. De Smet, K. Keller, R. Hänsel, R.F. Chandler)

(1,3,11)-triyne-(5,7,9) (up to 0.2 mg%) as major components. Other root constituents of *Arctium lappa* are γ-guanidino-*n*-butyric acid [9], and sulphur-containing acetylenic compounds, such as arctinones, arctinols, arctinal and arctic acids [10].

Burdock **leaves** contain inulin, tannin, mucilage and traces of essential oil [3]. Yochkova et al. [11] identified the triterpene alcohols α- and β-amyrin, lupeol, phytol, taraxasterol and ψ-taraxasterol in free and esterified state as well as the sterols stigmasterol and sitosterol in the leaves of *A. lappa*.

Burdock **fruits** contain fatty oil, lappaurin (a yellow substance), arctiin (glycosidic bitter principle) and lappanaesthin (an anesthetic substance), resin, and wax [3,4]. Yamanouchi et al. [12] isolated arctin, arctigenin and matairesinol as well as two new sesquilignan derivatives from the fruits of *A. lappa*.

Surewicz-Szewczyk [13] found 21.4% and 22.1% of fatty oil in the **seeds** of *A. minus* and *A. tomentosum*, respectively. Predominant fatty acids were linoleic acid (resp. 67.0% and 67.8%), oleic acid (resp. 20.3% and 15.4%), palmitic acid (resp. 9.0% and 9.6%) and linolenic acid (resp. 1.7% and 5.7%). Morris et al. [14] recovered 9.9% of *trans*-3,*cis*-9,*cis*-12-octadecatrienoic acid from the seed oil of *A. minus*.

Pharmacology and Uses

Burdock root has been recommended as a blood purifier and has been used externally to treat various chronic skin conditions, including psoriasis and acne. It is also claimed to have diuretic and diaphoretic properties [3,5,7]. In France the roots of *Arctium lappa* are permitted as a herbal drug for internal use, and its leaves may be applied topically [15]. In Germany, however, burdock root is considered an obsolete herb, which occurs primarily in homoeopathic products [2]. The German health authorities have not accepted burdock root as a herbal drug, because no therapeutic efficacy has been proven [7].

Burdock root extracts are claimed to have antitumor activity [16] and a lowering effect on the blood sugar level [3,6] in experimental animals. Kit et al. [17] reported a relatively weak hypoglycemic effect in alloxane-treated rats following a subcutaneously administered tincture of burdock root. In a recent study, oral administration of burdock **leaves** did not affect glucose homeostasis in normal mice, and it aggravated the hyperglycemia, polydipsia and loss of body weight in streptozotocin diabetic mice [18].

The young leaves of burdock may be eaten as greens [5], and the roots of a cultivated form of *A. lappa*, formerly known as *A. edulis* or *Lappa edulis*, are used as vegetables in Japan [3].

Adverse Reaction Profile

General Animal Data

The oils from seeds of *Arctium minus* and *A. tomentosum* did not exert toxic effects in mice when administered in oral or subcutaneous doses of 0.1–0.7 ml (*A. minus*) or 0.1–0.2 ml (*A. tomentosum*) [13].

A special veterinary risk of burdock is the so-called "burr tongue" that is commonly seen in long-haired breeds of dogs, and occasionally cats, running free in areas where burdock grows. The hair-like shafts forming the outer layers of the burdock bur have a hook on their tip by which the bur may stick to the coats of animals. When the animal tries to remove the bur by licking and chewing, some of the shafts may penetrate the mucous membrane of the mouth and tongue, leading to fibrous granuluation of the penetrated tissue [19,20].

General Human Data

As far as is known, the use of burdock root is not associated with major health hazards [7]. The principal risk appears to be anticholinergic poisoning due to adulteration or contamination with belladonna root (*Atropa belladonna*) [5,6]. The actual presence of toxic amounts of atropine [21–23] or belladonna root [23] in burdock root tea preparations has been repeatedly reported in the literature.

Dermatological Reactions

The rough hairs of burdock can produce mechanical irritation of the skin. There is no conclusive evidence that the leaves can produce contact dermatitis [25].

Daily treatment of shaved guinea pig skin with oil from burdock seeds for a period of one week did not produce any changes except for slight flushing of the treated area on the first day [13].

Ocular Reactions

The outer layers of the burdock bur are formed by hair-like shafts that characteristically hook on to clothing. Within the bur and attached to the seed pods are innumerable tiny barbed needles. These needles cause serious ocular reactions by imbedding in the conjunctiva or more rarely in the cornea. Due to their extremely small size, they may be overlooked when the physician is unfamiliar with burdock ophthalmia. Patients may complain of foreign body sensation. Conjunctival hyperemia and lid edema soon occur, and visual acuity decreases with the development of corneal edema and damage. The presence of linear scratch marks running in random directions on the cornea is a characteristic sign that should always suggest burdock ophthalmia [26–28].

As the projecting needle tip causes direct abrasion of the cornea during eyelid movement, burdock ophthalmia undoubtedly involves mechanical damage [27]. However, animal experiments by Bruhn [26] suggest that the toxicity of a water-soluble noxious agent also plays a role. This author obtained severe reactions of ocular tissues by injecting an aqueous extract from burdock hairs into the upper corneal layer. Such reactions were not observed following the injection of an oily extract.

Fertility, Pregnancy and Lactation

A crude extract of *Arctium lappa* prepared by boiling unspecified plant parts in water did not affect fertility of female mice, when injected subcutaneously twice a day for five days [29].

No data have been recovered from the literature on the effects of burdock preparations during pregnancy and lactation.

Mutagenicity and Carcinogenicity

Morimoto et al. [30] screened aqueous and methanolic extracts from fruits of *Arctium lappa* for mutagenicity in *Salmonella typhimurium* strains TA 98 and TA 100 and *Bacillus subtilis* strains H17 Rec^+ and M45 Rec^-. The aqueous extract gave a positive response in *Salmonella typhimurium* TA 98 only in the presence of S9 mix, whereas the methanolic extract was positive in the *Bacillus subtilis* rec-assay. No mutagenicity was observed by Yamamoto et al. [31] who tested an aqueous or methanolic extract from *Arctium* fruits in *Salmonella typhimurium* TA 98 and TA 100 in the absence or presence of rat liver S-9 mix.

Burdock has been repeatedly associated with antimutagenic activity [32–34]. Burdock root yields a desmutagenic factor with a molecular weight >300 000, which might be a lignin-like compound containing about 10% sugar [32,33]. Another interesting observation is that an ethanolic extract from the fruit of *Arctium lappa* inhibits the aflatoxin production by *Aspergillus parasiticus* [35].

Carcinogenicity data on burdock rhizomes come from a study by Hirono et al. [36]. This Japanese research group treated 6 male and 6 female rats with a diet containing 33% of rhizomes of burdock for 120 days without detecting tumors in any animal.

References

1. Lindner MW (1949) Lappa spec., die Klettenarten. Pharmazie 4:231–242
2. Schulte KE, Rücker G, Boehme R (1967) Polyacetylene als Inhaltsstoffe der Klettenwurzeln. Arzneim Forsch 17:829–833
3. List PH, Hörhammer L (1972) Hagers Handbuch der Pharmazeutischen Praxis. 4th edn. Dritter Band: Chemikalien und Drogen (Am-Ch). Berlin: Springer-Verlag, pp 173–177
4. Hoppe HA (1975) Drogenkunde. Band 1. Angiospermen. 8. Auflage. Berlin: Walter de Gruyter, pp 102–104
5. Tyler VE (1987) The New Honest Herbal. A sensible guide to herbs and related remedies. 2nd edn. Philadelphia: George F. Stickley Company, pp 49–50
6. Willuhn G (1989) Klettenwurzel. In: Wichtl M, ed. Teedrogen. Ein Handbuch für die Praxis auf wissenschaftlicher Grundlage. 2. Auflage. Stuttgart: Wissenschaftliche Verlagsgesellschaft, pp 278–280
7. Anonymous (1990) Bardanae radix (Klettenwurzel). Bundes Anzeiger nr.22a from 01.02.1990
8. Washino T, Iwabuchi H, Yoshikura M, Obata S (1985) Volatile constituents of Arctium lappa. Chem Abstr 103:52880b
9. Yamada Y, Hagiwara K, Iguchi K, Uchibe T (1975) γ-guanidino-*n*-butyric acid from *Arctium lappa*. Phytochemistry 14:582
10. Washino T, Yoshikura M, Obata S (1986) New sulfur-containing acetylenic compounds from *Arctium lappa*. Agric Biol Chem 50:263–269
11. Yochkova YI, Mladenova KA, Zaharieva EB, Dinkov N, Hashalov KL (1989) Triterpene alcohols and sterols of *Arctium lappa*. Compt Rend Acad Bulg Sci 42(10):43–45
12. Yamanouchi S, Takido M, Sankawa U, Shibata S (1976) On the constituents of the fruit of *Arctium lappa*. Yakugaku Zasshi 96:1492–1493
13. Surewicz-Szewczyk H (1970) Pharmacochemical investigations on the oil from seeds of *Arctium minus* (Hill) Bernh. and *Arctium tomentosum* Mill. (Compositae). Diss Pharm Pharmacol 22(6):427–430
14. Morris LJ, Marshall MO, Hammond EW (1968) The *trans*-3-enoic acids of *Aster alpinus* and *Arctium minus* seed oils. Lipids 3:91–95
15. Anonymous (1990) Avis aux fabricants concernant les demandes d'autorisation de mise sur le marché des médicaments à base de plantes. Bulletin Officiel no. 90/22 bis. Paris: Ministère des Affairs Sociales et de la Solidarité
16. Dombrádi CA, Földeák S (1966) Screening report on the antitumor activity of purified *Arctium lappa* extracts. Tumori 52:173–175
17. Kit SM, Boichuk RV, Khananayev LI, Ozarkiv TT (1972) A study of the hypoglycemic effect of some Pricarpatye plants in the experiment. Farm Zh 27(4):61–65
18. Swanston-Flatt SK, Day C, Flatt PR, Gould BJ, Bailey CJ (1989) Glycaemic effects of traditional European plant treatments for diabetes. Studies in normal and streptozotocin diabetic mice. Diabetes Res 10:69–73
19. Thivierge G (1973) Granular stomatitis in dogs due to burdock. Can Vet J 14(4): 96–97
20. Georgi ME, Harper P, Hyypio PA, Pritchard DK, Scherline ED (1982) Pappus bristles: the cause of burdock stomatitis in dogs. Cornell Vet 72:43–48
21. Bryson PD, Watanabe AS, Rumack BH, Murphy RC (1978) Burdock root tea poisoning. Case report involving a commercial preparation. JAMA 239:2157
22. Bryson PD (1978) Burdock root tea poisoning. JAMA 240:1586
23. Rhoads PM, Tong TG, Banner Jr W, Anderson R (1984–85) Anticholinergic poisonings associated with commercial burdock root tea. Clin Toxicol 22:581–584
24. Anonymous (1984) Belladonna-haltige Klettenwurzeltees in Frankreich. Dtsch Apoth Ztg 124:390
25. Mitchell J, Rook A (1979) Botanical dermatology. Plants and plant products injurious to the skin. Greengrass: Vancouver pp 187–188

26. Bruhn AM (1938) Klinische und experimentelle Untersuchungen über Augenschädigungen durch Klettenhaare. Klin Monatsbl Augenh 101:730–741
27. Havener WH, Falls HF, McReynolds WU (1955) Burdock bur ophthalmia. Arch Ophthalmol 53:260–263
28. Breed FB, Kuwabara T (1966) Burdock ophthalmia. Arch Ophthalmol 75:16–20
29. Matsui AS, Rogers J, Woo YK, Cutting WC (1976) Effects of some natural products on fertility in mice. Med Pharmacol Exp Int J Exp Med 16:414–424
30. Morimoto I, Watanabe F, Osawa T, Okitsu T (1982) Mutagenicity screening of crude drugs with *Bacillus subtilis* rec-assay and *Salmonella*/microsome reversion assay. Mutat Res 97:81–102
31. Yamamoto H, Mizutani T, Nomura H (1982) Studies on the mutagenicity of crude drug extracts. I. Yakugaku Zasshi 102:596–601
32. Morita K, Kada T, Namiki M (1984) A desmutagenic factor isolated from burdock (*Arctium lappa* Linne). Mutat Res 129:25–31
33. Morita K, Nishijima Y, Kada T (1985) Chemical nature of a desmutagenic factor from burdock (*Arctium lappa*). Agric Biol Chem 49:925–932
34. Shinohara K, Kuroki S, Miwa M, Kong Z-L, Hosoda H (1988) Antimutagenicity of dialysates of vegetables and fruits. Agric Biol Chem 52:1369–1375
35. Bahk J, Marth EH (1983) Aflatoxin production is inhibited by selected herbal drugs. Mycopathologia 83:129–134
36. Hirono I, Mori H, Kato K, Ushimaru Y, Kato T, Haga M (1977) Safety examination of some edible plants, part 2. J Environ Pathol Toxicol 1:71–74

Borago Officinalis

P.A.G.M. De Smet

Botany

The garden herb *Borago officinalis* L. (Boraginaceae) is commonly known as borage (E.), Boretsch (G), and bourrache (F.). Other English names include burrage, bee bread, ox's tongue, and cool tankard. The herb may also be referred to as bugloss in herbalistic sources, but this vernacular name is confusing, as it is also used for *Anchusa officinalis* (bugloss), *Lycopsis arvensis* (small bugloss), and *Echium vulgare* (viper's bugloss) [1–3].

Chemistry

The herb of borage contains 11% of mucilage, which yields glucose, galactose, and arabinose as principal sugars, when it is hydrolyzed [4]. Other herb constituents include allantoin, tannins (up to 3%), silicic acid, organic acids, and potassium nitrate [3,5,6].

Extraction of the seeds provides 13–33% of oil, which consists primarily of glycerides of unsaturated fatty acids, in particular oleic acid (17–19%), linoleic acid (37–39%), and γ-linolenic acid (20–22%). The γ-linolenic acid content is adversely affected by storage at room temperature without protection from light [7].

Swiss researchers have isolated seven pyrrolizidine alkaloids from the herb of *Borago officinalis*. Gravimetric analysis of three herb samples yielded crude alkaloid fractions of 20–26 mg/kg of free bases and 0–16 mg/kg of *N*-oxides, but GC analysis of these samples showed alkaloid levels of 2–8 mg/kg. The following individual alkaloids were detected: lycopsamine (16–39%), intermedine (<1%), 7-acetyllycopsamine (9–31%), 7-acetylintermedine (≤2%), amabiline (13–35%), supinine (12–36%) and an unidentified alkaloid with a molecular weight of 289 (2–20%) [8,9].

The presence of lycopsamine in borage (together with either amabiline or cynaustine and four other alkaloids) was also reported by an American research team. This group obtained a crude alkaloid fraction of 97 mg/kg from a bulk sample of dried plant fragments [10]. The American team also

Adverse Effects of Herbal Drugs, Vol. 2
(ed. by P.A.G.M. De Smet, K. Keller, R. Hänsel, R.F. Chandler)

analyzed borage flowers, seeds and seed oil [11]. The only pyrrolizidine constituent found in the flowers was the saturated alkaloid thesinine. Mature borage seeds yielded a crude alkaloid fraction in the range of 300 mg/kg. The major seed alkaloid was thesinine, with amabiline as a minor component. Immature seeds were also found to contain thesinine, but amabiline could not be demonstrated in this material. Samples of borage seed oil yielded only a small crude base fraction, and no pyrrolizidine alkaloids were recovered; amabiline was absent down to the level of 5 mg/kg [11].

Borago officinalis is able to produce trace amounts of hydrocyanic acid. Hegnauer [12] reported a maximum yield of 15 mg HCN/kg from young non-flowering plants collected early in June. In contrast, flowering plants collected at the end of June generated only 1.2 mg HCN/kg, with no HCN being detected in the inflorescences. The cyanophoric principle was later shown by Van Valen [13] to be the cyanogenic glucoside dhurrin. He recovered 35 mg of dhurrin from 100 g of fresh seedlings and basal leaves of older plants [13].

Pharmacology and Uses

Infusions of borage leaves or flowers have a long tradition in folk medicine. Their reputed virtues include emollient, diuretic, diaphoretic, febrifuge, galactogogue, calmative, blood purifying and vitalizing properties. The fresh herb has been used in the form of a poultice to treat wounds and inflammatory swellings, and it has also been made into an eyewash [1–3,8]. Suganda et al. [14] tested the activity of an ethanolic extract of *Borago officinalis* against human herpes virus and human poliovirus *in vitro*. No antiviral effect was demonstrated.

Infusions of the dried herb are also valued as salad admixtures with a refreshing effect and as summer drinks [3]. The herb may also be eaten like spinach, either raw or cooked [6].

As the seed oil of borage is rich in γ-linolenic acid, it is being promoted as an alternative dieatry supplement to evening primrose oil [3]. Pullman-Mooar and co-workers [15] administered borage seed oil (9 capsules per day, each containing 0.5 g of oil) to patients with active rheumatoid arthritis in an open uncontrolled study. They observed an apparent clinical benefit that could have been related in part to reduced generation of arachidonic acid oxygenation products.

Pharmacokinetics

Following ingestion of borage seed oil, the constituent γ-linolenic acid is converted to dihomo-γ-linolenic acid, the fatty acid precursor of monoenoic prostaglandins, such as prostaglandin E_1 [15].

Adverse Reaction Profile

A general review of the adverse reaction profile of medicinal plants containing pyrrolizidine alkaloids was provided in the first volume of this book series [16].

General Animal Data

Hannig [17] fed guinea pigs for 5 weeks by oral gavage with the dried herb, a 15% decoction, and the homoeopathic original tincture without observing adverse effects other than hepatic steatosis. In the mouse, a dose of 0.1 ml of borage seed oil per day by oral gavage did not produce adverse effects other than a weak laxative effect.

General Human Data

The presence of pyrrolizidine alkaloids (PAs) in borage has led several authors to caution against the excessive or prolonged use of the herb [2,3,6]. The internal use of borage flowers is still permitted in France [18], but in Germany the health authorities have recently rejected the medicinal use of both the herb and the flowers, because there is insufficient evidence of therapeutic usefulness and because of the risks involved [19].

The recommended daily dosage of borage herb is 2–4 cups of tea that have each been prepared from 2 g of herb. As was pointed out in the section on Chemistry, the herb yields 2–8 mg/kg of PAs. If these alkaloids pass completely into the tea, they will result in an exposure to 8–64 μg per day [8,9]. Such an exposure exceeds the limit of >1 μg of unsaturated PAs per day that has been established by the German Federal Health Office for the internal intake of unsaturated PAs [20]. The German limit for exposure to PAs is likewise exceeded by the use of commercially available borage juices. As these juices contain 0.4–1.2 mg/kg of PAs and should be taken in daily amounts of 3–4 tablespoons full, they will provide 12–48 μg of PAs per day [9].

Samples of borage seed oil were reported to be devoid of unsaturated PAs down to the level of 5 μg/g. This finding is less reassuring than it may seem to be at first sight. It means that, when users are taking 2–4 capsules with 500 mg of borage seed oil each per day, they will be exposed to less than 5–10 μg of unsaturated PAs per day. However, to meet the German demand that botanical drugs should not provide more than 1 μg of unsaturated PAs per day, when employed internally, the analytical assay used to prove the absence of unsaturated PAs in borage seed oil should be sensitive down to 0.5–1 μg/g. Because of this concern, Kruger [21] recently submitted two samples of borage seed oil, one a crude oil and the second one a processed oil (bleached), to a laboratory that could analyze unsaturated PAs with sufficient sensitivity. According to Kruger [21], alkaloids were not found at a 0.5 μg/g detection limit (using GC with electron capture detector) but the analytical details of this study have not been published.

Studies of borage seed oil in small series of subjects have not shown apparent adverse effects (other than softening of stools and an occasional sensation of bloastedness) from the daily ingestion of 5.5 g for 28 days [22] or 4.5 g for 12 weeks [15].

Dermatological Reactions

The herbalistic literature claims, without any reference to a properly documented clinical case, that fresh borage leaves may cause contact dermatitis in sensitive individuals [2]. Perhaps the origin of this statement goes back to the late 19th century, when J.C. White recorded, on basis of information supplied by a dealer in medicinal plants, that the short bristly hairs on the leaves of borage are irritant to the hands [23].

Gastrointestinal Reactions

See the section on general human data for data on borage seed oil.

Fertility, Pregnancy and Lactation

Graham and Noble [24] reported in the fifties that pregnant mare's serum is inactivated by incubation with aqueous *Lithospermum* extracts, and that this antigonadotrophic effect *in vitro* can also be produced by extracts of *Borago officinalis*. The responsible agent has never been identified, however, and the clinical relevancy of the observation has remained unclear till the present day.

No specific data have been recovered from the literature regarding the use of borage during pregnancy and lactation. A general discussion about the use of medicinal plants containing pyrrolizidine alkaloids during pregnancy and lactation was provided in the first volume of this book series [16].

Mutagenicity and Carcinogenicity

A general discussion about the mutagenicity and carcinogenicity of medicinal plants containing pyrrolizidine alkaloids was provided in the first volume of this book series [16]. See also the general human data in this monograph.

Bunce et al. [25] administered diets enriched with vegetal oils to female rats pretreated with 7,12-dimethylbenz(a)anthracene. The incidence of mammary tumours in the group fed with 20% of borage oil (87.5%) was quite comparable to that in the group given 20% of corn oil (88%).

References

1. Gessner O, Orzechowski G (1974). Gift- und Arzneipflanzen von Mitteleuropa. 3. Auflage. Heidelberg: Carl Winter Universitätsverlag, pp 408–409
2. Lust J (1974) The Herb Book. Toronto: Bantam Books, p 132
3. Awang DVC (1990) Borage. Can Pharm J 123:121–126
4. Franz G (1969) Untersuchungen über die Schleimpolysaccharide von *Tussilago farfara* L., *Symphytum officinalis* L., *Borago officinalis* L. und *Viola tricolor* L. Planta Med 17:217–220
5. Hegnauer R (1964) Chemotaxonomie der Pflanzen. Band 3: Dicotyledoneae, I. Teil. Von Acanthaceae bis Cyrillaceae. Basel: Birkhäuser Verlag, pp 297–301
6. Tyler VE (1987) The New Honest Herbal. A sensible guide to herbs and related remedies. 2nd edn. Philadelphia: George F. Stickley Company, pp 40–41
7. Carnat AP, Laurent P, Lamaison JL (1988) L'huile de graines de bourrache (Borago officinalis L.): une source interessante d'acide gamma-linolenique. J Pharm Belg 43:359–363
8. Lüthy J, Brauchli J, Zweifel U, Schmid P, Schlatter Ch (1984) Pyrrolizidin-Alkaloide in Arzneipflanzen der Boraginaceen: Borago officinalis L. und Pulmonaria officinalis L. Pharm Acta Helv 59:242–246
9. Brauchli-Theotokis J (1987) Zur toxikologischen Beurteilung der Pyrrolizidin-Alkaloide in den Arzneipflanzen Symphytum officinale und Borago officinalis. Zürich: Eidgenössische Technische Hochschule
10. Larson KM, Roby MR, Stermitz FR (1984) Unsaturated pyrrolizidines from borage (*Borago officinalis*), a common garden herb. J Nat Prod 47:747–748
11. Dodson CD, Stermitz FR (1986) Pyrrolizidine alkaloids from borage (*Borago officinalis*) seeds and flowers. J Nat Prod 49:727–728
12. Hegnauer R (1958) Over de verspreiding van blauwzuur bij vaatplanten. Pharm Weekbl 93:801–819
13. Van Valen F (1979) Contribution to the knowledge of cyanogenesis in Angiosperms. 12. Communication. Cyanogenesis in *Boraginaceae*. Proc K Ned Akad Wet Serie C Biol Med Sci 82:171–176
14. Suganda AG, Amoros M, Girre L, Fauconnier B (1983) Effets inhibiteurs de quelques extraits bruts et semipurifiés de plantes indigènes françaises sur la multiplication de l'herpesvirus humain 1 et du poliovirus humain 2 en culture cellulaire. J Nat Prod 46:626–632
15. Pullman-Mooar S, Laposata M, Lem D, Holman RT, Leventhal LJ, DeMarco D, Zurier RB (1990) Alteration of the cellular fatty acid profile and the production of eicosanoids in human monocytes by gamma-linolenic acid. Arthr Rheum 33: 1526–1533
16. Westendorf J (1992) Pyrrolizidine alkaloids – general discussion. In: De Smet PAGM, Keller K, Hänsel R, Chandler RF (ed) (1992) Adverse Effects of Herbal Drugs. Volume 1. Heidelberg: Springer-Verlag, pp 193–205
17. Hanning E (1950) *Borago officinalis* als Heil- und Gewürzpflanze in kritisch-experimenteller Betrachtung. Pharmazie 5:35–40
18. Anonymous (1990) Avis aux fabricants concernant les demandes d'autorisation de mise sur le marché des médicaments à base de plantes. Bulletin Officiel no.90/22 bis. Paris: Ministère des Affairs Sociales et de la Solidarité
19. Anonymous (1991) Monographie: Borago (Boretsch). Bundes Anzeiger nr.127, 12 July 1991

20. Anonymous (1990) Vorinformation Pyrrolizidinalkaloidhaltige Humanarzneimittel. Pharm Ztg 135:2532–2533, 2623–2624
21. Kruger R (1991) POS Pilot Plant Corp., Saskatoon (Canada). Personal communication June, 1991
22. Mills DE, Prkachin KM, Harvey KA, Ward RP (1989) Dietary fatty acid supplementation alters stress reactivity and performance in man. J Hum Hypertens 3:111–116
23. Mitchell J, Rook A (1979) Botanical dermatology. Plants and plant products injurious to the skin. Greengrass: Vancouver, p 140
24. Graham RCB, Noble RL (1955) Comparison of *in vitro* acitivity of various species of *Lithospermum* and other plants to inactivate gonadotrophin. Endocrinology 56: 239–247
25. Bunce OR, Wade AE, Abou-El-Ela SH, Prasse KW (1989) The effect of varying dietary levels and types of omega 6 and omega 3 fatty acids on mammary tumorigenesis in rats. Fed Am Soc Exp Biol J 3:A470

Caulophyllum Thalictroides

P.A.G.M. De Smet

Botany

Caulophyllum thalictroides (L.) Michx. (syn. *Leontice thalictroides* L., *Leontopetalon thalictroides* Hill.) belongs to the family Berberidaceae. Vernacular names include blue cohosh, pappoose root, papoose root, squaw root, blueberry (E); Löwenblatt, Frauenwurzel (G); and cohoche bleu (F). The plant part used medicinally is the root [1–5].

Chemistry

Flom et al. [6] analysed the roots and rhizomes, and obtained 5.9 mg/g of crude quaternary alkaloid chloride and 2.2 mg/g of crude tertiary alkaloids. The quaternary fraction yielded the aporphine alkaloid magnoflorine, whereas the tertiary fraction yielded the lupine alkaloids methylcytisine (= caulophylline), baptifoline, and anagyrine, as well as three unidentified alkaloids. Recovered amounts were 0.33 mg/g of methylcytisine, 0.20 mg/g of baptifoline, and 0.12 mg/g of anagyrine.

The rhizome and roots were also shown to contain the glycosides caulophyllosaponin and caulosaponin [7]. In one study, approximately 1 mg/g of caulosaponin was obtained [8]. According to Hegnauer [9], caulophyllosaponin is probably the primary saponin, which yields caulosaponin (=leontin) on partial hydrolysis. Further hydrolysis of caulosaponin yields the triterpenoid sapogenin hederagenin [6,10].

Additional substances isolated from the rhizome and roots of the blue cohosh include essential oil, citrullol and a mixture of fatty acids [7].

Secondary sources claim that methylcytisine and glycosides also occur in the leaves and seeds of the plant [5,11]. These claims go back to an unreferenced statement by Hardin and Arena [12].

Pharmacology and Uses

Methylcytisine was found to produce similar pharmacological effects as cytisine in various animal tests, but in most tests active doses were 10 to 20

Adverse Effects of Herbal Drugs, Vol. 2
(ed. by P.A.G.M. De Smet, K. Keller, R. Hänsel, R.F. Chandler)

times higher than those of cytisine. Methylcytisine also resembles nicotine in its peripheral effects, but its central activity may be different from that of nicotine, since the convulsions produced by methylcytisine in mice differ from those produce by nicotine [13,14]. Methylcytisine shows a hyperglycemic action, when given intravenously to rabbits in doses of 20–40 mg/kg [13].

Caulosaponin was found to constrict the coronary vessels of the rat heart and the carotid arteries of cattle and hogs. It also showed an oxytocic action on the rat uterus and a spasmogenic effect on the isolated intestine of rodents. The aglycone of caulosaponin produced a similar uterine action [8].

The root of the blue cohosh has been primarily employed as an antispasmodic, emmenagogue (to stimulate menstrual flow), and parturifacient (to speed childbirth). Reportedly, it has also been used for various other purposes, such as diuresis, diaphoresis, and the treatment of rheumatism [1–5]. It is also employed as a homoeopathic remedy for uterine dysfunction during labour or menstruation [15].

The roasted seeds are said to have found use as a coffee substitute [1,12].

Adverse Reaction Profile

General Animal Data

Acute toxicity testing of methylcytisine in mice yielded LD_{50} values of 21 mg/kg intravenously, 51 mg/kg intraperitoneally, and >500 mg/kg orally [14].

Power and Salway [7] gave caulosaponin and caulophyllosaponin to small cats, in oral doses of 0.1 g each, without observing any symptom other than a mild purgative action after several hours.

Ferguson and Edwards [8] reported intravenous LD_{50} values for caulosaponin of 11.8 mg/kg in mice and 20.3 mg/kg in rats. Small doses produced a depression while larger doses caused increased activity, ataxia, and terminal clonic convulsions. Death appeared to be due to asphyxia. Daily administration of 5 mg/kg subcutaneously to rats for sixty days did not produce symptoms of toxicity or gross pathology of the heart, liver, spleen, intestine, kidney, or uterus. Microscopic examination showed slight edema of the epithelium of renal tubuli, and a thickening in the arterial walls in the spleen. Caulosaponin showed a toxic action on animal cardiac muscle, probably due to its action on coronary vessels.

General Human Data

The dust of the root is extremely irritating to mucous membranes [2,16].

The blue fruits (which are actually naked seeds surrounded by their fleshy coat) are considered poisonous, especially when eaten by children [3,11].

Hardin and Arena [12] state, without references, that children have been poisoned by eating the seeds whereas roasted seeds can be used safely as coffee substitute. According to Millspaugh [2], *Caulophyllum* may cause pain in the small joints, as well as fleeting rheumatic pains in the extremities, but he does not support these allegations with a reference.

Dermatological Reactions

Dermatitis may develop from handling the rootstock [3,16].

Endocrine Reactions

Treatment of rats with a low-potency homoeopathic *Caulophyllum* preparation has been associated with histological changes in the thyroids [17,18].

Gastrointestinal Reactions

It is said that the leaves and seeds can cause severe stomach pains when ingested [12].

Ocular Reactions

Instillation of an 0.5% solution of caulosaponin in propylene glycol into the rabbit's eye resulted in marked inflammation, whereas only slight inflammation was produced by propylene glycole alone [8].

Fertility, Pregnancy and Lactation

The root is considered an abortifacient [11,19]. An alcoholic extract of blue cohosh was found to put the isolated uterus of the guinea pig into a state of tonic contraction [19], and caulosaponin shows an oxytocic action on the rat uterus *in vivo* [8]. Treatment of rats with a homoeopathic *Caulophyllum* preparation of low potency produced follicular and endometrial changes suggestive of an inhibitory effect on ovulation [17], and administration of this preparation to pregnant rats was found to interrupt implantation [18].

The alkaloid anagyrine, which occurs in the root of *Caulophyllum thalictroides*, is held responsible for a congential deformity called "crooked calf disease", which is caused by maternal ingestion of lupine. Experimental feeding of *Lupinus* extracts reproduced this disease in bovine stock whereas such an effect was not found in sheep or hamsters. The severity of the deformities in the calves was directly related to the concentration of anagyrine in the extracts tested, with about 30 mg/kg producing a severe effect [20]. There is also a case report about congenital malformations (marked anemia, skeletal dysplasia, and vascular anomaly) in a human infant, which could have resulted from the maternal use early during pregnancy of goat milk contaminated with anagyrine. The skeletal deformities of the infant were similar to those observed in crooked calf disease [21].

Mutagenicity, Cytotoxicity and Carcinogenicity

Triterpenoid glycosides from the root of *Caulophyllum robustum* M., caulosides B and C, were shown to have cytotoxic activity in developing sea urchin embryos [22,23].

Data about the mutagenic, cytotoxic or carcinogenic potential of *Caulophyllum thalictroides* have not been recovered from the literature.

References

1. List PH, Hörhammer L (1972) Hagers Handbuch der Pharmazeutischen Praxis. 4th edn. Dritter Band: Chemikalien und Drogen (Am-Ch). Berlin: Springer-Verlag, pp 776–777
2. Millspaugh CF (1974) American Medicinal Plants. New York: Dover Publications, pp 57–60
3. Weiner MA (1980) Weiner's herbal. The guide to herb medicine. New York: Stein and Day, p 70
4. Tyler VE (1987) The New Honest Herbal. A sensible guide to herbs and related remedies. 2nd edn. Philadelphia: George F. Stickley Company, pp 36–37
5. Der Marderosian A, Liberti LE (1988) Natural product medicine. A scientific guide to foods, drugs, cosmetics. Philadelphia: George F. Stickley Company, pp 262–263
6. Flom MS, Doskotch RW, Beal JL (1967) Isolation and characterization of alkaloids from *Caulophyllum thalictroides*. J Pharm Sci 56:1515–1517
7. Power FB, Salway AH (1913) The constituents of the rhizome and roots of *Caulophyllum thalictroides*. J Chem Soc 103:191–209
8. Ferguson HC, Edwards LD (1954) A pharmacological study of a crystalline glycoside of *Caulophyllum thalictroides*. J Am Pharm Sci Ed 43:16–21
9. Hegnauer R (1964) Chemotaxonomie der Pflanzen. Band 3: Dicotyledoneae: Acanthaceae – Cyrillaceae. Basel: Birkhäuser Verlag, p 248
10. McShefferty J, Stenlake JB (1956) Caulosapogenin and its identity with hederagenin. J Chem Soc 449:2314–2316
11. Lewis WH, Elvin-Lewis MPF (1977) Medical botany. Plants affecting man's health. New York: John Wiley & Sons, p 31 and p 325
12. Hardin JW, Arena JM (1974) Human poisoning from active and cultivated plants. 2nd edn. Durham: Duke University Press, pp 60–61
13. Scott CC, Chen KK (1943) The pharmacological action of N-methylcytisine. J Pharmacol Exp Ther 79:334–339
14. Barlow RB, McLeod LJ (1969) Some studies on cytisine and its methylated derivatives. Br J Pharmacol 35:161–174
15. Moskowitz R (1990) Two childbirth remedies. Br Homoeopath J 79:206–211
16. Mitchell J, Rook A (1979) Botanical dermatology. Plants and plant products injurious to the skin. Greengrass: Vancouver, p 434

17. Chandrasekhar K, Sarma GHR (1974) Observations on the effect of low and high doses of *Caulophyllum* on the ovaries and the consequential changes in the uterus and thyroid in rats. J Reprod Fertil 38:236–237
18. Chandrasekhar K, Vishwanath CR (1974) Studies on the effect of *Caulophyllum* on implantation in rats. J Reprod Fertil 38:245–246
19. Pilcher JD, Delzell WR, Burman GE (1916) The action of various "female" remedies of the excised uterus of the guinea-pig. JAMA 67:490–492
20. Keeler RF (1984) Teratogens in plants. J Animal Sci 58:1029–1039
21. Ortega JA, Lazerson J (1987) Anagyrine-induced red cell aplasia, vascular anomaly, and skeletal dysplasia. J Pediatr 111:87–89
22. Anisimov MM, Shentsova EB, Shcheglov VV et al. (1978) Mechanism of cytotoxic action of some triterpene glycosides. Toxicon 16:207–218
23. Anisimov MM, Popov AM, Dzizenko CN (1979) The effect of lipids from sea urchin embryos on cytotoxic activity of certain triterpene glycosides. Toxicon 17:319–321

Eleutherococcus Senticosus

U. Sonnenborn and R. Hänsel

Botany

Like *Panax ginseng* and its congeners (see our monograph on *Panax ginseng* in the preceding volume), *Eleutherococcus senticosus* (Ruprecht et Maximowicz) ex Maxim. belongs to the family Araliaceae. Another synonym frequently used in the international literature, and preferred by Asian scientists, is *Acanthopanax senticosus* (Ruprecht et Maximowicz) Harms. The plant is also known by the more popular names Siberian ginseng, taiga root, eleuthero, thorny ginseng, touch-me-not, and devil's shrub. In the USSR, the plant is called Eleutherokokk koljucij. In China and in Japan it is known as Wujiapi or Ciwujia [1–5].

E. senticosus is a slender, thorny shrub which grows exclusively in the taiga zone of the Far East (southeastern part of the USSR, northern China, Korea, and Japan) [1,2,4]. In contrast to *Panax ginseng*, it can easily be found growing wild in these parts of the world even today. It grows naturally in a cold, moderate climate and represents a normal part of the underwood of the East Asian mixed and coniferous forests [1].

The genus *Eleutherococcus* (*Acanthopanax*) comprises 15 polymorphous species of which *E. senticosus* is the most prominent and most important plant used as a drug source today. *E. senticosus* drugs sold on the world market generally originate from the USSR, although they may to a far lesser extent also stem from China and Korea [2,4,6]. Differences in composition and morphology of the crude drug can be observed between drugs from Russia and those from the other countries [4]. The Russian drug mainly consists of pieces of the rhizome of the plant, and only a little root material will be detected. On the contrary, the Korean drug mainly consists of root material, and rhizome material is rarely found. The Chinese crude drug is of intermediate appearance.

Falsifications of the *Eleutherococcus* drug, as described for *Panax ginseng*, have not been observed up to now. On the other hand, *E. senticosus* itself may be found occasionally as a *Panax ginseng* substitute in ginseng products [7].

Adverse Effects of Herbal Drugs, Vol. 2
(ed. by P.A.G.M. De Smet, K. Keller, R. Hänsel, R.F. Chandler)

E. senticosus was first established as an official medicinal plant in the USSR in 1962. In the western countries, it did not become popular until the early 1970s. In the USA, the Soviet pharmacopoeial liquid extract was introduced in 1971 [2].

Up to now *E. senticosus* is an official drug in the Russian pharmacopoea only, where it is listed as "Extractum radicis et rhizomatis Eleutherococcus" [2,4]. It is distributed and exported worldwide from Russia rarely as a dried crude drug, but rather mostly as an ethanolic extract, containing about 33% of alcohol. Similar to *P. ginseng*, *Eleutherococcus* products on the pharmaceutical and the health food markets of different countries are distributed in the form of tablets, capsules, teas, syrups, fluid extracts, and tonics [8]. *Eleutherococcus* products are sold either as single or as combination preparations mixed with other medicinal herbs, vitamins, and/or minerals. In the USA and Canada, in Australia, and in several European countries, these preparations are widely promoted in health food stores, not necessarily in pharmacies, and not necessarily as the pharmacopoeial product [2].

Chemistry

In the last 20 years, a number of chemical compounds with different pharmacological activities have been isolated from *E. senticosus*, mainly terpenoidal derivatives such as the triterpene saponins and also lignans, coumarins, phenylpropanes, steroids, carbohydrates, xanthones, and flavones [2,4,9–22]. All these constituents are ubiquitous in the plant kingdom and are thus not exclusively characteristic for *Eleutherococcus senticosus*. What possibly may be looked upon as typical for *E. senticosus* is the coexistence of triterpenoidal saponins and their prosapogenins, lignans, coumarins, phenylcarbonic acids, and xanthones in the same crude drug [20–22]. Unfortunately, compounds of such different chemical classes have been classified as "eleutherosides" by Russian phytochemists. This may be confusing to others, especially when compared to *P. ginseng*, where the ginsenosides as typical and exclusive constituents all belong to the same chemical group of substances. To diminish these problems, Wagner [20] proposed dividing the major eleutherosides into just two classes:

1. the triterpenoidal saponins, which are oleanolic acid glycosides (eleutherosides I, K, L, and M), and
2. the phenylpropane derivatives (eleutherosides B, B_1, D, and E), most of which are also glycosylated.

The total amount of eleutherosides of *E. senticosus* is in the range of 0.6% to 0.9% (w/w) in the roots and of 0.6% to 1.5% in the stems of the plant [17,18]. The ratio of eleutherosides A–G has been determined to be 8:30:10:12:4:2:1 by Ovodov and colleagues [19].

In contrast to *P. ginseng* roots, the triterpenoidal saponins of *E. senticosus* are only minor constituents of the rhizome of this plant, but are typical constituents of its leaves [16]. Eleutheroside I (syn. mussein B or mubenin B) and eleutheroside K (syn. β-hederin) are oleanolic acid derivatives with one disaccharide side chain composed of rhamnose and arabinose. Eleutheroside L and eleutheroside M (syn. hederasaponin B) possess an additional trisaccharide side chain at the carboxyl function. By means of TLC analysis, Lui and Staba [12] and Wagner and Wurmböck [15] have shown that *Panax*-type ginsenosides cannot be detected in the roots of *E. senticosus*. According to Obermeier [21], the oleanolic acid glycosides are not present in the commercially available *Eleutherococcus* fluid extract either.

The simplest main eleutheroside is the phenylpropane eleutheroside B (syn. syringin). Direct derivatives are the coumarins, where the side chain of the phenylpropane is closed to a second ring structure (e.g., eleutheroside B_1, syn. isofraxidineglucoside). The biosynthetic addition of two phenylpropane building blocks yields the basic structure of the lignans (e.g., eleutherosides D and E, two different stereochemical forms of syringaresinol-diglucoside).

Ro et al. [13] isolated the lignan glycoside liriodendrin (syn. lirioresinol-β-diglucoside) from *Eleutherococcus* root cortex which exhibited anabolic activity in mice (stimulation of ^{14}C-leucine incorporation into liver proteins).

In 26 samples collected in Hokkaido (Japan), Anetai and coworkers [22] recently determined the quantitative ratio of some pharmacologically active constituents of *E. senticosus*: eleutheroside B (I), chlorogenic acid (II), glucosyl-isofraxidin (III), syringaresinol-glucoside (IV), and isofraxidin (V). They found a mean ratio of 98.5 (I):604.4 (II):17.5 (III):79.2 (IV):3.8 (V) mg of the above-mentioned substances per 100 g plant material. Great variations (up to ninefold) of the content of the different compounds were noted between individual samples.

In addition to the classical eleutherosides (see above), other compounds have been isolated from *E. senticosus* as well:

- Besides eleutheroside A (syn. daucosterol) and the lignans ariensin and syringin, Chung and Kim [23] isolated the diterpenoid isopimara-9[11], 15-dien-19-ol and the polyacetylene compound falcarindiol from the Korean subspecies of *E. senticosus*.
- Wagner and coworkers [24,25] purified immunologically active polysaccharides from *E. senticosus*: a glucan of M_r 150000 and a heteroxylan of M_r 30000 Dalton. Similar compounds which stimulated interferon synthesis were isolated by Yang and Liu [26]. Zhu et al. [27] isolated a polysaccharide fraction from *E. senticosus* which provoked an increase of serum type-specific antibody levels in mice.
- Recently, Yun-Choi et al. [28] detected the platelet aggregation-inhibiting substance 3,4-dihydroxybenzoic acid (DBA) in *E. senticosus*.

Eleutherococcus senticosus (Siberian ginseng) is often compared to and equated with *Panax ginseng* (Korean ginseng). However, this is only partially substantiated, because from the phytochemical point of view both drugs exhibit more differences than similarities.

Pharmacology and Uses

Quite a few original reports now exist, mainly from Russia, which deal with pharmacological and toxicological aspects of *Eleutherococcus senticosus*. However, since most of them are written in the Russian language and have been published nearly exclusively in Russian journals, they are thus not readily available to Western scientists [1, 2].

Although, if compared to *Panax ginseng, Eleutherococcus* is a "newcomer" on the pharmaceutical and health food markets, there are already numerous review articles and monographs available on the pharmacology, toxicology, and clinical use of this drug [1–6,8–10,29–35].

An in-depth analysis of pharmacological, toxicological, and clinical studies on *E. senticosus* has been presented by Farnsworth and colleagues [2], reviewing the data available up to 1985.

In contrast to *P. ginseng*, only few studies on pharmacology of purified compounds from *E. senticosus* have been done so far [11,13,24–28,36–39]. Most studies deal with alcoholic extracts from this plant.

The main principle of pharmacological activity of *E. senticosus* seems to be that of a so-called adaptogen [2,4,9,10,30,31,34,35], and it is thus commonly used in a more preventive than a curative way. In this respect, it is rather similar to *P. ginseng* [2–4,8,30–33]. *Eleutherococcus* extracts have been shown to exhibit cytoprotective effects *in vitro* and antitoxic effects on experimental animals [9,22,40,41]. In addition, antistress properties and an antifatigue effect of the drug have been described [1,2,11,30,31,42,43].

As is the case with *P. ginseng*, the actions of *E. senticosus* may be partially explained by its antioxidant [44], but more likely by its immunomodulatory activities [24,25,45–54]. The enhancement of the unspecific branch of the immune system by the *Eleutherococcus* drug may explain the preventive and curative effects seen in Russian studies in the 1970s on larger patient groups with respiratory tract infections [48,51,52] or dysentery [53] (for a detailed review see reference 2).

Adverse Reaction Profile

General Animal Data

According to several workers, the toxicity of *E. senticosus* extracts seems to be extremely low [2,8,9,33–35,55]. LD_{50} values are reported to be in the range of about 30 g per kg body weight in mice for the powdered root [2,8]. The oral LD_{50} value of the 33% ethanolic extract was about 14.5 g/kg body weight in mice [2]. Medon and coworkers [56] showed that a single dose of 3 g freeze-dried root extract did not cause death in mice. Toxic effects at very high dosages (sedation, ataxia, tremor, or vomiting) are thought to be more readily due to the alcohol content of the extract than to a toxic effect of the *Eleutherococcus* compounds themselves [34].

Daily feeding of the 33% ethanolic extract by gastric intubation to male and female rats for a period of 2 months exhibited no significant effects on urine output and content, counts of white or red blood cells, hemoglobin content, adrenal ascorbic acid and cholesterol levels, liver glycogen content, and on animal weight [57]. The daily dosage applied was reported to be equivalent to 10 mg/kg of total eleutherosides (2 ml/kg of a 5% solution containing eleutherosides B, B_1, C, D, and E).

Golotin and colleagues [58] showed that feeding of 5 ml/kg of the 33% ethanolic extract in drinking water to rats for a total of 320 days did not cause toxic effects or deaths.

No adverse effects of *Eleutherococcus* root extracts on animal growth were observed in feeding experiments with minks, sheep, rabbits, and piglets, where the extracts had been mixed with the standard diet [2,8].

General Human Data

Problems with adverse reactions to *Eleutherococcus senticosus* are difficult to retrieve from the literature, because in some of the case reports and studies available, especially in those from Western countries, they may often be headed, and thus in this way be disguised, by the title "ginseng" (e.g., 7].

Until now, allergic reactions to *E. senticosus* have not been observed [2,8,50].

Since *Eleutherococcus* has been reported to increase the feeling of strength and well-being, Schmidt [59] has speculated upon the danger that older, weakened, and convalescent patients might overstrain themselves, when taking the drug. However, clinical studies or case reports about such an effect of *Eleutherococcus* intake are not available.

Cardiovascular Reactions

Unspecified ginseng products have more than once been associated with hypertensive reactions (for details, see our monograph on *Panax ginseng* in the preceding volume).

A report from Russia [43] states that *Eleutherococcus* should not be given to patients with high blood pressure in excess of 180/90 mm Hg.

In a clinical study conducted in Russia on 64 atherosclerotic patients [54 male, 10 female, aged 50 to 60] the following adverse drug reactions were noted in an unspecified proportion of patients: extrasystole, hypertonia, shifts in heart rhythm, and tachycardia [2]. The patients had taken 4.5 to 6.0 ml of the official ethanolic *Eleutherococcus* extract per day for a period of 25 to 35 days. This regimen had been repeated six to eight times with intervals of 3 to 4 months between the treatment periods.

In another Russian study on 55 patients (26 male, 29 female, aged 20 to 50) with rheumatic heart lesions, two patients experienced hypertension, pericardial pain, and palpitations together with pressure headaches when ingesting 3 ml daily of the ethanolic root extract for a total of 28 days [60].

Central Nervous System Reactions

Insomnia has been observed in some patients in clinical trials in Russia [2].

Dermatological Reactions

Dermatological side effects (skin eruptions) were noted in an open clinical study by Siegel [7] on ginseng users in California, where an unknown number of patients had been taking *Eleutherococcus* instead of *Panax ginseng*. However, since an uncontrolled use of uncontrolled products was allowed, no valid data can be drawn from this study (for details see our monograph on *Panax ginseng* in the previous volume).

Endocrine Reactions

As reported by Punnonen and Lukola [61], estrogenic effects were experienced by a Finnish postmenopausal woman who had been taken "Rumanian" ginseng tablets. It is not known what kind of Araliaceae was the source of the drug, since "Rumanian" ginseng does not exist as a botanical species. It may be speculated that the tablets contained *Eleutherococcus senticosus*, because an affinity to estrogen receptors of a methanolic extract from the tablets was detected by the authors. Such an affinity to estrogenic binding sites of methanolic extracts from *E. senticosus*, but not from *P. ginseng*, has been shown by Pearce and colleagues [62].

Gastrointestinal Reactions

Gastrointestinal side effects (morning diarrhoea) in an unspecified number of ginseng users in the USA were reported in 1979 by Siegel [7]. However, it is not known what kind of ginseng or *Eleutherococcus* prescriptions these patients had been taking (for details see our monograph on *Panax ginseng* in the previous volume).

Metabolic Reactions

Hikino and colleagues [63] showed that intraperitoneal injection of an aqueous extract from *Eleutherococcus senticosus* roots remarkably reduced blood sugar levels in mice. Fractionation of the extract yielded seven glycans, eleutherans A, B, C, D, E, F, and G, which exerted marked hypoglycemic, insulin-like effects in normal and alloxan-induced hyperglycemic mice.

Drug Interactions

In 1984, Medon and coworkers [64] showed that *E. senticosus* extracts produced inhibition of hexobarbital metabolism in mouse liver *in vitro* and increased hexobarbital-induced sleeping time *in vivo* when administered i.p. to mice.

Fertility, Pregnancy, and Lactation

Effects on fertility or effects during lactation have not been reported for humans. In a recent report by Koren et al. [65], maternal use of Canadian ginseng tablets with "pure Siberian ginseng" during pregnancy was tentatively associated with neonatal androgenization. In an additional letter to the same journal [66], Koren later postulated that the implicated herbal product contained a substance which acted like testosterone and suppressed endogenous testosterone synthesis in the mother. In a comment to these reports, however, Awang [67] from the Canadian Bureau of Drug Research questioned whether the implicated herbal remedy really contained *E. senticosus*.[1]

No teratogenic effects were noted on the offspring of Wistar rats at a dose of 10 mg daily of total eleutherosides per kilogram body weight for a period of 16 days [57]. In addition, no teratogenic effects and no adverse effects on offspring by *Eleutherococcus* extracts have been observed, when either pregnant sheep or pregnant mink received the drug mixed with the standard diet [2,8]. According to Curtze [34], teratogenicity studies on rats (13.5 ml of the fluid extract per kilogram body weight during the sixth to fifteenth day of pregnancy) did not reveal any negative effects on dams or fetuses. Similar studies on rabbits could not be carried out, because the dams died at the above dosage because of alcohol intoxication.

[1] See the note added in proof on p. 316

Mutagenicity and Carcinogenicity

Eleutherococcus is commonly used in Russia in oncological hospital departments to increase the tolerance of the patients to the adverse effects of chemotherapy and radiation therapy [42,49,50]. However, no human data on carcinogenicity of *Eleutherococcus* are available.

In vitro experiments, using the *Salmonella typhimurium* assay and the micronucleus test in mice, and *in vivo* experiments on rats did not reveal any mutagenic potential of this drug [55]. On the contrary, desmutagenic effects were observed in *Drosophila* [41].

In rats, no carcinogenic potential of *Eleutherococcus* was detected [55], whereas anticancer effects were noted in experimental animals with transplanted tumours [40,41,47].

References

1. Baranov AI (1982) Medicinal uses of Ginseng and related plants in the Soviet Union: recent trends in the Soviet literature. J Ethnopharmacol 6:339–353
2. Farnsworth NR, Kinghorn AD, Soejarto DD, Waller DP (1985) Siberian Ginseng (Eleutherococcus senticosus): Current status as an adaptogen. In: Wagner H, Hikino H, Farnsworth NR (eds) Economic and Medicinal Plant Research vol 1. London: Academic Press, pp 217–284
3. Phillipson JD, Anderson LA (1984) Ginseng – quality, safety and efficacy? Pharm J 232:161–165
4. Steinegger E, Hänsel R (1988) Lehrbuch der Pharmakognosie und Phytopharmazie 4. Auflage. Berlin: Springer-Verlag, pp 612–628
5. Tyler VE, Brady LR, Robbers JE (1988) Pharmacognosy 9th ed. Philadelphia: Lea & Febiger, p 471
6. Sprecher E (1977) Problematik moderner Drogen: Ginseng – Taigawurzel – Teufelskralle. In: Schriftenreihe der Bundesapothekerkammer, Vol. 5, Gelbe Reihe: XV. Internationaler Fortbildungskurs für praktische und wissenschaftliche Pharmazie. Meran: Bundesapothekerkammer, pp 71–95
7. Siegel RK (1979) Ginseng abuse syndrome – Problems with the Panacea. JAMA 241:1614–1615
8. Baldwin CA, Anderson LA, Phillipson JD (1986) What pharmacists should know about ginseng. Pharm J 583–586
9. Brekhman II, Dardymov IV (1969) New substances of plant origin which increase nonspecific resistance. Ann Rev Pharmacol 9:419–430
10. Brekhman II, Kirillov OI (1968) Ginseng and Eleutherococcus as sources of a new type of drugs. Rast Resur 4:3–13
11. Hahn DR, Kasai R, Kim JH et al. (1986) The glycosides of Araliaceous drugs and their biological activities. Saengyak Hakhoechi 17:78–84
12. Lui JHC, Staba EJ (1980) Ginsenosides of various ginseng plants and selected products. Lloydia 43:340–346
13. Ro HS, Lee SY, Han BH (1977) Studies on the lignan glycoside of Acanthopanax cortex. J Pharm Soc Korea 21:81–86
14. Shih C (1981) Study on chemical constituents in Acanthopanax senticosus Harms. Yao Hsueh T'ung Pao 16:53
15. Wagner H, Wurmböck A (1977) Chemie, Pharmakologie und Dünnschichtchromatographie der Ginseng- und Eleutherococcus-Droge. Dtsch Apoth Ztg 117:743–748

16. Wagner H, Heur YH, Obermeier A et al. (1982) Die DC- und HPLC-Analyse der Eleutherococcus Droge. Planta Med 44:193–198
17. Lapchik VF, Frolova GM, Ovodov YS (1967) Quantitative determination of Eleutherococcus senticosus glycosides. Rast Resur 5:455–457
18. Lapchik VF, Ovodov YS (1969) Determining the amount of biologically active substances in the raw material and drug preparations of Eleutherococcus senticosus. Visn Kyyivsk Univ Ser Biol 11:105–108
19. Ovodov YS, Ovodova RG, Solo'veva TF et al. (1965) Glycosides from Eleutherococcus. I. Isolation and some properties of eleutherosides band E. Khim Prirodn Soedin Akad Nauk Uz SSSR 1:3–7
20. Wagner H (1980) Analytik von Eleutherococcus-Extrakten. Naturheilpraxis 8:928–930
21. Obermeier A (1980) Zur Analytik der Ginseng- und Eleutherococcusdroge. Dissertation. Munich: University of Munich
22. Anetai M, Jamagishi T, Kaneshima H (1987) Quantitative determination of pharmacologically active constituents in the stems of Acanthopanax senticosus collected in Hokkaido. Hokkaidoritsu Eisei Kenkyushoho 37:85–87
23. Chung BS, Kim YH (1986) Studies on the constituents of Acanthopanax koreanum. Saengyak Hakhoechi 17:62–66
24. Fang JN, Proksch A, Wagner H (1985) Immunologically active polysaccharides of Acanthopanax senticosus. Phytochemistry 24:2619–2622
25. Wagner H, Proksch A, Riess-Maurer I et al. (1985) Immunstimulierend wirkende Polysaccharide (Heteroglykane) aus höheren Pflanzen. Arzneim Forsch 35:1069–1075
26. Yang JC, Liu JS (1986) Dynamic study of the interferon-stimulating effect of a polysaccharide of Acanthopanax senticosus on leukemic cell culture. Chung Hsi I Chieh Ho Tsa Chih 6:231–233
27. Zhu C, Tu G, Shen M (1982) Effect of polysaccharide from Acanthopanax senticosus on mouse serum type-specific antibodies. Yaoxue Tongbao 17:178
28. Yun-Choi HS, Kim JH, Lee JR (1987) Potential inhibitors of platelet aggregation from plant sources, III. J Nat Prod 50:1059–1064
29. Anton R (1987) Reflexions sur quelques nouvelles acquisitions en phytotherapie. J Pharm Belg 42:138–151
30. Fulder S (1980) The drug that builds Russians. New Scientist 21:576–579
31. Fulder S (1981) Ginseng and the hypothalamic-pituitary control of stress. Am J Chin Med 9:112–118
32. Minor JR (1979) Ginseng: fact or fiction? Hosp Formul 14:186–192
33. Owen RT (1981) Ginseng: A pharmacological profile. Drugs of Today 17:343–351
34. Curtze A (1980) Die Arzneipflanze Eleutherococcus senticosus Maxim. in der Bundesrepublik Deutschland. Der Kassenarzt 20:497–503
35. Vogt HH (1981) Eleutherococcus senticosus – Konkurrent für Ginseng. Naturwiss Rundschau 34:305–306
36. Anisimov MM, Suprunov NI, Prokofeva NG (1972) Effect of compounds isolated from Araliaceae family plants on the *in vitro* biosynthesis of protein. Rast. Resur 8:378–380
37. Brekhman II, Dardymov IV (1969) Pharmacological investigation of glycosides from Ginseng und Eleutherococcus. Lloydia 32:46–51
38. Nakagawa S, Yoshida S, Hirao Y et al. (1985) Cytoprotective activity of components of garlic, ginseng and ciwujia on hepatocyte injury induced by carbon tetrachloride *in vitro*. Hiroshima J Med Sci 34:303–309
39. Yang J, Xu H, Liu J (1984) Interferon induction by Acanthopanax senticosus polysaccharide and by sodium carboxymethyl starch in S 801 and S 7811 cell culture. Zhonghua Weishengwuxue He Mianyixue Zazhi 4:329–330
40. Monakhov BV (1965) Effect of an extract of the roots of Eleutherococcus senticosus on toxicity and antitumor activity of cyclophosphane. Vopr Oncol 11:60–63
41. Sakharova TA, Revazova YA, Barenboim GM (1985) The effect of Eleutherococcus extract on the induction of recessive lethal mutations by cyclophosphane and N-nitrosomorpholine in Drosophila. Khim-Farm Zh 19:539–540

42. Gvamichava AR, Khatiashvili TM, Khudzhadze RG et al. (1966) First results of the use of Eleutherococcus in the combined treatment of breast carcinoma. Lek Sredestva Dal'nego Vostoka 7:231–235
43. Dalinger OI (1986) The effect of an extract of Eleutherococcus on the cardiovascular system and some measures of the ability to work of older persons. Central nervous stimulants – Tomsk: 112–114
44. Mikaelyan EM, Mkhitaryan VG (1986) Antioxidant properties of Eleutherococcus. Biol Zh Arm 39:593–597
45. Barenboim GM, Sterlina AG, Bebyakova NV et al. (1986) Investigation of the pharmacokinetics and mechanism of action of Eleutherococcus glycosides. VIII. Investigation of natural killer activation by the Eleutherococcus extract. Khim-Farm Zh 28:914–917
46. Moskalik KG (1973) Change in the functional state of the reticulo-endothelial system and the phagocytic activity of blood leukocytes in rats with Pliss lymphosarcoma in the postoperative state under the effect of some adaptogens. Oncologiya, Kiev 4:170–173
47. Stukov AN (1966) Combined action of Eleutherococcus senticosus and sarcolysin on lymphosarcoma LIO-I in mice. Vopr Oncol 12:57–60
48. Barkan AI, Gaiduchenya LI, Makarenko YA (1980) Effect of Eleutherococcus on the morbidity of viral respiratory infections among children in organized collectives. Pediatrya (Moscow) 4:65–66
49. Khatiashvili TM (1968) Experimental use of fluid extract from Eleutherococcus in combined treatment of patients with carcinoma of the lip and oral cavity. B.A./RRM 6:7572
50. Kupin VI, Polevaya EV, Sorokin AM (1986) Use of Eleutherococcal extract to increase immunological reactivity in oncological patients. Vop Oncol (Leningrad) 32:21–26
51. Lyubomudrov VE, Fidel'man VG, Shikanov ME, Vankhanen GA (1971) Treatment of miners with chronic bronchitis. Vrach Delo 10:66–69
52. Lyubomudrov VE, Osadchuk VS, Shikanov ME, Vankhanen GA (1972) Acceleration of acclimatization in sanatorium climato-therapy of miners with chronic bronchitis and pneumoconiosis. Vopr Kurortol Fizioter Lech Fiz Kul't 37:130–132
53. Vereshchagin IA, Geskina OD, Bukhteeva RR (1982) Increasing of antibiotic therapy efficacy with adaptogens in children suffering from dysentery and Proteus infections. Antibiotiki 27:65–69
54. Bohn B, Nebe CT, Birr C (1987) Flow-cytometric studies with Eleutherococcus senticosus extract as an immunomodulatory agent. Arzneim Forsch 37:1193–1196
55. Hirosue T, Matsuzawa M, Kawai H et al. (1986) Mutagenicity and subacute toxicity of Acanthopanax senticosus extracts in rats. J Food Hyg Soc Jpn 27:380–386
56. Medon PJ, Thompson EB, Farnsworth NR (1981) Hypoglycemic effect and toxicity of Eleutherococcus senticosus following acute and chronic administration in mice. Acta Pharmacol Sin 2:281–285
57. Dardymov IV, Suprunov NI, Sokolenko LA (1972) Absence of toxicity of Eleutherococcus glycosides during administration for two months. Lek Sredestva Dal'nego Vostoka 11:66–69
58. Golotin VG, Brekhman II, Dobryakova AI, Li SE (1972) Influence of Ginseng and Eleutherococcus extracts on life expectancy of white rats. Lek Sredestva Dal'nego Vostoka 11:37–41
59. Schmidt M (1984) Ginseng – Alles heilendes Wundermittel? Dtsch Apoth Ztg 124:1397–1398
60. Mikunis RI, Serkova VK, Shirkova TA (1966) The effect of Eleutherococcus on some biochemical parameters of the blood in the combined treatment of patients with rheumatic lesions of the heart. Lek Sredestva Dal'nego Vostoka 7:227–230
61. Punnonen R, Lukola A (1980) Oestrogen-like effect of ginseng. Brit Med J 281:1110
62. Pearce PT, Zois I, Wynne KN, Funder JW (1982) Panax ginseng and Eleutherococcus senticosus extracts – *in vitro* studies on binding to steroid receptors. Endocrinol Jpn 29:567–573

63. Hikino H, Takahashi M, Otake K, Konno C (1986) Isolation and hypoglycemic activity of eleutherans A, B, C, D, E, F, and G: glycans of Eleutherococcus senticosus roots. J Nat Prod 49:293–297
64. Medon PJ, Ferguson PW, Watson CF (1984) Effects of Eleutherococcus senticosus extracts on hexobarbital metabolism *in vivo* and *in vitro*. J Ethnopharmacol 10:235–241
65. Koren G, Randor S, Martin S, Danneman D (1990) Maternal ginseng use associated with neonatal androgenization. JAMA 264:2866
66. Koren G (1991) Maternal use of ginseng and neonatal androgenization. JAMA 265:1828
67. Awang DVC (1991) Maternal use of ginseng and neonatal androgenization. JAMA 265:1828

Eupatorium Species

H.J. Woerdenbag

Botany

The genus *Eupatorium* belongs to the Eupatorieae, one of the thirteen tribes of the Asteraceae [1]. In the Index Kewensis over one thousand *Eupatorium* species are listed [2], but recently the genus has been taxonomically revised to contain 44 species [3]. It shows a rather classic arctotertiary distribution; representatives are found mainly in eastern North America, eastern Asia, along the western Asian mountains and in Europe. The greatest number occur in North America [4].

In this monograph *Eupatorium* species are discussed, relevant because of their use in (herbal) medicine, in relationship with pharmacological and toxicological aspects. Special attention is paid to the pyrrolizidine alkaloids that are present in many members of the genus *Eupatorium* (Table 1).

The monograph will primarily focus on the medicinal species *E. cannabinum* and *E. perfoliatum*, both reviewed by Madaus [5], as well as on the stock-poisoning *E. rugosum*. Data from other *Eupatorium* species are summarized in table format (Table 2).

The United States Food and Drug Administration (FDA) designated *E. rugosum* as a herb that should not be used in medicines [6]. However, *E. perfoliatum* but not *E. rugosum* has been widely used in American folk medicine [7]. Perhaps the FDA classified the former species as unsafe, because it is very hard to distinguish it from other species [8].

Latin synonyms for *Eupatorium cannabinum* L. are *E. nodiflorum* Wall., *Hepatorium vulgare*, *H. adulterinum* and *H. cannabinum*. The plant is known under a large number of vernacular names: English: waterhemp, hemp agrimony, thoroughwort, sweet mandlin, water mandlin, Dutch agrimony and Dutch Eupatorium; German: Wasserhanf, Wasserdost, Gemeiner Wasserdost, Kunigundenkraut, Hanfartiges Kunigundenkraut, Leberkraut, Hirschklee, Alpenkraut, Donnerkraut, Dostenkraut and Drachenkraut; French: eupatoire, à feuilles de chanvre, herbe de Sainte Cunégonde, chanvrin, origan de marais [5,9,10].

For *Eupatorium perfoliatum* L. the Latin synonyms *E. connatum* Michx., *E. glandulosum* Michx. and *E. virginicum* exist [11]. The following verna-

Adverse Effects of Herbal Drugs, Vol. 2
(ed. by P.A.G.M. De Smet, K. Keller, R. Hänsel, R.F. Chandler)

cular names are used for this plant: English: boneset, feverwort, vegetable antimony, sweating plant, Indian sage, agueweed; French: eupatoire perfoliée, herbe à la fièvre; German: Durchwachsener Wasserhanf [12,13].

Latin synonyms for *E. rugosum* Houtt. are *E. ageratoides* L.f. and *E. urticaefolium* Reichard non L.f.. This species is commonly known as white snakeroot and richweed [12,14]. It should be noted that the term "snakeroot" has not solely been applied to *E. rugosum*, but to a wider range of plants [15].

Chemistry

Eupatorium species are chemically characterized by the presence of sesquiterpene lactones, flavonoids, pyrrolizidine alkaloids, triterpenes and essential oil. Most sesquiterpene lactones belong to the germacranolides, fewer have a guaianolide structure, but other types are found as well. Large differences between the various species occur; in some species sesquiterpene lactones are abundant, yet others lack them completely [16]. The sesquiterpene lactones are usually highly oxygenated and the flavonoids highly methoxylated. The pyrrolizidine alkaloids, containing a necine base, are often esterified with trachelanthic or viridifloric acid [17–19]. The occurrence of toxic pyrrolizidine alkaloids in *Eupatorium* species is reviewed in Table 1.

Eupatorium cannabinum L., has been investigated profoundly. It contains sesquiterpene lactones, essential oil, flavonoids and alkaloids [33,34]. The principal sesquiterpene lactone is the germacranolide eupatoriopicrin [35,36]. The dried herb contains about 0.4% of this compound [10], that also occurs in the roots [37]. Further germacranolides are eupatolide [38], eucannabinolide (= hiyodorilactone A) [39] chromolaenide (= hiyodorilactone B), eupasimplicin B, 5′-dehydroxyeupatoriopicrin, hiyodorilactone E [40], 3β-hydroxyeupatoriopicrin, eupatoriopicrin 19-O-acetate, eupatoriopicrin 19-O-linolenoate, sachalinin and 8β-acetoxy-2α-hydroxycustunolide [41]. Guaianolides found are eupachifolin C [40] and 2-acetyl-8β-[4,5-dihydroxytigloyloxy]-preeupatundin [41]. The accumulation of sesquiterpene lactones with hydroxylated tiglates at C8 is very common for this species [41].

In subterranean as well as in aerial parts pyrrolizidine alkaloids are present. Echinatine and its β-acetyl-, isobutyryl-, isovaleryl- and angelyl/tiglyl esters as well as supinine and its β-isobutyryl-, isovaleryl- and angelyl/tiglyl esters, in different stereoisomerical forms have been found (Table 1). In addition, turneforcidine, a pyrrolizidine alkaloid with a saturated necin moiety, is present in roots and rhizomes. The alkaloids may be present in the plant material as their N-oxides [21–24].

Table 1. Toxic pyrrolizidine alkaloids (PA) in *Eupatorium* species

E. album	
medicinal use[a]	–
plant part	unspecified
toxic PA:	no
reference:	20
E. altissimum	
medicinal use[a]:	–
plant part:	root
toxic PA:	rinderine angelylheliotridine
reference:	20
E. cannabinum	
medicinal use[a]:	+
plant part:	whole plant
toxic PA:	echinatine, supinine and -derivatives approx. 0.03% on dry weight[b]
reference:	21–24
E. chinense	
medicinal use[a]:	see Table 2
plant part:	root
toxic PA:	approx. 0.002% on dry weight[b]
reference:	25,26
E. compositifolium	
medicinal use[a]:	–
plant part:	unspecified
toxic PA:	intermedine, lycopsamine
reference:	20,27
E. cuneifolium	
medicinal use[a]:	+
plant part:	unspecified
toxic PA:	traces
reference:	20
E. fortunei	
medicinal use[a]:	+
plant part:	stalk, leaf
toxic PA:	unidentified approx. 0.01% on dry weight[b]
reference:	25,26
E. japonicum	
medicinal use[a]:	+
plant part:	stalk, leaf
toxic PA:	approx. 0.005% on dry weight[b]
reference:	25,26
E. perfoliatum	
medicinal use[a]:	+
plant part:	unspecified
toxic PA:	no
reference:	28

Table 1. *Continued*

E. purpureum	
medicinal use[a]:	+
plant part:	whole plant
toxic PA:	echinatine, trachelanthamine in roots probably echinatine in aerial parts
reference:	27,29
E. rotundifolium	
medicinal use[a]:	see Table 2
plant part:	root
toxic PA:	echinatine and derivatives of echinatine, trachelanthamine and echimidine
reference:	19
E. serotinum	
medicinal use[a]:	+
plant part:	aerial
toxic PA:	supinine, rinderine
reference:	27,30
E. stoechadosmum	
medicinal use[a]:	+
plant part:	root
toxic PA:	lindelofine, supinine
reference:	27,31

[a] Based on Penso's Index Plantarum Medicum [32]: + = included; − = not included. Note that several species are mentioned for their (traditional) use in other sources (see Table 2).
[b] These contents have been calculated from the (raw) data given in the literature.

Flavonoids in *E. cannabinum* are astragalin, hispidulin, kaempferol, quercetin, hyperoside, isoquercitrin, kaempferol-3-rutinoside, rutin and eupafolin [42–46].

The essential oil (about 0.3% v/w) contains mono- and sesquiterpenes, including a large number of esters, and some phenylpropane derivatives [22,41,42,44,47].

Other compounds isolated from this species are: euparin and other 6-hydroxytremetone derivatives, coumarin, choline, lutein, cannaclerodanolide, (E)-hex-1-enoic acid, the plant acids caffeic, ferulic and chlorogenic acid, derivatives of ascorbic and p-coumaric acid, the triterpenes eupacannol, taraxasterol, taraxasterone, campestrol, dammaradienyl acetate, sitosterol and stigmasterol, the monosaccharides fructose, glucose, rhamnose, rutinose and inositol, fructosanes and polysaccharides, and the acetylene compound pentaynene [17,37,41,42,44,47–52]. Root cultures of this plant accumulate a variety of benzofuran derivatives [52].

Eupatorium perfoliatum L. contains the flavonoids astragalin, eupatorin, hyperoside, rutin, kaempferol, kaempferol rutinoside and quercetin [54–

56], terpenes [57], the sterols sitosterol and stigmasterol, triterpenes, α-amyrin, 3β-hydroxy-ursa-20-ene, dotriacontane [58], the germacranolides euperfolin and euperfolitin, the guaianolides eufoliatin, eufoliatorin (a dilactone guaianolide), dihydroeuperfolid and euperfolid [18,59], traces of pentaynene, a sesquiterpene alcohol, iso-humulene, an euparin derivative [18,60] and polysaccharides [49]. Finally, the plant contains alkaloids that have not been characterized so far [61].

Eupatorium rugosum Houtt. contains the benzofurans euparin, tremetol, toxol and the flavonoids rutin and kaempferol-3-rutinoside [17,62,63]. Tremetol is a crude toxin, consisting of four components, of which tremetone, dehydrotremetone and hydroxytremetone have been characterized. Furthermore, a sesquiterpene and sterols have been found [64,65].

For the chemistry of other *Eupatorium* species, see Table 2.

Table 2. Survey of *Eupatorium* species, other than *E. cannabinum*, *E. perfoliatum* and *E. rugosum*: synonyms, vernacular names, constituents, pharmacology and uses

Eupatorium adenophorum L.
Vernacular name: Crofton weed.
Constituents: The plant contains cadinenes (sesquiterpenes), isohexacosane, n-hexacosanic acid, β-amyrin, stigmasterol, lupeol, taraxasterol, epifriedelinol and salvigenin (5-hydroxy-4′,6,7-trimethoxyflavone) [66–68].
Pharmacology and uses: The plant is used in India as an antiseptic and a blood coagulant. A decoction is recommended to treat jaundice and ulcers [66]. Cadinenes possess insect antifeedant properties [68].

Eupatorium album L.
Constituents: In aerial parts the flavonoids eupatorin (5,3′-dihydroxy-6,7,4′-trimethoxyflavone) [18], rutin (quercetin 3-rutinoside) and kaempferol 3-rutinoside [54] and the diterpenes, eupatalbin and eupatoralbin have been found [69,70]. The sesquiterpene lactone fraction is small [69] and the plant is devoid of pyrrolizidine alkaloids [20].

Eupatorium altissimum L.
Vernacular name: Thoroughwort
Constituents: In above ground parts the flavones eupatorin and 5-hydroxy-6,7,3′,4′-tetramethoxyflavone [71], a glucosidic germacradienolide [72], germacranolides [73], guaianolides and heliangolides [74] occur. The roots contain pyrrolizidine alkaloids [20].
Pharmacology and uses: The flavonoids possess moderate cytotoxic activity *in vitro* [71].

Eupatorium aromaticum L.
Vernacular names: Pool root, wild hoarhound, smaller wild snakeroot, white sanicle (E), Wohlriechender Wasserhanf, Weiße Schlangenwurzel (G), eupatoire aromatique (F) [9,75].
Constituents: Roots contain coumarin [11].
Pharmacology and use: Rootstock is reputed to have diuretic, antispasmodic, and aromatic properties [75]. The plant is used in homoeopathy against aphths [76].

Eupatorium capillifolium (Lam.) Small.
Vernacular names: Dog fennel, hogweed [9,75].
Constituents: Astragalin (kaempferol-3-β-glucoside), hyperoside (quercetin-3-β-galactoside) [54], 3,4′-dihydroxy-5,7-dimethoxyflavanone, 3,5,4′-trihydroxy-7-methoxyflavanone [77], dimethyl ether of thymohydroquinone, phellandrene, borneol,

Table 2. *Continued*

limonene, taraxasterol and its esters, the sesquiterpene costic acid and alkaloids have been found [78–80]. The plant contains no sesquiterpene lactones [81].
Pharmacology and uses: Costic acid possesses antibacterial activity [80]. The herb is put over floors to keep off insects [75].

Eupatorium chinense L.
Vernacular names: (China) Lan-tsao [25], Hua Zelan [26].
Constituents: The guaianolides peroxyeupahakonin A and B, eupahakonin A and B, eupahakonenin A and B, eupachifolin A, B, C, D and E and eupahakonesin are present [82,83]. The leaves contain taraxasterol, taraxasteryl palmitate and taraxasteryl acetate [84]. In the roots low concentrations of yet unidentified pyrrolizidine alkaloids are present [25].
Pharmacology and uses: In Southern China used to alleviate syndromes caused by summer heat and wetness, including headache, fatigue, feeling of fullness in the stomach, anorexia, nausea, vomiting and diarrhoea. Serves as a diuretic and anthelmintic, and is used in the treatment of diphteria [25,85].

Eupatorium cuneifolium Willd.
Constituents: The plant contains the germacranolides eupacunin, eupacunoxin, eupatocunin, eupatocunoxin and eupatocunolin [86–88] as well as the flavonoids hispidulin, eupafolin, kaempferol, quercetin, hyperoside and astragalin [18,54,89]. Trace amounts of pyrrolizidine alkaloids are present [20].
Pharmacology and uses: Traditionally used for the treatment of cancer [88]. Flavonoids possess moderate cytotoxicity *in vitro* [89]. Cystostatic activities of the sesquiterpene lactones have been described [86,87].

Eupatorium formosanum Hay.
Constituents: Above-ground parts contain the germacranolides eupatolide [90,91], eupaformonin [92,93] and eupaformosanin [94].
Pharmacology and uses: Applied in Formosan folk medicine because of antileukemic, antipyretic and anti-inflammatory activities [90] and traditionally used for the treatment of cancer [88]. Cytostatic activities of the sesquiterpene lactones have been described [90–94]. Eupatolide and eupaformosanin possess anti-inflammatory activity [95,96]. Eupatolide lacks antimicrobial [97] and antimalarial activities [98]. Eupaformosanin inhibited aerobic basal respiration and oxidative phosphorylation processes as well as deoxyribonucleic acid polymerase and thymidylate synthetase activities in mice and rats [99].

Eupatorium fortunei Turcz.
Vernacular names: (Japan) Fujibakama [25]; (China) Pei Lan [26].
Constituents: The germacranolides eupafortunin, eupatolide and eupatoriopicrin, fumaric and succinic acid, mannitol, taraxasterol, taraxasteryl acetate, taraxasteryl palmitate, p-cymol, neryl acetate, a thymol methylester and euparin are present [84,100,101]. Low concentrations of yet unidentified pyrrolizidine alkaloids have been found in leaves and stalks [25].
Pharmacology and uses: In Chinese medicine applied for the treatment of dropsical swelling of diabetes, as a diuretic, antipyretic and emmenagogue [101]. Eupatolide and eupatoriopicrin possess cytotoxic properties. Eupatoriopicrin reduced cellular glutathione levels, caused DNA breaks and membrane damage [102].

Eupatorium hyssopifolium L.
Constituents: The plant contains the germacranolides eupahyssopin, eupassopilin, custunolid derivatives and eupassofilin, a sesquiterpene lactone with an unusual lipid ester side chain [18,103,104], the flavonoids kaempferol, kaempferol-3-rutinoside, quercetin and quercetin-3-glucoside [17,54], germacrene D, dammadienylacetate, a nerol derivative and 1-oxolongipinene derivatives [18].
Pharmacology and uses: Eupahyssopin possessed immunostimulating [105] as well as antiinflammatory [95,96] and cytotoxic [103] activities. It lowered serum cholesterol and

Table 2. *Continued*

serum triglycerides in mice, to be ascribed to inhibition of enzymes of the lipid synthesis [106]. Eupahyssopin inhibited the synthesis of DNA, RNA, protein and cholesterol in mice, as well as aerobic basal respiration, oxidative phosphorylation, deoxyribonucleic acid polymerase and thymidylate synthetase activities in mice and rats [99,107].

Eupatorium japonicum Thumb.
Vernacular names: (China) Tse-lan [25], Zelan [26].
Constituents: The guaianolide euponin has been isolated [108]. The essential oil mainly consists of mono- and sesquiterpenes [109]. Leaves and stalks contain minor amounts of pyrrolizidine alkaloids [25].
Pharmacology and uses: In Southern China used to alleviate syndromes caused by summer heat and wetness, including headache, fatigue, feeling of fullness in the stomach, anorexia, nausea, vomiting and diarrhoea. Applied as an analgesic agent and a nervous sedative [25,85]. Euponin inhibits insect development [108].

Eupatorium odoratum L.
Vernacular name: Christmas bush [9].
Constituents: The triterpene alcohols lupeol, epoxylupeol, β-amyrin, the flavononoids salvigenin, sakuranetin, isosakuranetin, kaempferide, betulenol, 3,5,7,3′-tetra-O-methylquercetagetin, tamarixetin and flavonoid glycosides based on sakuranetin and isosakuranetin, the sesquiterpenes eupatol and eupatene, the chalcone odoratin, sitosterol, ceryl alcohol and p-anisic acid have been found [17,110–114].
Pharmacology and uses: In Nepal juice of leaves is used to treat cuts and wounds [115]. Serves in the Himalayas as a fish poison. Known as a "fever plant" in Puerto Rica. Used in Nigeria for its toxicity to anthropods and higher animals. In Nigerian ethnomedicine the plant is topically applied to arrest bleeding and to promote wound healing. A decoction of its leaves is valued to cure malaria and as a cough remidy. Extracts possess antibacterial activity [111,114].

Eupatorium purpureum L.
Synonyms: *E. maculatum* L., *E. ternifolium* Ell. Sketch [11,116].
Vernacular names: Joe-Pye Weed, gravel root (E), Roter Wasserhanf (G).
Constituents: Eupatorin, euparin, saponins [11], terpenes [57] and pyrrolizidine alkaloids [27,29].
Pharmacology and uses: The plant is used in homoeopathy against fever, sickness and vomiting [76,117–119].

Eupatorium riparium Regel
Vernacular name: Mistflower
Constituents: The plant contains germacrene D, taraxasteryl palmitate, taraxasteryl acetate, taraxasterol, epi-friedelinol, stigmasterol, dammadienylacetate, benzofurans and chromenes, such as ageratoriparin, ripariochroment A, methylripariochromen A, acetovanillochromene, eupatoriochromene and eupatoriochromene derivatives [50,120–122].

Eupatorium rotundifolium L.
Constituents: The guaianolides euparotin, euparotin acetate, eupatoroxin, 10-epi-eupatoroxin, eupatundin, the chlorine containing sesquiterpene lactones eupachlorin, eupachlorin acetate and eupachloroxin, 5α-hydroxy-eupasseifolid B, 5α-hydroxy-8β-angeloyloxypreeupatundin [123–126], pyrrolizidine alkaloids [19], isohumulene [18] and hispidulin [17] are present. Chlorhydrine has been found [125], but may be an artifact [18].
Pharmacology and uses: Traditionally used for the treatment of cancer [88]. For the sesquiterpene lactones cytostatic activities have been described [123–125].

Eupatorium sachalinense Makino
Constituents: The germacranolides hiyodorilactone-A, -B, -C [127], -D, -E, -F [128], the

Table 2. *Continued*

sesquiterpene lactone peroxide peroxysachalinin, sachalinin, sachalin and eupatoriopicrin [128] have been found.
Pharmacology and uses: Cytostatic activities have been described for the plant's sesquiterpene lactones [127,128].

Eupatorium semiserratum DC.
Constituents: Aerial parts contain the flavones eupatorin, salvigenin, pectolinarigenin, hispidulin, eupatilin, eupatoretin and eupatin as well as the germacranolides eupasserin and deacetyleupasserin [17,88,89,130,131].
Pharmacology and uses: Traditionally used for the treatment of cancer [88]. Cytostatic activities of the sesquiterpene lactones have been described [131]. The flavonoids possess moderate cytotoxicity *in vitro* [89].

Eupatorium serotinum Michx.
Constituents: Germacranolides, such as euserotin, costunolide derivatives and parthenolide derivatives occur, and the flavonoids pectolinargenin, vicenin-2, hyperoside and hispidulin, pyrrolizidine alkaloids, germacrene D, α-humulene, β-cubebene derivatives, stigmasterol and longipinene derivatives are present [17,30,132–136].

Eupatorium stoechadosmum Hance
Constituents: Coumarins, quinones, eupatin and pyrrolizidine alkaloids have been found [17,31]. The essential oil contains thymohydroquinone dimethylether, selinadiene, β-caryophyllene, β-elemene, and several other mono- and sesquiterpenes [137].
Pharmacology and uses: The plant is used for incense and in Vietnam as a diuretic and to treat bile diseases. Root decoction is an antidote to poisoning and regulates menstruation [9,31,137].

Eupatorium subhastatum Hooker et Arnott
Constituents: The flavonoids eriodictyol, eupafolin, quercetin, kaempferol, quercetin-3-galactoside, quercetin-3-glucoside, quercetin-3-rhamnoside, quercetin-3-rutinoside, acacetin, hispidulin, rutin, eupatorin, 5,7,3′,4′-tetrahydroxy-6-methoxyflavanone [138,139], as well as the biflavone 4′4‴-dimethylcupressuflavone [140] and protocatechinic acid have been found [139].
Pharmacology and uses: The flavonoids possess antioxidant and free radical scavenging properties [141].

Eupatorium triplinerve Vahl.
Synonym: *Eupatorium ayapana* Vent [142].
Constituents: The plant contains thymohydrochinone dimethylester, α-terpinene, borneol, bornyl acetate, linalool, α-phellandrene, sabinene, herniarin, ayapanin (7-methoxy coumarin), ayapin (6,7-methylenedeoxy coumarin) and carotene [11,17,142].
Pharmacology and uses: In Ayurvedic medicine an aqueous extract of leaves and shoots is a cardiac stimulant. A leaf decoction possesses a hemostatic effect that is ascribed to coumarin derivatives. Hot infusion of the herb is a tonic, expectorant and diaphoretic, and serves in large quantities as laxative and emetic [74,142,143].

Pharmacology and Uses

Extracts of *E. cannabinum* have been used against liver, biliary and spleen diseases, diarrhoea, snake poisoning, ulcers, to promote wound healing, as a diuretic, a febrifuge, an anthelmintic and as a repellent for poisonous animals [5]. Nowadays leaves (harvested before flowering) and roots (in spring and in autumn) are used in popular medicine because of supposed depurative, choleretic, laxative, appetizing, stimulating and wound healing properties [11,33,34].

E. perfoliatum has been employed in the treatment of fevers, bronchial affections, migraine [5] and for the treatment of intestinal worms [61]. American Indians used its leaves and flowering tops for the treatment of colds, catarrh, influenza, rheumatism, and all kinds of fever. The plant has been a popular remedy for malaria [7,61,144] and is still in use for the allevation of fevers and for the relief of constipation. The pharmacologic properties of *E. perfoliatum* have been classified as diaphoretic and laxative in normal doses, and emetic and cathartic in large dose [13]. Tyler [7] considers *E. perfoliatum* to be ineffective to break up colds and flu, but effective in inducing sweating.

Both *E. cannabinum* and *E. perfoliatum* are used in phytotherapy. Extracts of these plants are said to stimulate bodily defence mechanisms against viral infections and to act against fever [145]. Both species are used in homoeopathy for a variety of ailments, including fever, liver and bile diseases and rheumatism [76,146]. In a clinical trial, published in 1981, the efficacy of the homoeopathic drug Eupatorium perfoliatum D2 in the treatment of common cold (flu) was tested and compared with acetylsalicylic acid. Both drugs were judged equally active, based on subjective complaints, body temperature and laboratory findings of patients [147]. The experimental setting was weak, however, as it did not include a dummy drug to assess placebo effects and as it was not a double-blind study.

From *E. cannabinum* and *E. perfoliatum* polysaccharide fractions have been isolated, consisting of water-soluble, acidic branched-chain heteroglycans, showing significant immunostimulating activities in the carbon clearance, granulocyte- and chemiluminescence tests [49,105,148–151]. These findings may support the use of extracts and homoeopathic preparations of these plants against fever [152].

The traditional indications of *E. cannabinum*, choleretic and hepatoprotective effects, have been investigated in laboratory animals: an aqueous extract induced hypercholeresis in the rat and possessed antinecrotic properties against carbon tetrachloride-induced hepatotoxicity in mice [153,154].

Flavonoids exhibit a broad range of biological activities, but in general of low intensity [155,156]. Flavonoid-containing extracts of *Eupatorium* species, as well as isolated flavones and flavonol glycosides have been shown to possess moderate cytotoxic activity *in vitro*, against cultured tumour cells [46,71,89]. In the case of *E. cannabinum*, they do not significantly contribute to the cytotoxic properties, because only small amounts are present in the plant material [46]. Eriodictyol, a flavone isolated from *E. subhastatum*, and several other flavonoids possess antioxidant and free radical scavenging properties, *in vitro* as well as *in vivo* [141].

The N-oxide of indicine has been studied for its use as an antitumour agent in humans [157], but appeared to be too toxic for clinical use.

Of sesquiterpene lactones a series of biological activities is known. As a general rule, an α-methylene γ-lactone functionality is necessary for their biological activity [158–160].

With the aim to obtain novel cytostatic agents from natural sources, many sesquiterpene lactones from *Eupatorium* species, including *E. cannabinum*, have been tested for cytotoxicity against cultured cell lines from rodent or human origin, and for antitumour activity in animal models [11,86,87,90–94,102,103,123–125,127,128,131,159,162–172].

The exact mechanism of the cytostatic action of sesquiterpene lactones is not yet fully understood. Due to the α-methylene γ-lactone group, sesquiterpene lactones are apt to react with biological nucleophiles, such as sulphydryl groups of enzymes, glutathione, proteins as well as parts of DNA. As a result, cellular enzyme activities and metabolism are inhibited [34,173–183]. In addition, sesquiterpene lactone-induced DNA lesions and membrane damage have been reported [184–186].

The present opinion is that no sesquiterpene lactone can be used clinically as a cytostatic, because of their rather non-specific action, resulting in too little discrimination between toxicity to tumour tissue and normal tissue [187]. Attempts to significantly increase the activity by chemical synthesis have, so far, been unsuccessful. Recently, evidence has been found that several sesquiterpene lactones display some selectivity and that their mechanism of action is more than a non-specific reaction with sulphydryl groups [160].

The heliangolide chromolaenide possesses slight antimicrobial activity [188]. Eufoliatin from *E. perfoliatum* possessed immunostimulating activity, but less than the polysaccharides from the same plant [149]. Thus, this sesquiterpene lactone is a low molecular weight compound with immunostimulating activity [105,189].

For details about the pharmacology, folk and homoeopathic uses of other *Eupatorium* species, see Table 2.

Adverse Reaction Profile

Pyrrolizidine alkaloids are found in several *Eupatorium* species (Table 1). They possess hepatotoxic and carcinogenic properties and may cause damage to kidney and lung. Therefore, they are principally hazardous if present in herbal teas or other botanical preparations. In addition, they may cause poisoning, disease and even cattle losses when ingested by these animals [19,24,29,190,191]. Especially pyrrolizidine alkaloids with an unsaturated necin moiety, esterified with a branched short-chain acid are potentially toxic [191]. The hepatoxicity and carcinogenicity of pyrrolizidine alkaloids are associated with the metabolism of these compounds by liver microsomal enzymes to reactive pyrrolic compounds, the dehydropyrrolizidines [192,193]. The acute hepatotoxicity is related to the amount of pyrrole metabolites formed in the liver [194–196].

General Animal Data

Determination of the acute toxicity of an ethanolic extract of *E. adenophorum* in mice yielded an $LD_{50} > 1000$ mg/kg after intraperitoneal administration [66]. As early as in 1937, it was reported that green parts of *E. chinense*, consumed daily by rabbits or guinea pigs caused chronic poisoning, with necrotic degeneration of the liver, tubular nephritis and glycosuria [85]. The researchers were unable to detect tremetol in this species.

The LD_{50} for eupatoriopicrin in mice lies between 20 and 40 mg/kg after intraperitoneal injection and was >40 mg/kg after intravenous administration [172]. Five days after an intravenous injection of 40 mg/kg eupatoriopicrin in mice, the amount of leucocytes dropped from 8000–10000 per ml blood (normal value) to 2300 per ml. The values were restored to normal within four weeks after administration [34].

Species of the genus *Eupatorium* are suspect of causing liver disease in animals. Pyrrolizidine alkaloids may be responsible for some of the poisonous effects, but also species devoid of these alkaloids can be potential hazards [20].

Ingestion of *E. adenophorum* caused severe respiratory diseases in horses in Queensland, Australia [197]. Coughing, rapid having respiration, decreased excercise tolerance and loss of condition were seen in infected animals. The flowering stage of the plant was more toxic than the non-flowering [198]. *E. riparium* induced similar toxic effects [199]. *E. adenophorum* and *E. riparium*, however, are not in use as herbal medicines.

E. rugosum is regarded as an important stock-poisoning plant. Grazing large amounts causes tremetol poisoning, resulting in characteristic trembles. Tremetol poisoning that can be lethal within 5–27 days [200] has been induced in cattle, a variety of laboratory animals and a human being. The lesions found include congestion and fatty degenerative changes, often extreme in liver and kidney. Hemorrhage has been found in the heart and the gastrointestinal tract. Tremetol is excreted slowly, except in the milk of lactating animals, and therefore is cumulative in animals consuming the plant [201].

Tremetol, as isolated from white snakeroot, was not toxic to *in vitro* cultured cells, but after microsomal activation cytotoxicity appeared. It is therefore likely that a P-450 enzyme converts tremetol into toxic metabolites [202].

Grazing toxic plants with sesquiterpene lactones containing an α-methylene γ-lactone can potentially disrupt a variety of metabolic pathways necessary for homoeostasis. Toxicity of sesquiterpene lactone poisoning in ruminants may, in part, be due to the degranulation of tissue mest cells, with the liberation of histamine and other physiologically active compounds [203].

A high nitrate content (300–1000 ppm) in *E. perfoliatum* and *E. purpureum* has been held responsible for the abortion in cattle that had eaten the plants [204,205].

General Human Data

All *Eupatorium* species, containing pyrrolizidine alkaloids are, in principle, hazardous for men. The pyrrolizidine alkaloids present in *E. cannabinum* should be considered toxic and as to its use as a medicinal plant one should be cautious. The present opinion is to be very careful using herbal medicines containing pyrrolizidine alkaloids, not only because of their high toxicity, but also because of the variability in concentrations [190,206,207].

The German health authorities have recently announced their intention to ban pyrrolizidine alkaloid-containing drugs. For internally used medicines the allowed daily intake is maximally 1 or 10 μg, dependent on the type of drug, and 100 μg for externally used preparations. Such pyrrolizidine alkaloid-containing drugs may not be used longer than six weeks per year. For the unlimited internal use of pyrrolizidine alkaloid-containing plants, a maximal daily dose of 0.1 μg of pyrrolizidine alkaloids has been established [28]. Homeopathic preparations of *E. cannabinum* may contain maximally 1 ppm pyrrolizidine alkaloids, calculated as echinatine [76].

As the literature is devoid of adverse incidents due to *E. perfoliatum*, Tyler [7] designates the plant as safe, when used in normal individuals, buth Roth et al. [55] list the plant as poisonous, due to the presence of the cytotoxic flavone eupatorin.

The United States Food and Drug Administration (FDA) considers *E. rugosum* as a poisonous plant, because of the presence of tremetol, combined with a resin acid, causing livestock poisoning and milk sickness [6].

Milk sickness is produced in humans by ingestion of milk, butter and possibly meat from animals poisoned by *E. rugosum* [6]. The symptoms of milk sickness are anorexia, severe constipation, violent vomiting and tremors [208,209]. This syndrome, caused by tremetol, is associated with metabolic disturbance characterized by severe ketoacidosis and changes in blood glucose levels [210].

During the 19th century many deaths were attributed to the consumption of toxic milk from animals that had eaten white snakeroot. With extensive clearing of the land and improved agronomy practices, the plant has faded from many grazing areas. Less home production of milk products and pooling of the milk guard against toxic effects. Nowadays, however, people are returning to consume raw milk products from their own animals. The incidence of milk sickness may therefore be rising again [211].

Dermatological Reactions

Many members of the Asteraceae are capable of provoking a wide range of dermatoses, mostly as a result of sensitization to sesquiterpene lactones [212]. Contact dermatitis may occur through conjugation of sesquiterpene lactones with sulphydryl groups of proteins in cells, resulting in complete antigens, capable of producing cell-mediated allergic reactions [158]. In addition, sesquiterpene lactones lacking an exocyclic α-methylene at the lactone ring, but possessing further unsaturated centres, such as a cyclopentenone ring or an epoxy group, may cause allergic contact dermatitis as well [213].

Dermatological reactions, due to *Eupatorium* species, have been reported for *E. altissimum*, especially at the blooming season [214], *E. cannabinum* [215], *E. capillifolium* [216] and *E. serotinum* [158,217]. From other *Eupatorium* species no reports concerning skin reactions are known, but because of their sesquiterpene lactone content many others are potentially allergenic. Cross-sensitivity to other plants, containing structurally similar sesquiterpene lactones, frequently occurs [212].

At present, there exists no effective treatment of this skin disease. The use of the amino acid L-cysteine in order to control dermatitis in guinea pigs, senstized to the sesquiterpene lactone helenin, has been reported recently. As the effect may be explained by a reaction of its sulphydryl group with the exocyclic methylene function of the free sesquiterpene lactone, and thereby reducing the amount of allergen that could potentially be formed, cysteine treatment may offer a promising way to control this type of allergy in humans [218].

Gastrointestinal Reactions

Large amounts of the tea or extracts of *E. perfoliatum* may induce diarrhoea and vomiting [12,13,200]. The hot version of teas is much more likely to cause vomiting than the cold [7]. The effect is to be ascribed to eupatorin, which is a strong emetic [8]. The diarrhoea occurs 6–7 hours after ingestion, together with severe sweating [200].

Symptoms of toxicity after ingestion of *E. rugosum*, a species that is very hard to distinguish from others, include weakness, reluctance to move, nausea, vomiting, loss of appetite, thirst and constipation. The plant's toxicity is reduced with drying [8].

Hepatic Reactions

Pyrrolizidine alkaloids, as present in many *Eupatorium* species, and tremetol in *E. rugosum*, are hepatotoxic [29,210]. In cases in which a drug may induce lipid peroxidation, as suggested for eupatoriopicrin [186], it could act synergistically with other compounds in the aggraviation of liver injury [219]. In this respect the co-occurrence of sesquiterpene lactones and pyrrolizidine alkaloids in many representatives of the genus *Eupatorium* species may be of importance for the toxicological evaluation.

Zhao et al. [25] studied the effect of extracts of roots of *E. chinense* and leaves and stalks of *E. fortunei* and *E. japonicum*, administered orally to mice, on the liver by measuring pyrrole metabolites. These *Eupatorium* species, containing very low levels of pyrrolizidine alkaloids, are used in traditional Chinese medicine. Pyrrole metabolites were detectable in liver tissue only when very large repeated doses were administered to the animals. In Chinese medicinal practice these herbs are usually prescribed in portions of about 10 g as an ingredient of herbal tea mixtures. It is usually taken as a single dose and repeated administration is seldom necessary. It would therefore be unlikely for such a dose to cause pyrrole accumulation in the liver, as was indeed found for other hepatotoxic herbs, containing considerably higher pyrrolizidine alkaloid levels.

However, *E. chinense*, *E. fortunei* and *E. japonicum* contain sufficient pyrrolizidine alkaloids to be genotoxic. The usual doses of 10 g yield 200, 1000 and 500 μg of toxic pyrrolizidine alkaloids, respectively (Table 1). These levels are much higher than the maximal pyrrolizidine alkaloid dose of 0.1 μg that has been established by the Bundesgesundheitsamt (BGA) for the unlimited internal use of pyrrolizidine alkaloid-containing plants. They also exceed the 1 μg per day that is permitted by the BGA for short-term use of maximal 6 weeks per year [28].

In traditional use, where the plant material is boiled in water, the toxicity of these *Eupatorium* species appears to be low, as only high percentages of pyrrolizidine alkaloids are extracted from the plant with more nonpolar solvents. After storage of *E. chinense* roots for one year the pyrrolizidine alkaloid content became drastically reduced [26].

Fertility, Pregnancy and Lactation

As the toxic principle of white snakeroot passes into the milk of cows eating it [211], suckling infants of mothers consuming the plant may be adversely affected.

According to the Bundesgesundheitsamt (BGA), pyrrolizidine alkaloid-containing drugs should not be used during pregnancy and lactation [28].

Mutagenicity and Carcinogenicity

No data have been recovered from the literature on the possible carcinogenicity and mutagenicity of *Eupatorium* species. However, pyrrolizidine alkaloids, as constituents of several representatives used as herbal remedies, possess carcinogenic properties [190].

In view of the rather non-specific mechanism of cytotoxic action of sesquiterpene lactones, carcinogenicity and mutagenicity may not be excluded. There could be a potential hazard to humans because of the presence of nucleotoxic, mutagenic and carcinogenic hydroaminoalcohol metabolites in herbal teas or other botanical remedies [25].

Euparin from *E. japonicum* as well as herniarin from *E. triplinerve* lacked mutagenic activity, determined in a modified Ames' method using *Salmonella typhymurium* strains TA 98 and TA 100, in the absence or presence of rat liver S-9 mix [220]. The same result has been reported for an aqueous and methanolic extract from "Eupatorii herba" [221]. The exact species involved in the latter study is not mentioned, but is likely to be *E. japonicum* as it is a Japanese communication.

References

1. Frohne D, Jensen U (1979) Systematik des Pflanzenreichs. Stuttgart New York: Gustav Fischer Verlag, pp 218–255
2. Hooker JD, Jackson BD (1960) Index Kewensis. Vol I. Oxford: Clarendon Press, pp 915–921
3. Robinson H, King RM (1985) Comments on the generic concepts of the Eupatorieae. Taxon 34:11–16
4. King RM, Robinson H (1970) *Eupatorium*, a composite genus of arcto-tertiary distribution. Taxon 19:769–774
5. Madaus G (1938) Lehrbuch der Biologischen Heilmittel. Leipzig: George Thieme Verlag, pp 1310–1318
6. Larkin T (1983) Herbs are often more toxic than magical. FDA Consumer 17 (October):5–10
7. Tyler VE (1987) The New Honest Herbal. Philadelphia: George F. Stickley Company, pp 38–39, 247
8. Spoerke Jr DG (1980) Herbal Medications. Santa Barbara: Woodbridge Press Publishing Co., pp 43–44
9. Von Reis Altschul S (1973) Drugs & Foods from Little-known Plants. Cambridge (Massachussetts): Harvard University Press, pp 299–303
10. Malingré ThM (1971) *Eupatorium cannabinum* L., een oud geneeskruid met nieuwe perspectieven. Pharm Weekbl 106:738–744
11. Hoppe HA (1975) Drogenkunde. Band 1. Angiospermen. Berlin: Walter de Gruyter, pp 482–484
12. Osol A, Farrar GE (1955) The Dispensatory of the United States of America. 25th Edition. Philadelphia: J.B. Lippincott Company, p 1687
13. Baker DM (1983) Boneset – an old Indian remedy still in use. Lawrence Rev Nat Prod 4:21–23
14. Zander R (1984) Handwörterbuch der Pflanzennamen. Encke F, Buchheim G, Seybold S, red. Stuttgart: Eugen Elmer GmbH & Co., p 225
15. Vogel VJ (1970) American Indian Medicine. Norman: University of Oklahoma Press, p 368
16. Bos R, Woerdenbag HJ, Drenth BFH (1986) HPLC screening of constituents from *Eupatorium* species by diode array detection [abstract]. Planta Med 52:532–533
17. Dominguex XA (1977) Eupatorieae-chemical review. In: Heywood VH, Harborne JB, Turner BL, red. The Biology and Chemistry of the Compositae. Vol. I. London New York San Francisco: Academic Press, pp 487–502
18. Bohlmann F, Mahanta PH, Suwita A, Suwita A, Natu AA, Zdero C, Dorner W, Ehlers D, Grenz M (1977) Neue Sesquiterpenlactone und andere Inhaltsstoffe aus Vertretern der *Eupatorium*-Gruppe. Phytochemistry 16:1973–1981
19. Hendriks H, Huizing HJ, Bruins AP (1988) Ammonium positive-ion and hydroxide negativeion chemical ionization gas chromatography-mass spectrometry for the identification of pyrrolizidine alkaloids in *Eupatorium rotundifolium* L. var. *ovatum*. J Chromatogr 428:352–356

20. Herz W, Kulanthaivel P, Subramanian PS, Culvenor CCJ, Edgar JA (1981) Alkaloids of *Conoclinium coelestinum* (L.) DC., *Eupatorium compositifolium* Walt., and *E. altissimum* L.: Isolation of crystalline intermedinine from *C. coelestinum*. Experientia 37:683
21. Pedersen E (1975) Echinatine and supinine: pyrrolizidine alkaloids from *Eupatorium cannabinum*. Phytochemistry 14:2086–2087
22. Hendriks H, Malingré ThM, Elema ET (1983) Pyrrolizidine alkaloids, flavonoids and volatile compounds in the genus *Eupatorium*. Pharm Weekbl Sci Ed 5:281–286
23. Hendriks H, Balraadjsing W, Huizing HJ, Bruins AP (1987) Investigation into the presence of pyrrolizidine alkaloids in *Eupatorium cannabinum* by means of positive and negative ion chemical ionization GC-MS. Planta Med 53:456–461
24. Huizing HJ, De Boer F, Hendriks H, Balraadjsing W, Bruins AP (1986) Positive and negative ion chemical ionization mass spectrometry of trimethylsilyl derivatives of pyrrolizidine alkaloids using NH_4^+ and OH^- as the reactant ions. Biomed Environment Mass Spectr 13:293–298
25. Zhao XL, Chan MY, Kumana CR, Ogle CW (1987) A comparative study on the pyrrolizidine alkaloid content and the pattern of hepatic pyrrolic metabolite accumulation in mice given extracts of *Eupatorium* plant species, *Crotalaria assamica* and an Indian herbal mixture. Am J Chin Med 15:59–67
26. Zhao XL, Chan MY, Ogle CW (1989) The identification of pyrrolizidine alkaoid-containing plants. A study on 20 herbs of the Compositae family. Am J Chin Med 17:71–78
27. Anonymous (1988) Pyrrolizidine Alkaloids. Environmental Health Criteria 80. Geneva: World Health Organization
28. Anonymous (1990) Vorinformation Pyrrolizidinalkaloid-haltige Humanarzneimittel. Pharm Ztg 135:2532–2533; 2623–2624
29. Smith LW, Culvenor CCJ (1981) Plant sources of hepatotoxic pyrrolizidine alkaloids. J Nat Prod 44:129–152
30. Locock RA, Beal JL, Doskotsch RW (1966) Alkaloid constituents of *Eupatorium serotinum*. J Nat Prod 29:201–205
31. Furuya T, Hikichi M (1973) Lidelofine and supinine: pyrrolizidine alkaloids from *Eupatorium stoechadosmum*. Phytochemistry 12:225
32. Penso G (1983) Index Plantarum Medicinalium Totius Mundi Eorumque Synonўmorum. Milano: Organizzazione Editoriale Medico Farmaceutica, pp 390–392
33. Woerdenbag HJ (1986) *Eupatorium cannabinum* L. A review emphasizing the sesquiterpene lactones and their biological activity. Pharm Weekbl Sci Ed 8:245–251
34. Woerdenbag HJ, Hendriks H, Bos R (1991) *Eupatorium cannabinum* L.-Der Wasserdost oder Wasserhanf. Neue Forschungen an einen alten Arzneipflanze. Z Phytother 12:28–34
35. Von Gizycki F (1951) *Eupatorium cannabinum* L., Wasserdost und Verwandte (III). Pharmazie 6:686–688
36. Dolejš L, Herout V (1962) On terpenes. CXLV. Constitution of eupatoriopicrin, a germacranolid from *Eupatorium cannabinum* L. Coll Czechoslov Chem Commun 27:2654–2661
37. Sagareishvili TG, Alaniya MD, Kemertelidze EP (1981) Nonpolar components of *Eupatorium cannabinum*. Khim Prir Soedan, pp 106–107
38. Droždž B, Bialek-Grygiel G (1971) Composition of lactone fraction of leaves and inflorescence of *Eupatorium cannabinum*. Diss Pharm Pharmacol 23:537–540
39. Droždž B, Grabarczyk H, Samek Z, Holub M, Herout V, Šorm F (1972) Sesquiterpene lactones from *Eupatorium cannabinum* L. Revision of the structure of eupatoriopicrin. Coll Czechoslov Chem Commum 37:1546–1554
40. Bos R, Hendriks H, Bruins AP, Schripsema J, Kloosterman J, Sipma G (1984) The presence of some sesquiterpene lactones in *Eupatorium cannabinum* L. [abstract]. Farm Tijdschr Belg 61:398
41. Zdero C, Bohlmann F (1987) Eupatoriopicrin 19-O-linolenoate and other constituents from *Eupatorium cannabinum*. Planta Med 53:169–172

42. Pagani T, Romussi G (1967) Sui constituenti dell' *Eupatorium cannabinum* var. *syriacum*. Farmaco Ed Prat 22:771–785
43. Aquino R, D'Agostino M, Domestico M, Senatore F (1988) Flavonoid glycosides from *Eupatorium cannabinum* subsp. *cannabinum*. Fitoterapia 59:236–238
44. Oswiecimska M, Sendra J (1972) *Eupatorium cannabinum* L., search for biologically active fraction. Diss Pharm Pharmacol 24:475–483
45. Stevanovic M, Solaja B, Dermanovic M, Milovanovic M (1986) Chemical investigations of the plant species of *Eupatorium cannabinum* L. (Compositae). J Serb Chem Soc 51:575–581
46. Elema ET, Schripsema J, Malingré ThM (1989) Flavones and flavonol glycosides from *Eupatorium cannabinam* L. Pharm Weekbl Sci Ed 11:161–164
47. Hendriks H, Bos R, Bruins AP (1985) Analysis of the essential oil of *Eupatorium cannabinum* by combined gas chromatography-mass spectrometry using electron impact and negative ion chemical ionization. Planta Med 51:541–542
48. Talaptra SK, Bhar Talaptra B (1974) Dammaradienyl acetate and taraxasterol from *Eupatorium cannabinum*. Mass spectrometric study of dammaradienyl acetate and its derivates. Aust J Chem 27:1137–1142
49. Vollmar A, Schäfer W, Wagner H (1986) Immunologically active polysaccharides of *Eupatorium cannbinum* and *Eupatorium perfoliatum*. Phytochemistry 25:377–381
50. Pagani F, Romussi G (1972) Derivati di fitoconstituenti dell' *Eupatorium cannabinum* L., var. *syriacum* (Jacq.) (Compositae). Nota II. Prodotti di ossidazione del $18\alpha,19\beta$ H-urs-20(30)-en-3β-olo (taraxasterole). Farmaco Ed Sci 27:1083–1090
51. Aquino R, D'Agostino M, De Simone F, Schettino O (1985) Metaboliti dell' *Eupatorium cannabinum*. Boll Soc Ital Biol Sper 61:1087–1091
52. Talaptra B, Mukhopadhyay R, Talaptra SK (1978) Chemical constituents of *Eupatorium riparium* Regel. J Ind Chem Soc 55:296–297
53. Siebertz R, Proksch P, Wray V, Witte L (1989) Accumulation and biosynthesis of benzofurans in root cultures of *Eupatorium cannabinum*. Phytochemistry 28:789–793
54. Wagner H, Iyengar MA, Hörhammer L, Herz W (1972) Flavonol-3-glucosides in eight *Eupatorium* species. Phytochemistry 11:1504–1505
55. Roth L, Daunderer M, Kormann K (1984) Giftpflanzen - Pflanzengifte. Landsberg München: Ecomed Verlagsgesellschaft mbH, pp IV-1-E, 16–17
56. Herz W, Gibaja S, Bhat SV, Srinivasan A (1972) Dihydroflavonols and other flavonids of *Eupatorium* species. Phytochemistry 11:2859–2863
57. Cassidy JM, Tomassini TCB, Knevel AM (1969) Terpene constituents from *Eupatorium* species. J Nat Prod 32:522
58. Dominguez XA, Quintanilla JAG, Rojas MP (1974) Sterols and triterpenes from *Eupatorium perfoliatum*. Phytochemistry 13:673–674
59. Herz W, Kalayanaraman PS, Ramakrishnan G, Blount JF (1977) Sesquiterpene lactones of *Eupatorium perfoliatum*. J Org Chem 42:2264–2271
60. Bohlmann F, Grenz M (1977) Über neue Inhaltsstoffe aus Vertretern der *Eupatorium*-Gruppe. Chem Ber 110:1321–1329
61. Locock RA (1990) Boneset *Eupatorium*. Can Pharm J 123:229–230
62. Lin TJ, Ramstad E, Heinstein P (1974) *In vivo* biosynthesis of isopentenyl-acetophenones in *Eupatorium rugosum*. Phytochemistry 13:1809–1815
63. Lin TJ, Heinstein P (1974) *In vitro* biosynthesis of isopentenylacetophenones in *Eupatorium rugosum*. Phytochemistry 13:1817–1823
64. Bonner WA, De Graw JI, Bowen DM, Shah VR (1961) Toxic constituents of "white snakeroot". Tetrahedron Lett 2:417–420
65. Bonner WA, De Graw JI (1962) Ketones from "white snakeroot" *Eupatorium urticaefolium*. Phytochemistry 18:1295–1309
66. Ansari S, Jain P, Tyagi RP, Joshi BC, Barar FSK (1983) Phytochemical and pharmacological studies of the aereal parts of *Eupatorium adenophorum* L. Herba Pol 29:93–96
67. Shukla VS, Barua NC, Chowdhury PK, Sharma RP (1983) Structure of a new and a degradated (des-isopropyl)-cadinene. Chem Ind 22:863–864

68. Bordoloi MJ, Shukla VS, Sharma RP (1985) Absolute stereochemistry of the insect antifeedant cadinene from *Eupatorium adenophorum*. Tetrahedron Lett 26:509–510
69. Herz W, Sharma RP (1976) New hydroxylated ent-kauranoic acids from *Eupatorium album*. J Org Chem 41:1021–1026
70. Herz W, Govindan SV, Blout JF (1979) Tetracyclic analogues of the rosane lactones from *Eupatorium album*. J Org Chem 44:2999–3003
71. Dobberstein RH, Tin-Wa M, Fong HHS, Crane FA, Farnsworth NR (1977) Flavonoid constituents from *Eupatorium altissimum* L. (Compositae). J Pharm Sci 66:600–602
72. Herz W, Ramakrishnan G, Murari R (1978) A glycosidic germacradienolide from *Eupatorium altissimum*. Phytochemistry 17:1953–1955
73. Jakupovic J, Sun H, Bohlmann F, King RM (1987) Further sesquiterpene lactones from *Eupatorium altissimum*. Planta Med 53:97–98
74. Boeker R, Jakupovic J, Bohlmann F, King RM, Robinson H (1986) Further heliangolides and guaianolides from *Eupatorium altissimum*. Phytochemistry 25:1669–1672
75. Uphof JCTh (1968) Dictionary of Economic Plants. Lehre: Verlag J. Cremer, p 214
76. Wiesenauer M (1989) Homöopathie für Apotheker und Ärzte. Stuttgart: Deutscher Apotheker Verlag
77. Herz W, Gibaja S, Bhat SV, Srinivasan A (1972) Dihydroflavonols and other flavonoids of *Eupatorium* species. Phytochemistry 12:2859–2863
78. Dominguez XA, Gutierrez M, Armenta N (1970) A chemical survey of seventeen medicinal Mexican plants. Planta Med 18:51–54
79. Dominguez XA, Gomez ME, Gomez PA, Villareal AN, Rombold C (1971) Physical data on the essential oils of five Compositae plants. Planta Med 19:52–54
80. Rao KV, Alvarez FM. Antibiotic principle of *Eupatorium capillifolium* (1981) J Nat Prod 44:252–256
81. Herz W, De Groote R, Murari R (1978) Sesquiterpene lactones of *Eupatorium recurvans*. J Org Chem 43:3559–3564
82. Ito K, Sakakibara Y, Haruna M (1982) Seven guaianolides from *Eupatorium chinense*. Phytochemistry 21:715–720
83. Ito K, Sakakibara Y, Haruna M (1979) New sesquiterpene lactones from *Eupatorium chinense* var. *simplicifolium* (Makino) Kitam. Chem Lett, pp 1473–1476
84. Yoshizaki M, Suzuki H, Sano K, Kimura K, Namba T (1974) Studies on Lan-so and Ze-lan. I. On the constituents of *Eupatorium* spp. Yakugaku Zasshi 94:338–342
85. Pak C, Read BE (1937) Chinese *Eupatorium*. Chin J Physiol 12:263–274
86. Kupchan SM, Maruyama M, Hemingway RJ, Hemingway JC, Shibuya S, Fujita T, Cradwick PD, Hardy ADU, Sim GA (1971) Eupacunin, a novel antileukemic sesquiterpene lactone from *Eupatorium cuneifolium*. J Am Chem Soc 93:4914–4916
87. Kupchan SM, Maruyama M, Hemingway RJ, Hemingway JC, Shibuya S, Fujita T (1973) Structural elucidation of novel tumor-inhibitory sesquiterpene lactones from *Eupatorium cuneifolium*. J Org Chem 38:2189–2196
88. Herz W, Govindan SV, Kuman N (1981) Sesquiterpene lactones and other constituents of *Eupatorium lancifolium* and *E. semiserratum*. Phytochemistry 20:1343–1347
89. Kupchan SM, Sigel CW, Hemingway RJ, Knox JR, Udayamurtha MS (1969) Tumor inhibitors XXXIII. Cytotoxic flavones from *Eupatorium* species. Tetrahedron 25:1603–1615
90. Lee KH, Huang HC, Huang ES, Furukawa H (1972) Antitumor agents II: eupatolide, a new cytotoxic principle from *Eupatorium formosanum* HAY. J Pharm Sci 61:629–631
91. McPhail AT, Onan KD (1975) Crystal and molecular structure of eupatolide, the major cytotoxic principle from *Eupatorium formosanum* HAY. J Chem Soc Perkin II, pp 1798–1801
92. McPhail AT, Onan KD, Lee KH, Ibuka T, Huang HC (1974) Structure and stereochemistry of eupaformonin, a novel cytotoxic sesquiterpene lactone from *Eupatorium formosanum* HAY. Tetrahedron Lett 16:3203–3206

93. McPhail AT, Onan KD (1976) Crystal and molecular structure of eupaformonin, a cytotoxic germacranolide from *Eupatorium formosanum* HAY. J Chem Soc Perkin II, pp 578–582
94. Lee KH, Kimura T, Haruna M, McPhail AT, Onan KD, Huang HC (1977) Structure and stereochemistry of eupaformosanin, a new antileukemic and antisarcoma germacranolide from *Eupatorium formosanum*. Phytochemistry 16:1068–1070
95. Hall IH, Lee KH, Starnes CO, Sumida Y, Wu RY, Waddell TG, Cochran JW, Gerhart KG (1979) Anti-inflammatory activity of sesquiterpene lactones and related compounds. J Pharm Sci 68:537–542
96. Hall IH, Starnes CO, Lee KH, Waddell TG (1980) Mode of action of sesquiterpene lactones as anti-inflammatory agents. J Pharm Sci 69:537–543
97. Lee KH, Ibuka T, Wu RY, Geissman TA (1977) Structure-antimicrobial activity relationship among the sesquiterpene lactones and related compounds. Phytochemistry 16:1177–1181
98. Tani S, Fukamiya N, Kiyokawa H, Musallam HA, Pick RO, Lee KH (1985) Antimalarial agents. 1. α-Santonin-derived cyclic peroxide as potential antimalarial agent. J Med Chem 28:1743–1744
99. Hall IH, Lee KH, Starnes CO, ElGebaly SA, Ibuka T, Wu YS, Kimura T, Haruna M (1978) Antitumor agents XX: Evaluation of α-methylene-γ-lactone-containing agents for inhibition of tumor growth, respiration, and nucleic acid synthesis. J Pharm Sci 67:1235–1239
100. Hegnauer R (1964) Chemotaxonomie der Pflanzen. Band 3. Basle Stuttgart: Birkhäuser Verlag, p 448
101. Haruna M, Sakakibara Y, Ito K (1986) Structure and confirmation of eupafortunin, a new germacrane type sesquiterpene lactone from *Eupatorium fortunei* Turcz. Chem Pharm Bull 34:5157–5160
102. Woerdenbag HJ (1989) A fundamental study on the cytostatic action of sesquiterpene lactones from *Eupatorium cannabinum* L. Pharm Weekbl Sci Ed 11:67–8
103. Lee KH, Kimura T, Okamoto M, Cowherd M, McPhail AT, Onan KD (1976) The structure and stereochemistry of eupahyssopin, a new antitumor germacranolide from *Eupatorium hyssopifolium*. Tetrahedron Lett 18:1051–1054
104. Herz W, Sharma RP (1976) Sesquiterpene lactones of *Eupatorium hyssopifolium*. A germacranolide with an unusual lipid ester side chain. J Org Chem 41:1051–1020
105. Wagner H (1984) Immunstimulantien aus Pilzen und höheren Pflanzen. In: Ölschläger H, red. Fortschritte in der Arzneimittelforschung. Stuttgart: Wissenschaftliche Verlagsgesellschaft mbH, pp 133–148
106. Hall IH, Lee KH, Starnes CO, Muraoka O, Sumida Y, Waddell TG (1980) Antihyperlipidemic activity of sesquiterpene lactones and related compounds. J Pharm Sci 69:694–697
107. Hall IH, Lee KH, ElGebaly SA (1978) Antitumor agents XXIX: Effects of eupahyssopin on nucleic acid, protein, anaerobic and aerobic metabolism of Ehrlich ascites tumor cells. J Pharm Sci 67:1232–1234
108. Nakajima S, Kawazu K (1978) Euponin: a new epoxy sesquiterpene lactone inhibiting insect development from *Eupatorium japonicum*. Heterocycles 10:117–121
109. Miyazawa M, Kameoka H (1977) The contituents of the essential oil from *Eupatorium japonica* Thumb. Yakugaku Zasshi 97:120–122
110. Talaptra SK, Bhar DS, Talaptra B (1974) Flavonoid and triterpenoid constituents of *Eupatorium odoratum*. Phytochemistry 13:284–285
111. Iwu MM, Chiori CO (1984) Antibacterial activity of *Eupatorium odoratum* extracts. Fitoterapia 55:354–356
112. Bose PK, Chakrabarti P, Chakravarti S, Dutta SP, Barua AK (1973) Flavonoid constituents of *Eupatorium odoratum*. Phytochemistry 12:667–668
113. Arene EO, Pettit GR, Ode RH (1978) The isolation of isosakuranetin methyl ether from *Eupatorium odoratum*. J Nat Prod 41:186–189

114. Metwally AM, Ekejiuba EC (1981) Methoxylated flavonols and flavonones from *Eupatorium odoratum*. Planta Med 42:403–405
115. Manandhar NP (1990) Traditional phytotherapy of Danuwar tribes of Kamlakhonj in Sindhuli district, Nepal. Fitoterapia 61:325–331
116. Tsuda Y, Marion L (1963) The alkaloids of *Eupatorium maculatum* L. (Queen-of-the-meadow). Can J Chem 41:1919–1923
117. Wiesenauer M (1990) Homöopathie in Kindesalter. Dtsch Apoth Ztg 130:1128
118. Wiesenauer M (1990) Globuli für unterwegs. Dtsch Apoth Ztg 130:1128–1129
119. Anonymous (1985) Homöopathisches Arzneibuch. 1. Ausgabe 1978, 4. Nachtrag. Stuttgart: Deutscher Apotheker Verlag; Frankfurt: Govi-Verlag GmbH, pp 181–182
120. Patra A, Mukhopadhyay AK, Mitra AK (1981) Constituents of *Eupatorium riparium* Regel. J Ind Chem Soc 58:1124–1125
121. Taylor DR, Wright JA (1971) Chromenes from *Eupatorium riparium*. Phytochemistry 10:1665–1667
122. Anthonson T (1969) New chromenes from *Eupatorium* species. Acta Chem Scand 23:3605–3607
123. Kupchan SM, Hemingway JC, Cassady JM, Knox JR, McPhail AT, Sim GA (1967) The isolation and structure elucidation of euparotin acetate, a novel guaianolide tumor inhibitor from *Eupatorium rotundifolium*. J Am Chem Soc 89:465–466
124. Kupchan SM, Kelsey JE, Maruyama M, Cassady JM (1968) Eupachlorin acetate, a novel chloro-sesquiterpenoid lactone tumor inhibitor from *Eupatorium rotundifolium*. Tetrahedron Lett 9:3517–3520
125. Kupchan SM, Kelsey JE, Maruyama M, Cassady JM, Hemingway JC, Knox JR (1969) Tumor inhibitors. XLI. Structure elucidation of tumor-inhibitory sesquiterpene lactones from *Eupatorium rotundifolium*. J Org Chem 34:3876–3883
126. Bohlmann F, Suwita A, King RM, Robinson H (1980) Neue Guajanolide aus *Eupatorium rotundifolium*. Phytochemistry 19:1233–1234
127. Takahashi T, Eto H, Ichimura T, Murae T (1978) Hiyodorilactones A and B, new tumor inhibitory germacradienolides from *Eupatorium sachalinense* Makino. Chem Lett, pp 1345–1348
128. Takahashi T, Ichimura T, Murae T (1979) Hiyodorilactones D, E, and F, new cytotoxic sesquiterpene lactones from *Eupatotorium sachalinense* Makino. Chem Pharm Bull 27:2539–2543
129. Ito K, Sakakibara Y, Haruna M (1979) New sesquiterpene lactones from *Eupatorium sachalinense* (Fr. Schmidt) Makino. Chem Lett, pp 1503–1506
130. Kupchan SM, Knox JR, Udayamurthy MS (1965) Tumor inhibitors VIII. Eupatorin, a new cytotoxic flavone from *Eupatorium semiserratum*. J Pharm Sci 54:929–930
131. Kupchan SM, Fujita T, Maruyama M, Britton RW (1973) The isolation and structure elucidation of eupasserin and deacetyleupasserin, new antileukemic sesquiterpene lactones from *Eupatorium semiserratum*. J Org Chem 38:1260–1264
132. Herz W, De Groote R, Murari R, Kumar N, Blount JF (1979) Sesquiterpene lactones of *Eupatorium serotinum*. J Org Chem 44:2784–2788
133. Bohlmann F, Zdero C, King RM, Robinson H (1985) Further germacranolides from *Eupatorium serotinum*. Planta Med 51:76–77
134. Wagner H, Iyengar MA, Düll P, Herz W (1972) Flavone O- und C-Glykoside in *Eupatorium serotinum*. Phytochemistry 11:1506
135. Bohlmann F, Jalupovic J, Vogel W (1982) 11-Hydroxy-α- and β-cububene from *Eupatorium serotinum*. Phytochemistry 21:1153–1154
136. Bohlmann F, Banerjee S, King RM, Robinson H (1984) Additional germacranolides from *Eupatorium serotinum*. Phytochemistry 23:1189–1190
137. Nguyêñ Xuân Duñg, Dôx Tât Loi (1991) Selection of traditional medicines for study. J Ethnopharmacol 32:57–70
138. Ferraro GE, Coussio JD (1973) Flavonoids from *Eupatorium subhastatum*. Phytochemistry 12:1825
139. Ferraro GE, Martino VS, Borrajo G, Coussio JD (1987) 5,7,3′,4′-Tetrahydroxy-6-methoxyflavone from *Eupatorium subhastatum*. Phytochemistry 26:3092–3093

140. Ferraro GE, Martino VS, Coussio JD (1988) 4′,4‴-Dimethylcuppressuflavone from *Eupatorium subhastatum*. J Nat Prod 51:586–587
141. Fraga CG, Martino VS, Ferraro GE, Coussio JD, Boveris A (1987) Flavonoids as antioxidants evaluated by *in vitro* and *in situ* liver chemiluminescence. Biochem Pharmacol 36:717–720
142. Kapoor LD (1990) Handbook of Ayurvedic Medicinal Plants. Boca Raton: CRC Press, Inc., p 181
143. Anonymous (1952) the Wealth of India. A Dictionary of Indian Raw Materials and Industrial Products. Vol. III. New Delhi: Council of Scientific & Industrial Research, pp 223–224
144. Hall Jr ThB (1974) *Eupatorium perfoliatum*. A plant with history. Mo Med 71:527–528
145. Weiß RF (1991) Lehrbuch der Phytotherapie. 7. Auflage. Stuttgart: Hippokrates Verlag, pp 298–299
146. Anonymous (1985) Homöopathisches Arzneibuch. 1. Ausgabe 1978, 3. Nachtrag. Stuttgart: Deutscher Apotheker Verlag; Frankfurt: Govi-Verlag GmbH, pp 163–164
147. Gassinger CA, Wünstel G, Netter P (1981) Klinische Prüfung zum Nachweis der therapeutischen Wirksamkeit des homöopathischen Arzneimittel Eupatorium perfoliatum D2 (Wasserhanf Composite) bei der Diagnose "grippaler Infekt". Arzneim Forsch/Drug Res 31(I):732–736
148. Wagner H, Proksch A, Riess-Maurer I, Vollmar A, Odenthal S, Stuppner H, Jurcic K, Le Turdu M, Fang JN (1985) Immunstimulierend wirkende Polysaccharide (Heteroglykane) aus höheren Pflanzen. Arzneim Forsch/Drug Res 35(II):1069–1075
149. Wagner H, Proksch A, Vollmar A, Kreuzkamp B, Bauer J (1985) *In vitro* Phagozytose Stimulierung durch isolierte Pflanzenstoffe gemessen im Phagozytose-Chemolumineszens-(CL)-Modell. Planta Med 51:139–144
150. Wagner H (1985) Neue Untersuchungen über die immunstimulierende Wirkung einiger pflanzlichen Homöopathika. Biol Med 14:399–407
151. Wagner H (1991) Pflanzliche Immunstimulanzien. Dtsch Apoth Ztg 131:117–126
152. Hänsel R, Haas R (1983) Pflanzliche Immunstimulanzien und Hyposensibilisierung mit Pflanzenstoffen. In: Hänsel R, Haas R, red. Therapie mit Phytoparmaka. Berlin-Heidelberg-New York-Tokyo: Springer-Verlag, pp 256–261
153. Lexa A, Fleurentin J, Lehr PR, Mortier F, Pruvost M, Pelt JM (1989) Choleretic and hepatoprotective properties of *Eupatorium cannabinum* in the rat. Planta Med 55:127–132
154. Lexa A, Fleurentin J, Younos C, Mortier F (1990) Study of antihepatotoxicity of *Eupatorium cannabinum* L. in mice. An adequate method of screening *in vivo* antihepatotoxic natural principles. Phytother Res 4:148–151
155. McClure JW (1975) Physiology and functions of flavonoids. In: Harborne JB, Mabry TJ, Mabry H, red. The Flavonoids. London: Chapman and Hall, pp 970–1055
156. Steinegger E, Hänsel R (1988) Flavone und Flavonoide. In: Steinegger E, Hänsel R, red. Lehrbuch der Pharmakognosie und Phytopharmazie. Berlin Heidelberg New York Paris Tokyo: Springer-Verlag, pp 389–411
157. Kovach JS, Ames MA, Powis G, Moertel CG, Hahn RG, Creagan ET (1979) Toxicity and pharmacokinetics of a pyrrolizidine alkaloid, indicine N-oxide, in humans. Cancer Res 39:4540–4545
158. Rodriguez E, Towers GHN, Mitchell JC (1976) Biological activities of sesquiterpene lactones (review). Phytochemistry 15:1573–1580
159. Picman AK (1986) Biological activities of sesquiterpene lactones. Biochem Syst Ecol 14:255–281
160. Willuhn G (1987) Sesquiterpenlactone, potentielle Leitsubstanzen für die Arzneistoffindung. Dtsch Apoth Ztg 127:2511–2517
161. Kupchan SM, Fessler DC, Eakin MA, Giacobbe TJ (1970) Reactions of alpha methylene lactone tumor inhibitors with model biological nucleophiles. Science 168:376–377

162. Lee KH, Huang ES, Piantadosi C, Pagano JS, Geissman TA (1971) Cytotoxicity of sesquiterpene lactones. Cancer Res 31:1649–1654
163. Kupchan SM, Eakin MA, Thomas AM (1971) Tumor inhibitors 69. Structure-cytotoxicity relationship among the sesquiterpene lactones. J Med Chem 14:1147–1152
164. Kupchan SM, Ashmore JW, Sneden AT (1978) Structure-activity relationships among *in vivo* active germacranolides. J Pharm Sci 67:865–867
165. Hładoń B, Droždž B, Grabarczyk H, Bobkiewicz T, Obszewski J (1975) Sesquiterpene lactones. Part XIII. Cytotoxic activity of eupatolide and eupatoriopicrin on human and animal malignant cells in tissue culture *in vitro*. Pol J Pharmacol Pharm 27:429–438
166. Woerdenbag HJ, Meijer C, Mulder NH, De Vries EGE, Hendriks H, Malingré ThM (1986) Evaluation of the *in vitro* cytotoxicity of some sesquiterpene lactones on a human lung carcinoma cell line using the fast green dye exclusion assay. Planta Med 52:112–114
167. Woerdenbag HJ, Hendriks H, Malingré ThM, Van Stralen R, Van den Berg KJ, Konings AWT (1988) *In vitro* cytotoxicity of sesquiterpene lactones from *Eupatorium cannabinum* L. and semi-synthetic derivatives from eupatoriopicrin. Phytother Res 2:109–114
168. Hładoń B, Droždž B, Holub M, Bobkiewicz T (1975) Sesquiterpene lactones. Part XVI. *In vitro* studies on cytotoxic properties of sesquiterpene lactones in tissue cultures of human and animal malignant cells. Arch Immunol Ther Exp 23:845–855
169. Hładoń B, Chodera A (1975) Sesquiterpene lactones XVII. Cytostatic and pharmacological activity. Arch Immunol Ther Exp 23:857–865
170. Woerdenbag HJ, Lemstra W, Hendriks H, Malingré ThM, Konings AWT (1987) Investigation of the anti-tumour action of eupatoriopicrin against the Lewis Lung tumour. Planta Med 53:318–322
171. Woerdenbag HJ, Malingré ThM, Lemstra W, Konings AWT (1987) Cytostatic activity of eupatoriopicrin in fibrosarcoma bearing mice. Phytotherapy Res 1:76–79
172. Woerdenbag HJ, Lemstra W, Malingré ThM, Konings AWT (1989) Enhanced cytostatic activity of the sesquiterpene lactone eupatoriopicrin after glutathione depletion. Br J Cancer 59:68–75
173. Lee KH, Hall IH, Mar EC, Starnes CO, ElGebaly S, Waddell TG, Hadgraft RI, Ruffner CG, Weidner I (1977) Sesquiterpene antitumor agents: inhibitors of cellular metabolism. Science 196:533–536
174. Arrick BA, Nathan CF, Cohn ZA (1983) Inhibition of glutathione synthesis augments lysis of murine tumor cells by sulfhydryl-reactive antineoplastics. J Clin Invest 71:258–267
175. Picman AK, Rodriguez E, Towers GHN (1979) Formation of adducts of parthenin and related sesquiterpene lactones with cysteine and glutathione. Chem-Biol Interact 28:83–89
176. Meister A, Anderson ME (1983) Glutathione. Annu Rev Biochem 52:711–760
177. Arrick BA, Nathan CF (1984) Glutathione metabolism as a determinant of therapeutic efficacy: a review. Cancer Res 44:4224–4232
178. Woerdenbag HJ, Malingré ThM, Lemstra W, Konings AWT (1988) Reduced levels of glutathione in liver and tumour tissue of the mouse after administration of eupatoriopicrin. Phytotherapy Res 2:80–84
179. Hładoń B, Droždž B, Holub M, Szafarek P, Klimaszewska O (1978) Sesquiterpene lactones (SL) part XXIV. Further studies on cytotoxic activities of SL in tissue culture of human cancer cells. Pol J Pharmacol Pharm 30:611–620
180. Woynarowski JM, Konopa J (1981) Inhibition of DNA biosynthesis in HeLa cells by cytotoxic and antitumor sesquiterpene lactones. Mol Pharmacol 19:97–102
181. Klimek D, Chmiel J, Baer W (1981) The effect of sesquiterpene lactones on the synthesis of nucleic acid in cultures of human lymphocytes stimulated by phytohemagglutinin. Arch Immunol Ther Exp 29:195–203

182. Baer W, Chmiel J, Gnojkowski J, Klimek D (1983) The effect of sesquiterpene lactones, eupatoriopicrin and hydroxyisonobilin, on the glycolytic metabolism of human lymphocytes. Int J Clin Pharmacol Ther Toxicol 21:41–46
183. Chagonda L, Lockey PM, Marples BA, Salt WG, Traynor JR (1989) Cytotoxic action of alpha-methylene lactones towards HeLa cells in culture. Phytother Res 3:196–200
184. Woynarowski JW, Beerman TA, Konopa J (1981) Induction of deoxyribonucleic acid damage in HeLa S3 cells by cytotoxic and antitumor sesquiterpene lactones. Biochem Pharmacol 30:3005–3007
185. Woerdenbag HJ, Van der Linde JCC, Kampinga HH, Malingré ThM, Konings AWT (1989) Induction of DNA damage in Ehrlich ascites tumour cells by exposure to eupatoriopicrin. Biochem Pharmacol 38:2279–2283
186. Woerdenbag HJ, Edwards ACM, Budé EJM, Malingré ThM, Konings AWT (1989) Eupatoriopicrin-induced lipid peroxidation in liver and tumour tissue of the mouse. Biochem Pharmacol 38:3115–3118
187. Hoffmann HMR, Rabe J (1985) Synthesis and biological activity of α-methylene-γ-butyrolactones. Angew Chem Int Ed Engl 24:94–110
188. Calzada J, Ciccio JF, Echandi G (1980) Antimicrobial activity of the heliangolide chromonaelide and related sesquiterpene lactones. Phytochemistry 19:967–968
189. Wagner H (1990) Was können pflanzliche Immunstimulanzien? Dtsch Apoth Ztg 130:1123–1125
190. Lüthy J (1990) Toxikologie von Arzneipflanzen mit Pyrrolizidinalkaloiden. Z Phytotherapie 11:23–24
191. Frohne D (1990) Sind pflanzliche Arzneimittel unschädlich? Nutzen ohne Risiko-oder Risiko ohne Nutzen? Dtsch Apoth Ztg 130:1861–1871
192. Mattocks AR (1968) Toxicity of pyrrolizidine alkaloids. Nature 217:723–728
193. Mattocks AR (1971) Hepatotoxic effects due to pyrrolizidine alkaloid N-oxides. Xenobiotica 1:563–565
194. Mattocks AR (1972) Acute hepatotoxicity and pyrrolic metabolite in rats dosed with pyrrolizdine alkaloids. Chem-Biol Interact 5:227–242
195. Westendorf J (1992) Pyrrolizidine alkaloids. In: De Smet PAGM, Hänsel R, Keller K, Chandler RF, red. Adverse Effects of Herbal Drugs. Volume 1. Berlin: Springer-Verlag, pp 193–205
196. Rizk AFM, Kamel A (1991) Toxicity, carcinogenecity, pharmacology, and other biological activities of pyrrolizidine alkaloids. In: Rizk AFM, red. Naturally Occurring Pyrrolizidine Alkaloids. Boca Raton Ann Arbor Boston: CRC Press, pp 211–226
197. O'Sullivan BM (1979) Crofton weed (*Eupatorium adenophorum*) toxicity in horses. Aust Vet J 55:19–21
198. O'Sullivan BM (1985) Investigations into crofton weed (*Eupatorium adenophorum*) toxicity in horses. Aust Vet J 62:30–32
199. Gibson JA, O'Sullivan BM (1984) Lung lesions in horses fed mist flower (*Eupatorium riparium*). Aust Vet J 61:271
200. Lewin L (1962) Gifte und Vergiftungen. Lehrbuch der Toxikologie. 5 Ausgabe. Ulm/Donau: Karl F. Haug Verlag, p 754
201. Olson CT, Keller WC, Gerken DF, Reed SM (1984) Suspected tremetol poisoning in horses. J Am Vet Med Assoc 185:1001–1003
202. Beier RC, Norman JO, Irvin TR, Witzel DA (1987) Microsomal activation of constituents of white snakeroot (*Eupatorium rugosum* Houtt) to form toxic products. Am J Vet Res 48:583–585
203. Elissalde MH, Ivie GW, Rowe LD, Elissalde GS (1983) Considerations of the structure of sesquiterpene lactones on biological activity: influence of the α-methylene-γ-lactone moiety on the mast cell degradation. Am J Vet Res 44:1894–1897
204. Sund JM, Wright MJ (1957) Weeds containing nitrate cause abortion in cattle. Agron J 49:278–279

205. Sund JM, Wright MJ (1959) Control weeds to prevent lowland abortion in cattle. Down to Earth 15:10–13
206. Lüthy J, Brauchli J, Zweifel U, Schmid P, Schlatter Ch (1984) Pyrrolizidin-Alkaloide in Arzneipflanzen der Boraginaceen: *Borago officinalis* L. und *Pulmonaria officinalis* L. Pharm Acta Helv 59:242–246
207. Röder E (1984) Pyrrolizidinalkaloide in Heilpflanzen. Dtsch Apoth Ztg 124:2300–2302
208. Jordan EO, Harris NM (1909) Milksickness. J Infect Diseases 6:401–491
209. Niederhofer RE (1985) The milk sickness. Drake on medical interpretation. JAMA 254:2123–2125
210. Wu CH, Lampe KF, Mende TJ (1973) Metabolic changes induced in chickens by the administration of tremetol. Biochem Pharmacol 22:2835–2841
211. Stotts R (1984) White snakeroot toxicity in dairy cattle. Vet Med 79:118–120
212. Schmidt RJ (1986) Compositae. Clin Dermatol 4:46–61
213. Hausen BM, Schmalle HW (1985) Structure-activity aspects of 4 allergenic sesquiterpene lactones lacking the exocyclic α-methylene at the lactone ring. Contact Dermat 13:329–333
214. Brier AJ (1940) Contact dermatitis from thurowort (*Eupatorium altissimum*). J Allergy 11:402–406
215. Evans FJ, Schmidt RJ (1980) Plants and plant products that induce contact dematitis. Planta Med 38:289–316
216. Mitchell J, Rook A (1979) Botanical Dermatology. Plants and Plant Products injurious to the skin. Vancouver: Greengrass, p 204
217. Shelmire B (1939) Contact dermatitis from weeds: patch testing with their oleoresins. JAMA 113:1085–1090
218. Picman J, Picman AK (1990) Treatment of dermatitis caused by the sesquiterpene lactone helenin. Pharmazie 45:57–59
219. Poli G, Albano E, Dianzani MU (1987) The role of lipid peroxidation in liver damage. Chem Phys Lipids 45:117–142
220. Nagao M, Morita N, Yahagi T, Shimizu M, Kuroyanagi M, Fukuoka M, Yoshihira K, Natori S, Fujino T, Sugimura T (1981) Mutagenicities of 61 flavonoids and 11 related compounds. Environ Mut 3:401–419
221. Yamamoto H, Mizutani T, Nomura H (1982) Studies on the mutagenicity of crude drug extracts I. Yakugaku Zasshi 102:596–601

Gossypol

H.J. Woerdenbag

Botany

Gossypol occurs in members of the genus *Gossypium,* which is one of 75 genera that belong to the Malvaceae. *Gossypium* species or cotton plants, of which 20–47 representatives are known (authorities differ on this subject), occur in tropical and subtropical regions all over the world. They are annual or perennial shrubs or small trees, which produce capsules containing numerous seeds.

Gossypium species have been used for the production of cotton since ancient times. Cotton consists of the epidermal trichomes of the seeds. Four cultivated *Gossypium* species are considered to be of economic importance. They include the Asian-African *G. arboreum* L. (= *G. neglectum* Tod.) and *G. herbaceum* L. (= *G. indicum* Lam.), as well as the American *G. barbadense* L. (= *G. vitiflorium* Lam.) and *G. hirsutum* L. Each of these species comprises a large number of varieties and races based on geographical distribution and associated with genetical features. Vernacular names for *G. herbaceum* are Indian cotton plant (E), Indische Baumwollstaude (G) and cotonnier de l'Inde (F). *G. hirsutum* is commonly known as American Upland cotton [1–5].

Cottonseed oil is expressed from the seeds of various *Gossypium* species and is used in food products and for pharmaceutical purposes [1,2]

Chemistry

Gossypol is a yellow polyphenolic bisesquiterpene that occurs in the subepidermal glands of *Gossypium* species. These glands are present in the leaves, stems, roots, flowers, and especially in the seeds of the plants [6]. The gossypol content depends on the species and variety as well as on the climate in which the plant was grown [4]. Gossypol is present in the kernels at concentrations of 0.4–2.0%. Seeds of *G. herbaceum* types contain low gossypol contents, and the seeds of *G. barbadense* are richest in gossypol [5]. The gossypol levels in different parts of *G. hirsutum* are: root 0.15%;

Adverse Effects of Herbal Drugs, Vol. 2
(ed. by P.A.G.M. De Smet, K. Keller, R. Hänsel, R.F. Chandler)

stem 0.003%; seed 0.74%; seed cake 0.097% [7]. Several glandless species only contain traces. Gossypol is present in homemade, unheated cottonseed oil, but is largely destroyed by moist heat treatment during processing of the commercial oil [8]. In addition to the yellowish gossypol, the red pigment gossypurin and the green pigment gossyverdurin have been found, with chemical structures similar to gossypol [6].

Gossypol exists in three tautomeric forms: the aldehyde, the ketone and the hemiacetal. Gossypol, isolated from cottonseed, is racemic. It can be separated into a (+)-isomer and a (−)-isomer that show different biological activities [10]. (+)-Gossypol has been isolated in good yields from *Thespesia populnea* (L). Soland. ex Correa (= *Hibiscus populneus* L.) (Malvaceae) [11]. No report is known on the presence of the (−)-isomer as the sole form in any plant [6,8,11].

In laboratory investigations and in clinical trials gossypol as well as the adducts gossypol acetic acid and gossypol formic acid have been used [9]. Until 1983 most studies focusing on its biological activity have been carried out with racemic gossypol. Subsequently, the separate isomers have also been studied [10].

Pharmacology and Uses

Several parts of the cotton plant have been or are still used in traditional medicine. In Ayurvedic medicine, root bark of *G. herbaceum* has been used as an emmenagogue and abortifacient, because of its uterine stimulant activities. The root also possesses slight narcotic action. The seeds are demulcent, laxative, expectorant, galactogogue and are used as a nervine tonic in headaches and brain affections. A decoction of the seed is given in dysentery and intermittent fevers. The oil is an embrocation for rheumatic diseases and dressing for herpes, scabies and wounds. A syrup of cotton flowers is given in hypochondriasis. A poultice of the leaves and seeds is applied to bruises, sores, swelling, burns and scalds [5,12,13]. The Chinese used cotton root bark for the treatment of chronic bronchitis and cough [6]. In homeopathy, preparations of *G. herbaceum* serve to treat several gynecological disorders [12,14].

Cottonseed oil is used in food products and pharmaceutically as a vehicle in injectable preparations. It is included in the Unites States Pharmacopeia [15]. Cottonseed oil emulsions have been given to humans as a source of energy or when a nitrogen-free diet was required [2]. The press cake of cotton seeds is used as a livestock feed [1].

Gossypol, isolated from cotton plants, has attracted particular interest since it was shown to exhibit an antifertility action in males. This activity was discovered by coincidence during the 1950s, when Chinese scientists associated a high prevalence of male infertility in several rural communes in China with the consumption of crude cottonseed oil, used for cooking purposes. Later it became clear that this effect was to be ascribed to gossypol [8,16].

Gossypol functions as a contraceptive, and has been studied for this purpose, especially in China. In men, the drug induces oligospermia or azoospermia and impairs sperm motility, resulting in infertility. In women, it causes amenorrhea and endometrical changes, which also render infertility. In addition, gossypol has been reported to be effective for the treatment of certain gynecological diseases, such as menorrhagia, leiomyona and endometrosis [1,8,17].

In China, clinical trials with racemic gossypol, administered orally to men, started in 1972. In several trials, an antifertility activity with an efficacy exceeding 99% was obtained by a loading dose of 20 mg per day for 60–70 days, followed by about 60 mg/week. This dose level is much smaller than the doses required for antifertility effects in most animal species, even in the most sensitive ones. The criterion used was a reduction of normal sperm concentration (40–250 × 10^6/ml) to less than 4 × 10^6/ml [6,9,17,18]. Despite its antispermatogenic activity after oral administration, it should be mentioned that it is difficult to inhibit spermatogenesis completely, and men have fathered children even with a sperm density as low as 1 × 10^6/ml [19]. The antifertility capacity of gossypol resides in the (−)-isomer. The (+)-form lacks this activity, but significantly contributes to the general toxic effects [20].

Among the first effects that are observed in the ejaculate after administration of gossypol are loss of sperm motility, gradual drop in sperm counts, an increase in malformed spermatozoa, ultrastructural abberations and the presence of immature, spermatogenic cells. Thus, spermatogenesis becomes dearranged [6,8].

The mechanism of antifertility action of gossypol is independent on the hormonal events of the hypothalamo-hypophyseal-gonadal axes. No effects on serum hormone levels have been found. The site of action appears to be local. Gossypol reduces the motility of the spermatocyte and affects several sperm enzymes. Particularly, energy producing enzymes are inhibited. Mitochondria are the cellular organelles of the spermatogenic cells that are most sensitive to gossypol. In these organelles, gossypol inhibits Na-K-ATP-ase and the sperm-specific enzyme lactate dehydrogenase-X (LDH-X), thereby disturbing the sperm-synthesizing capacity of the testes [21]. However, the latter effect, as the *in vivo* mechanism of antifertility action of gossypol, seems controversial, is it has been found that LDH-X was not inhibited in rats *in vivo*, but only *in vitro* [22]. In addition, gossypol affects the spermatid stages of the spermatogenesis, thus influencing sperm maturation. Further, enzymes that are involved in the fertilization process, such as acrosin, are inhibited. It has been reported than an effect on prostaglandins might participate in the antispermatogenic action of gossypol [6,8,9,17].

When incubated with ejaculates, at a concentration of 0.1 ng/ml, gossypol lowered sperm motility by 90%, thereby inhibiting the fertilizing capacity

[23]. Because of its direct effect on sperm cells, gossypol may be applied directly to the vagina, as a topical contraceptive.

Gossypol is cytotoxic to a wide range of human and animal tumor cell lines, grown *in vitro. In vivo,* mammary tumor growth in rats was inhibited. In addition, gossypol possesses antiviral and antitrypanosomal activity, an interferon-inducing effect and insecticidal properties [6,8,24,25]. In mice, a dose-related and selective depression of humoral immune response has been observed [26]. The (−)-enantiomer of gossypol has been shown to possess an inhibitory effect on human immunodeficiency virus (HIV) replication [27,28], and may be a potential drug for the treatment of AIDS (acquired immune deficiency syndrome) [29]. As gossypol induced a significant decrease in the body weight in experimental animals, it has been suggested that this compound might be used to treat obesity [6].

Pharmacokinetics

The apparent stereoselective action of gossypol may be due to dispositional or pharmacodynamic differences. After oral administration to rats, gossypol absorption from the gastrointestinal tract was slow and poor. The (+)-isomer was even absorbed slower than the (−)-form. In the case of (−)-gossypol, levels of the free form were higher in the heart, kidney, lungs and testes than of the (+)-isomer [30]. Most of the absorbed gossypol undergoes biotransformation in the liver and is excreted via the bile, probably as an iron complex, into the feces [6,9]. Only small amounts are found in the urine [31].

In rats and in dogs, the elimination half life of (+)-gossypol was much longer than of (−)-gossypol. This difference may be due to the lower rate of binding to tissue proteins of the (−)-isomer, since the volume of distribution of (−)-gossypol is much smaller than that of the (+)-isomer. The pharmacokinetics of the racemate were basically similar to those of (+)-gossypol [10,32].

The pharmacokinetics of gossypol in humans have only been documented recently. After oral administration, the elimination half life of the racemate was 286 h, of the (+)-isomer 133 h and of the (−)-isomer 4.6 h. Thus, the half life of (+)-gossypol was 29 times that of (−)-gossypol. The average peak plasma concentration, clearance and the AUC (area under the drug concentration – time curve) of (+)-gossypol were significantly greater than of the (−)-isomer [32]. Several weeks were needed to reach equilibrium conditions and only low concentrations have been found in peripheral tissues, such as the tests, where it takes a long time to build up appropriate concentrations [6]. Recall that the desired biological activity, viz. the antifertility effect, resides in the nonaccumulating (−)-isomer.

Introduced vaginally, gossypol has been designated potentially safe, because it was only slightly absorbed in the form of a gossypol-PVP (polyvinyl pyrolidon) tablet [8,17].

Adverse Reaction Profile

The toxic actions of gossypol can be summarized as follows [31,33]. Acute toxicity is characterized by circulatory failure and subacute toxicity by the formation of lung edema. Symptoms of chronic toxicity are feeling sick and undernourishment. Several compounds with structures similar to gossypol, such as gossypurpurin and gossyverdurin as well as their degradation products, are also toxic. Many side effects have been associated with impurities in the gossypol preparations used. Other pigments, found in cottonseed products (although in lower quantities) have been found to be more toxic than gossypol itself [31,33].

Gossypol possesses a stereoselective toxicity. A selective component causes the antispermatogenic effect (due to the (−)-isomer), and a nonselective component is responsible for the remaining tissue toxicity (mainly due to the (+)-isomer). Thus, by administration of the (−)-isomer a better therapeutic ratio may be achieved than with the racemate [10,16].

Gossypol is chemically reactive, easily oxidized, and photosensitive [6,7,11,16]. For proper testing, pure, stabilized gossypol should be used. When orally administered, interactions with other compounds or with the diet, should be prevented. In the studies done so far, these requirements have not always been met [6].

The two aldehyde groups of gossypol can easily bind to proteins, via aldehyde-amino group linkage. This feature may be the basis of nonspecific biological responses to the drug. In addition, biological systems that require a divalent cation for their activity may be inhibited due to its chelating capacity and gossypol may become deactivated due to chelate formation [6]. Gossypolone, the *in vivo* oxidation product of gossypol that also possesses a spermicidal effect, may form a redox system with its corresponding hemiquinone, resulting in free radical generation. Free radicals may cause cellular alterations that ultimately lead to tissue damage. Racemic gossypol stimulated free radical formation when incubated with either rat liver or kidney microsomes, but not with those of the heart or testes [9,10].

In order to overcome the adverse effects of gossypol (see below), a number of derivatives and metal chelates have been prepared, but none of these compounds seemed better than gossypol, although gossypol formic acid had been said to possess fewer side effects than gossypol and gossypol acetic acid [9,10]. A lower dosage of gossypol (e.g. 15 mg/day) is currently under re-evaluation [34].

General Animal Data

Cottonseeds are a by-product of cotton production and have been used as a feed supplement for livestock, because of their richness in proteins. Animals, however, often became intoxicated and died. High dietary levels of gossypol, >0.18%, are known to be toxic to ruminants, but even very low levels, <0.04%, have been reported to be toxic to young calves and lambs [35]. Swine, poultry and dogs are most sensitive to the toxic effects of a cottonseed meal [36]. Intoxicated animals showed difficulty in breathing and became lethargic due to muscular weakness. Frequently, a froth was seen in the mouth. The cardiovascular system became compromised and edema developed. Just prior to death, generalized convulsions and cyanosis were seen. Autopsy showed edema of the lungs and liver, venous congestion, myocarditis, liver necrosis, nephritis, hemmorrhagic areas with lesions in the intestine, and gastroenteritis.

After administration of gossypol, the signs of toxicity are quite similar to those of cottonseed intoxication. Death is usually caused by pulmonary edema or circulatory failure and damage to liver and kidneys has been found [6]. Cardiotoxicity was observed in experimental gossypol intoxication of dogs with gossypol. The cardiotoxicity was attributed to an effect on the endothelium of the heart and to myocardial changes. In addition, axonal fragmentation, demyelination of peripheral nerves and degeneration of cerebellar neurons was revealed [37].

Toxicosis caused by gossypol, due to prolonged feeding of cottonseed meals to animals is believed to be a result of several events. Gossypol binds to amino acids, particularly lysine, thereby making lysine unavailable for protein synthesis and ultimately leading to hypoproteinemia and severe edema. Due to chelation of iron in the gastrointestinal tract and in the liver, iron deficiency is caused. Furthermore, gossypol inhibits the release of oxygen from hemoglobin. Finally, still poorly understood effects on membranes and specific enzymes, such as inhibition of adenosine triphosphatase, oxidative phosphorylation, and electron transport, have been reported [36].

The response to gossypol with respect to its antifertility action as well as to its toxicological effects in animals is species- and in some cases strain-dependent. Rats, hamsters and monkeys are far more tolerant to gossypol than dogs, guinea pigs and rabbits. In rats minor lesions occur in the liver, heart and kidneys at doses exceeding those necessary for antifertility action. Monkeys are tolerant to the toxic effects of gossypol, but only moderately sensitive to its antispermatogenic action. In dogs lethal liver and heart damage (myocardial necrosis) occur at doses that do not have an antispermatogenic effect. Rabbits are sensitive to the toxic, but not to the antispermatogenic effect. Generally, a low therapeutic index has been found [6,9,16].

A decrease in weight of animals has been reported after administration of (+)- and (±)-gossypol. The effect was larger with the racemate than with the (+)-isomer. In rats, gossyverdurin was more toxic than gossypol [6].

It has been found that (+)-gossypol possesses lower acute toxicity than (−)-gossypol following intraperitoneal administration to mice [20]. However, the elimination half life of the (+)-isomer is much longer than that of the (−)-isomer, so that subchronic toxicity testing of both isomers may show a different picture. No experimental data have been recovered on this point.

General Human Data

The most important disadvantages of gossypol are its slow onset of action and the risks of sterility and hypokalemia, all being more or less related to the dosage schedule [32].

A high percentage of side effects has been reported in humans, although generally mild and sometimes subjective. Side effects included changes in appetite, dryness of the mouth, fatigue, diarrhea, elevation of serum glutamic pyruvic acid transaminase (SGPT) levels, tendency to sleepiness, edema, dyspnea, neuritis and loss of libido. A significant decrease of serum potassium levels has been found at the time fatigue occurred [38].

In a Chinese clinical study reporting on the effects after long-term administration (6–10 years) of gossypol acetic acid to a group of 32 men [39], SGPT levels were found to be increased in a few cases. This effect persisted for more than a year. In addition, the positive rate of Et formation of peripheral blood lymphocytes was remarkably decreased and after cessation of the therapy for 6–12 months, it had still not returned to normal. Also, serum IgG levels were decreased. The shorter the duration of gossypol administration, the higher the sperm recovery rate was. It would therefore be advisable, according to the authors, that the duration of the drug intake should not exceed 2 years, in order to avoid infertility.

During the intravenous infusion of cottonseed oil emulsions, dyspnea, cyanosis, myalgia, nausea, vomiting headache, lumbar pains, flushing and hypotension have been reported. Patients receiving the emulsions over prolonged periods may exhibit the "overload syndrome", manifested by bone-marrow depression, anemia, thrombocytopenia, thrombotic episodes, jaundice, and persistent hyperlipidemia. The effects are reversible on discontinuing the infusion [40].

After parenteral administration of gossypol, edema, irritation and inflammatory reactions occur at the site of injection [6].

Dermatological Reactions

Cotton dust and cotton bracts may evoke an anti-inflammatory stimulus to the human skin [41]. Exposure of the face, hands and other parts of the body to gossypol-containing cottonseed oil may cause a local burning sensation. These symptoms, called "burning fever", have also been observed after consumption of the oil [8].

Gastrointestinal Reactions

After oral administration, gossypol may have serious effects on the gastrointestinal tract, most frequently when the drug is administered over a longer period of time. Tissue congestion, mucosal sloughing, necrosis of the mucosa and hemorrhage of the intestinal wall may lead to anorexia and weight loss [6]. Some persons taking gossypol experienced transient nausea, loss of appetite and diarrhea [19]. In order to overcome these side effects, enteric coated tablets have been used in a Chinese clinical trial. Both the systemic side effects and the antifertility activity were much less than with ordinary tablets [9].

Oral administration of gossypol acetic acid to male rats, 10 mg/kg body weight/day for 15 days, caused a significant reduction in the uptake of glucose, alanine, leucine and calcium in the small intestine. It also interfered with enzyme systems involved in the digestion, such as sucrase, lactase, maltase and alkaline phosphatase [42].

Hepatic Reactions

After administration, gossypol is preferentially distributed to the liver. From animal studies, it has become clear that gossypol and its derivatives are capable of causing damage to liver cells, including necrosis and increased serum liver enzymes [37].

In rats, prolongation of the pentobarbital sleeping time, increase of SGPT level, decrease of the cytochrome P-450 and glutathione contents in the liver, inhibition of the liver metabolizing enzymes cytochrome-C-reductase, aminopyrine-N-demethylase, aniline hydroxylase, catechol-O-transferase, α-naphthylacetate esterase, catalase and glutathione-S-transferase, as well as induction of the activity of β-glucuronidase have been found. These findings suggest that gossypol can inhibit hepatic detoxification mechanisms. Reactive oxygen species, such as the superoxide anion radical and hydrogen peroxide may be generated, resulting in lipid peroxidation as well as inhibition of calcium sequestration in microsomes. In addition, damage to structure of liver cells has been found in electron microscopical studies. Gossypol could irreversibly bind to microsomal proteins [17,43,44].

The gossypol-induced liver toxicity is likely to limit the human use of this compound [17], although no literature data have been found to support this.

Metabolic Reactions

Fatigue and muscular weakness may be the prodromal symptoms of a subsequent hypokalemic paralytic attack [38]. Hypokalemia is a serious side effect and a major reason for concern. It has been the most important stumbling block to the general application of gossypol as an infertility agent. The effect is due to renal potassium loss. The mechanism is not clear as yet but has been associated with adrenal suppressive actions of gossypol and with inhibition of mitochondrial Na-K-ATP-ase. It has been reported by several authors that supplementation with a potassium salt causes prompt and complete recovery [2,6,8,9,38]. From a controlled, randomized study, however, it appeared that supplementation with a potassium salt, while using gossypol, did not cause a reversal of the effect of gossypol on serum potassium levels, and the potassium blocking agent triamterene did not prevent loss of serum potassium [45].

Pulmonary Reactions

Gossypol inhibited the myotropic activity of lung parenchyma of guinea-pigs *in vitro* and appeared to be a potent inhibitor of leukotriene- and PAF-acether-induced contractions. It has been suggested that gossypol may influence the arachidonic acid metabolism in the lung by interfering with the formation of cyclo-oxygenase products [46].

Inhalation of cotton bracts or dust may cause bronchial hyperresponsiveness in humans and has been associated with the lung disease, byssinosis. Symptoms are wheezing, chest thightness, shortness of breath and reversible changes in lung functions. This type of airway hyperresponsiveness is probably ascribed to inflammatory processes [41]. Inhalation of seeds of *G. herbaceum* may cause hay fever and asthma [12].

Drug Interactions

The absorption of orally given gossypol is disturbed by bivalent cations and proteins, influencing both the toxic and pharmacologic effects. In the development of a gossypol formulation, this has been a serious problem [6].

Because gossypol is a potent inhibitor of the hepatic microsomal drug system *in vivo,* the function of hepatic drug metabolizing enzymes may be decreased [44]. See also the section on hepatic reactions.

Fertility, Pregnancy and Lactation

In rats, slight damage has been found in the germinal epithelium of the testes after oral administration of 30 mg/kg/day of (+)-gossypol for 4 weeks [20]. A single intratesticular injection of 200 μg (−)-gossypol caused a 70% decrease of sperm count, along with marked atrophy of the testes. The (+)-isomer caused neither decrease in sperm count, nor atrophy [10].

Histological and histochemical studies in rats, that were given gossypol acetic acid orally for a longer period, revealed changes in the corpus epididymis. The tubular lumen became narrowed with thickened pseudostratified epithelium, and a reduction of the amount of spermatozoa was found. There was an increase in esterase, alkaline phosphatase, acid phosphatase and ATP-ase activity. These changes increased in intensity with the duration of the treatment [47].

In mice, gossypol was not teratogenic, but could interfere with fetal implantation and it possessed embryocidal effects at high doses, which were also toxic to the dams [26]. Embryocidal effects have also been found in rats after administration of gossypol, in the range of 25–100 mg/kg/day [48]. In rats, a small number of malformed fetuses was found after intraperitoneal administration of 10 mg/kg cottonseed oil, whereas 5 mg/kg did not reveal teratogenic effects [49]. It is not clear from this study whether the cottonseed oil used contained gossypol.

Based on another study with rats, it was suggested that gossypol may damage genetic material. Gossypol-treated males were allowed to mate with untreated female animals, at several time points after gossypol treatment. The ratio of dead fetuses to the number of implantation sites, determined on the 13th day of pregnancy, was significantly higher for the gossypol-treated animals than for the untreated animals. The effect, however, was transient, as it decreased with the length of the post-regimen period [9]. Gossypol has been shown to exhibit anti-implantation and pregnancy-interrupting actions in rats [50].

Bovine embryos, cultured with different concentrations of gossypol acetic acid, revealed a dose-dependent detrimental action of this compound on early embryo development and suggested a direct action on the embryo itself [37].

It is not clear whether these effects are mediated by the parent compound or its metabolites, or whether these findings have any clinical relevance [26]. There is no evidence so far that routinely used clinical dosages affect genetic material in humans [9].

In women, gossypol causes amenorrhea and endometrical changes, resulting in infertility. After gossypol withdrawal, menstruation is resumed [17]. Because of its antiprogesterone and anticorpus luteum activity, gossypol may cause abortion in pregnant women [33]. Decreased libido and impotence in men have been observed in individual cases [9,40].

In men, normal sperm density is generally restored within several months after cessation of the anticonceptive therapy with gossypol, although it may remain suppressed for a longer period. Even permanent suppression of sperm counts may occur after cessation of therapy and should be regarded as a major disadvantage of gossypol. The persistence of oligospermia is strongly related to the magnitude of the doses and the duration of the gossypol therapy [9,19,32].

In a Chines study [51], the degree and time of recovery of spermatogenesis was followed in 46 men, after cessation of gossypol administration. Usually, a loading dose of 20 mg/day had been given for 8–11 weeks, followed by a maintenance dose of 50 mg/week. The duration of gossypol treatment ranged from 0.6–9.2 years and the cumulative dose from 2.5–27.5 g. At the time of cessation, 87% of the men were azoospermic. After a median recovery time of 1.1 years, 61% had recovered to sperm counts of $\geqslant 20 \times 10^6$/ml. After a median follow-up period of 1.9 years, 39% had still not recovered to this threshold and of these 39%, 22% remained azoospermic.

In 19 men, 3–10 years after cessation of gossypol treatment and 2–9 years after recovery of normal sperm density, it appeared that sperm function was still lower compared with a non-treated control group [52]. This may have been a result of persistent gossypol-mediated damage to the testes. In response to Sertoli cell damage, an increased amount of follicle stimulating hormone (FSH) is released. In the treated group, blood FSH levels were indeed significantly enhanced.

Mutagenicity and Carcinogenicity

Gossypol has been tested in the Ames *Salmonella*-microsomal test in order to determine whether the drug exerts its contraceptive or toxic effects by interaction with genetic material. No mutagenic effects have been found in five standard test strains of *Salmonella typhimurium,* either with or without the inclusion of rat liver metabolic enzyme fractions [9,53].

At concentrations of 1, 5 and 10 μg/ml, gossypol did not induce chromosome breakage in cultured Chinese hamster cells, with and without the presence of a metabolic activation system (rat liver S9 mix). In human lymphocyte cultures neither an increase in the frequention of chromosome breakage, nor polyploidy has been found [54]. However, gossypol-induced chromosomal aberrations and mutagenicity in mice have been reported [55].

Gossypol induced a dose-related increase of DNA strand breaks in human skin fibroblasts *in vitro,* at concentrations of 5–40 μg/ml. These breaks may be ascribed to a direct interaction with cellular DNA. As gossypol is readily oxidized to the hemiquinone gossypolone, a redox system is formed, in which free radicals are generated that may damage the DNA indirectly [56].

In mice skin-painting tests, gossypol showed tumor-inducing and tumor-promoting properties. Other data on the possible carcinogenicity of gossypol are not available [9].

References

1. Evans WC (1989) Trease and Evans' Pharmacognosy, 13th edn. London: Ballière Tindall, pp 346, 519–520
2. Reynolds JEF, Parfitt K, Parsons AV, Sweetman SC (ed) (1989) Martindale The Extra Pharmacopoeia. 29th edn. London: The Pharmaceutical Press, pp 1561, 1576

3. Frohne D, Jensen U (1979) Systematik des Pflanzenreichs, 2. Aufl. Stuttgart, New York: Gustav Fischer Verlag, pp 137–138
4. Hegnauer R (1969) Chemosystematik der Pflanzen. Band 5. Basle: Birkhäuser Verlag, pp 29–46
5. Anonymous (1956) The Wealth of India. A Dictionary of Indian Raw Materials and Industrial Products. Vol. IV. New Delhi: Council of Scientific & Industrial Research, pp 170–251
6. Waller DP, Zaveveld LJD, Farnsworth NR (1985) Gossypol: pharmacology and current status as a male contraceptive. In: Wagner H, Hikino H, Farnsworth NR (ed) Economic and Medicinal Plant Research. London: Academic Press, pp 87–112
7. Wang MZ (1987) Analysis of gossypol by high performance liquid chromatography. J Ethnopharmacol 20:1–11
8. Wu DF (1989) An overview of the clinical pharmacology and therapeutic potential of gossypol as a male contraceptive agent and in gynaecological disease. Drugs 38:333–341
9. Qian SZ, Wang ZG (1984) Gossypol: a potential antifertility agent for males. Ann Rev Pharmacol Toxicol 24:329–360
10. Yu YW (1987) Probing into the mechanism of action, metabolism and toxicity of gossypol by studying its (+)- and (−)-stereoisomers. J Ethnopharmacol 20:65–78
11. Huang L, Zheng DK, Si YK (1987) Resolution of racemic gossypol. J Ethnopharmacol 20:13–20
12. Madaus G (1938) Lehrbuch der biologischen heilmittel. Band II. Leipzig: Georg Thieme Verlag, pp 1477–1480
13. Kapoor LD (1990) Handbook of Ayurvedic Medicinal Plants. Boca Raton: CRC Press, p 198
14. Wiesenauer M (1989) Homöopathie für Apotheker und Ärzte. Stuttgart: Deutscher Apotheker Verlag, pp 3/78, 4/56
15. Anonymous (1990) The United States Pharmacopeia XXII / The National Formulary XVII. Rockville: Unites States Pharmacopeial Convention, pp 1737, 1921
16. Anonymous (1984) Gossypol prospects. Lancet I, 1108–1109
17. Max B (1984) Cafetaria contraception in China: some pharmacological novelties. TIPS 5:362–363
18. National Coordinating Group on Male Antifertility Agents (1978) Gossypol – a new antifertility agent for males. Chin Med J 91:417–428
19. Wilson JD (1990) Androgens. In: Gilman AG, Rall TW, Nies AS, Taylor P (ed) Goodman and Gilman's The Pharmacological Basis of Therapeutics. 8th edn. New York: Pergamon Press, pp 1413–1430
20. Wang NG, Zhou Guan MH, Lei HP (1987) Effect of (−)- and (+)-gossypol on fertility in male rats. J Ethnopharmacol 20:21–24
21. Lee CY, Malling HV (1981) Selective inhibition of sperm-specific lactate dehydrogenase-X by an antifertility agent, gossypol. Fed Proc 40:718
22. Yao KQ, Gu QM, Lei HP (1987) Effect of (±)-, (+)- and (−)-gossypol on the lactate dehydrogenase-X activity in rat testis. J Ethnopharmacol 20:25–29
23. Ridley AJ, Blasco L (1981) Testosterone and gossypol effects on human sperm motility. Fertil Steril 36:638–642
24. Montamat EE, Burgos C, De Burgos NMG, Rovari LE, Blanco A, Segura EL (1982) Inhibitory action of gossypol on enzymes and growth of *Trypanosoma cruzi*. Science 218:288–289
25. Wichman K, Vaheri A, Luukkainen T (1982) Inhibitory herpes simplex virus type-2 infection in human epithelial cells by gossypol, a potent spermicidal and contraceptive agent. Am J Obstet Gynecol 142:593–594
26. Sein GM, Phil M (1986) The embryotoxic and immunodepressive effects of gossypol. Am J Chin Med 14:110–115
27. Lin TS, Shinozi R, Griffith B, August EM, Eriksson BFH, Zhang DK, Huang L, Prosoff WH (1989) Selective inhibition of human immunodeficiency virus type 1 replication by the (−)- but not the (+)-enantiomer of gossypol. Antimicrob Agents Chemother 33:2149–2151

28. Polsky B, Segal SJ, Baron PA, Gold JNM, Ueno H, Armstrong D (1989) Inactivation of human immunodeficiency virus *in vitro* by gossypol. Contraception 39:579–587
29. Vlietinck AJ, Vanden Berghe DA (1991) Can ethnopharmacology contribute to the development of antiviral drugs? J Ethnopharmacol 32:141–153
30. Chen QQ, Chen H, Lei HP (1987) Comparative study on the metabolism of optical gossypol in rats. J Ethnopharmacol 20:31–37
31. Abou-Donia MB (1976) Physiological effect and metabolism of gossypol. Res Rev 61:125–161
32. Wu DF, Yu YW, Tang ZM, Wang MZ (1986) Pharmacokinetics of (±)-, (+)-, and (−)-gossypol in humans and dogs. Clin Pharmacol Ther 39:613–618
33. Steinegger E, Hänsel R (1988) Lehrbuch der Pharmakognosie und Phytopharmazie. 4. Aufl. Berlin: Springer-Verlag, pp 55, 101
34. Xiao PG, Wang NG (1991) Can ethnopharmacology contribute to the development of antifertility drugs? J Ethnopharmacol 32:167–177
35. Morgan SE (1989) Gossypol as a toxicant in livestock. Vet Clin North Am Food Anim Pract 5:251–262
36. Haschek WM, Beasley VR, Buck WB, Finnell JH (1989) Cottonseed meal (gossypol) toxicosis in a swine herd. J Am Vet Med Assoc 195:613–615
37. Patton CS, Legendre AM, Gompf RE, Walker MA (1985) Heart failure caused by gossypol poisoning in two dogs. J Am Vet Med Assoc 195:625–627
38. Liu GZ, Ch'iu Lyle K, Cao J (1987) Clinical trial of gossypol as a male contraceptive drug. Part I. Efficacy study. Fertil Steril 48:459–461
39. Duo X, Cai WJ, Zhu BH, Dong CJ, Zheng ZC, Gao ZQ (1988) Clinical safety of long-term administration of gossypol in 32 cases. Contraception 37:129–135
40. Reynolds JEF, Prasad AB (ed) (1982) Martindale The Extra Pharmacopoeia. 28th edn. London: The Pharmaceutical Press, p 696
41. Witek Jr JT, Mazzara CA, Zuskin E, Beck GJ, Buck MG, Schachter EN (1988) Bronchial responsiveness after inhalation of cotton bark extract. Am Rev Respir Dis 138:1579–1583
42. Chadha S, Sanyal SN, Kanwar U (1988) Effects of gossypol acetic acid on the absorptive and digestive functions of rat intestine. Biochem Int 17:1117–1133
43. Wang Y, Lei HP (1987) Hepatotoxicity of gossypol in rats. J Ethnopharmacol 20:53–64
44. Johansen RL, Misra HP (1990) Effects of gossypol on the hepatic drug metabolizing system in rats. Contraception 42:683–690
45. Liu GZ, Ch'iu-Hinton K, Cao JA, Zhu CX, Li BY (1988) Effects of K salts or a potassium blocker on gossypol-related hypokalemia. Contraception 37:111–117
46. Touvay C, Vilain B, Sirois P, Soufir M, Braquet P (1987) Gossypol: a potent inhibitor of PAF-acether- and leukotriene-induced contractions of guinea pig lung parenchyma strips. J Pharm Pharmacol 39:454–458
47. Zhou LF, Qi SQ, Lei HP (1987) Effect of gossypol acetic acid on the epididymis: histochemical and scanning electron microscope studies. J Ethnopharmacol 20: 39–43
48. Barcellona PS, Campana A, De Martino C (1984) The embryotoxicity of gossypol in the rat. IRCS Med Sci 12:19–20
49. Singh AR, Lawrence WH, Autian J (1972) Teratogenicity of phthalate esters in rats. J Pharm Sci 61:51–55
50. Wang NG, Guan MZ, Lei HP (1987) Effect of gossypol acetic acid on rat luteal cell *in vitro*. J Ethnopharmacol 20:45–51
51. Meng GD, Zhu JC, Chen ZW, Wong LT, Zhang GY, Hu YZ, Ding JH, Wang XH, Qian SZ, Wang C, Manchin D, Pinol A, Waites GMH (1988) Recovery of sperm production following the cessation of gossypol treatment: a two-centre study in China. Int J Androl 11:1–11
52. Zhong CQ, Lui QL, Tang YJ, Wang Y, Shi FJ, Qian SZ (1990) Study on sperm function in men long after cessation of gossypol treatment. Contraception 41:617–622
53. De Peyster A, Wang YY (1979) Gossypol – Proposed contraceptive for men passes the Ames test. New Eng J Med 301:275–276

54. Liang JC, Ye WS (1985) Clastogenicity of a male contraceptive, gossypol, in mammalian cell cultures with and without the metabolic activation by S9 mix. Environ Res 36:138–143
55. Yang YH, Sheih SP (1982) Studies on the gossypol effect on chromosome aberration and SCE in mice. Acta Anat Sin 13:215–250
56. Nordenskjöld M, Lambert M (1984) Gossypol induces DNA strand breaks in human fibroblasts and sister chromatid exchanges in human lymphocytes *in vitro*. J Med Genet 21:129–132

Hedera Helix

P.A.G.M. De Smet

Botany

Hedera helix L. (family Araliaceae) is cultivated in many parts of the world as an ornamental plant. The leaves are also used for medicinal purposes. Vernacular names are ivy (E); Efeu or Eppig (G); and lierre commun or lierre grimpant (F) [1,2]. The term ivy refers mainly to three subspecies of *H. helix*, namely ssp. *helix*, ssp. *canariensis*, and ssp. *poetarum*. The subspecies *helix* is generally known as common ivy or English ivy. The ssp. *canariensis* is sometimes presented in the literature as a separate species, *H. canariensis* Willd. It is named Canary Island ivy in Great Britain and Algerian ivy in the United States [3–5]. Its variety *variegata* is known as variegated Algerian ivy [6].

Many other plants are called ivies without being related to *Hedera* plants [3]. A notable example is the poison ivy, *Toxicodendron radicans*, which belongs to the Anacardiaceae [5].

Chemistry

The leaves of *H. helix* contain saponins which have either hederagenin or oleanolic acid as their aglycone [7–12]. Wagner and Reger [9] found hederacoside C, hederacoside B, α-hederin and hederasaponin X as genuine saponins. The total level in dried leaves ranged from 25 to 57 mg/g with hederacoside C as the major saponin (up to 48 mg/g). Analysis of trade samples of ivy extracts showed that hederacoside C may partially hydrolyse during preparation and/or storage of commercial products. Elias and coworkers [12,13] have isolated and identified several other hederasaponins from the leaves of *H. helix*.

According to Mayer et al. [10], particularly high levels of saponins occur in the fruits of ivy. Hostettmann [14] isolated four triterpenoid saponins from the fresh berries and identified all of them as hederagenin glycosides.

Adverse Effects of Herbal Drugs, Vol. 2
(ed. by P.A.G.M. De Smet, K. Keller, R. Hänsel, R.F. Chandler)

An Egyptian research group reported the presence of the alkaloid emetine in four Egyptian varieties of *H. helix* (var. *baltica*, var. *hibernica*, var. *marginata* and var. *erecta*) [15]. Subsequently, minor amounts of emetine and cephaeline were recovered from European samples in an Austrian study [10].

The leaves of *H. helix* (ssp. *helix* and ssp. *canariensis*) contain the allergenic principles falcarinol and didehydrofalcarinol. These polyacetylenic compounds show remarkable variation in concentration and ratio, depending on such factors as the time of collection [5,16]. Gafner et al. [6] assessed the falcarinol content in the stems (with petioles) of three common varieties of ivy and recovered 0.8–2.7 mg/g from English ivy, 0.6–1.4 mg/g from Algerian ivy and 1.6 mg/g from variegated Algerian ivy. Additional polyacetylenes isolated from *H. helix* are falcarinone, an oxidation product of falcarinol [17], and the unstable 11,12-dehydrofalcarinol [6].

The leaves of *H. helix* also contain germacrene B and β-elemene [18], and rutin has been demonstrated in juvenile twigs [19].

Pharmacology and Uses

Ivy leaf extracts are used in respiratory diseases, such as bronchitis and influenza, because of their reputed expectorant, secretolytic, and spasmolytic properties [2,5,9,10]. One brand preparation is even standardised on its spasmolytic effect on the isolated ileum of the guinea pig: 1 g of standardised extract should have the same activity as 10 mg of papaverine [10]. Ivy leaf extracts are also incorporated into topical preparations, e.g., for the treatment of cellulitis [5,11].

Lanza et al. [1] tested aqueous extracts from ivy seeds *in vivo* and *in vitro*. They observed a transient fall in arterial blood pressure after intravenous administration to rats and a biphasic response (spasmolysis followed by spasmogenesis) in isolated rat intestine.

Saponins from *H. helix* have been reported to show antibacterial effects against Gram-positive and Gram-negative bacteria [20,21], antifungal activity against *Candida albicans* or dermatophytes [20,22,23], antileishmanial effects [24], and anthelminthic activity against the liver flukes of sheep [22,25]. Antimutagenic properties not due to bactericidal or bacteriostatic action [26], antitumor effects [27] and antimitotic activity [28] have also been described.

Hostettmann [14] compared the molluscicidal effects of different ivy extracts and found that a crude leaf extract was less active than a crude methanolic extract of the berries. He isolated four saponins from the berries, all of which showed a strong molluscicidal action against the bilharziasis-transmitting snail *Biomphalaria glabrata*.

Pharmacokinetics

It is assumed in the literature that hederasaponins are poorly absorbed following oral administration [29]. Some evidence in support of this assertion comes from experiments by Vogel and Marek [30] who found a more than 7.7-fold difference between the i.v. and p.o. LD_{50}-values of saponin from the leaf of *H. helix* in the rat.

Adverse Reaction Profile

General Animal Data

Lanza et al. [1] studied the acute oral toxicity of several ivy extracts in rats. A hydroalcoholic extract from the seeds (2.8–4.7 g/kg) produce apathy, diarrhoea, hemorrhage and death, whereas hydroalcoholic extracts from the leaves (3.0–4.1 g/kg) or from the fresh berries deprived of their seeds (2.8 g/kg) merely produced diarrhoea. Diarrhoea was also the only symptom when an aqeuous extract from the seed (3.0–3.9 g/kg) was given, and no effects were seen with an aqueous extract from the berries (3.0 g/kg).

Vogel and Marek [30] found LD_{50}-values of 13 mg/kg i.v. and >100 mg/kg p.o. for saponin from the leaf of *H. helix* in rats. Timon-David et al. [23] reported oral LD_{50} values for α-hederin and hederacoside C of >4 g/kg in the mouse. For α-hederin, they established an intraperitoneal LD_{50} in the mouse of 1.8 g/kg.

General Human Data

As far as is known, major side effects have not been observed in clinical studies on standardised ivy leaf preparations [10]. Toxic effects due to the presence of emetine and cephaeline are unlikely, in view of the low concentrations isolated [10]. There is only one clinical report on poisoning by ivy leaf. This case involved a 3.5-year-old boy, who presented with mild delirium alternating with stupor, clonic convulsions, visual hallucinations, convulsions, intense scarlet-like rash, rapid pulse, dilated pupils and raised temperature following the consumption of a considerable amount of leaves of the ordinary common ivy. His symptoms subsided following gastric lavage [31].

The berries of ivy are considered poisonous, especially for children [3]. Their ingestion may lead to nausea, diarrhoea and vomiting [10], and fatal intoxications were reported in the 19th century [1]. Two or three berries may be sufficient to induce gastric spasms, vomiting, facial reddening and somnolence in small children [29].

Allergic Reactions

See the section on dermatological reactions.

Dermatological Reactions

H. helix is a powerful irritant and, to a lesser degree, a contact sensitizer [5]. According to Goldman et al. [32], ivy may cause dermatitis not only from its leaves and stems but also from its roots. Over the years, at least 60 ivy-induced cases of irritant or allergic contact dermatitis have been described, most of which developed after ivy pruning [5,33]. The reaction may be sufficiently severe to warrant hospitalization [4]. In at least ten cases, positive patch tests with negative results in controls suggested an allergic reaction to *Hedera* plants, e.g., *H. helix* ssp. *helix* or *H. helix* ssp. *canariensis* [3–5,33–36]. After Roed-Petersen [34] had observed four patients with positive reactions to ivy, she tested 138 consecutive patients and found three more positive reactions.

Hausen et al. [5] identified the poylacetylenic compounds falcarinol and didehydrofalcarinol as the major allergens in ivy. The former substance is the main sensitizer, giving positive reactions at a test concentration as low as 0.3 mg/g. It has also irritating properties. Didehydrofalcarinol elicited a positive reaction in part of ivy-sensitive test subjects at a concentration of 10 mg/g. Gafner et al. [6] performed a human maximization test with falcarinol. In this test, ten of twenty subjects became sensitized to 10 mg/g, with seven of these reacting to only 0.5 mg/g. Gafner and colleagues [6] also recovered an additional allergen from *Hedera*, viz. 11,12-dehydrofalcarinol. The allergenic potency of this unstable compound was slightly lower than that of falcarinol. Hansen et al. [37] did not obtain positive reactions to falcarindiol, falcarinone or dehydrofalcarinone in a patient allergic to falcarinol.

Falcarinol can be found in cosmetics containing ivy extracts. Although its concentration in these products may be too low to induce contact allergy during usage, it cannot be excluded that its level might be sufficient to elicit an allergic response in patients with a pre-existing ivy allergy [5].

Falcarinol also occurs in various other plants, such as *Panax ginseng*, *Daucus carota* and *Schefflera arboricola* [37–39]. It has also been found in celery roots in concentrations ranging from less than 0.02 mg/g to 1.4 mg/g. The highest levels were recovered from celery plants that had been grown in *Fusarium* infected soil [6].

Ocular Reactions

Saponin from the leaf of *H. helix* produced irritation of the rabbit eye at a minimal concentration of 1:10000 in a physiological salt solution [30].

Fertility, Pregnancy and Lactation

Pant et al. [40] reported that nepalins (i.e., hederagenin glycosides occurring in the inflorescence of *Hedera nepalensis*) have an immobilizing effect on human spermatozoa.

No data have been recovered from the literature concerning the effects of *H. helix* on fertility or concerning its effects during pregnancy or lactation.

Mutagenicity and Carcinogenicity

No data concerning mutagenicity or carcinogenicity have been recovered from the literature, except for the finding that α-hederin and two other saponins isolated from the dried leaves of *H. helix* did not show mutagenicity in the *Salmonella typhimurium* tester strain TA98 with or without the presence of S9 mix [26].

References

1. Lanza JP, Steinmetz MD, Pellegrin E, Mourgue M (1980) Actions toxique et pharmacodynamique sur le rat d'extraits de lierre grimpant (*Hedera helix* L.). Plant Med Phytothér 14:221–229
2. Willuhn G (1989) Efeublätter. In: Wichtl M (ed.) (1989) Teedrogen. Ein Handbuch für die Praxis auf wissenschaftlicher Grundlage. 2. Auflage. Stuttgart: Wissenschaftliche Verlagsgesellschaft, pp 139–141
3. Dorsey CS (1957) Contact dermatitis from Algerian ivy. AMA Arch Dermatol 75:671–675
4. Boyle J, Harman RMH (1985) Contact dermatitis to Hedera helix (common ivy). Contact Dermatitis 12:111–112
5. Hausen BM, Bröhan J, König WA, Faasch H, Hahn H, Bruhn G (1987) Allergic and irritant contact dermatitis from falcarinol and didehydrofalcarinol in common ivy (*Hedera helix* L.). Contact Dermatitis 17:1–9
6. Gafner F, Epstein W, Reynolds G, Rodriguez E (1988) Human maximization test of falcarinol, the principal contact allergen of English ivy and Algerian ivy (*Hedera helix*, *H. canariensis*). Contact Dermatitis 19:125–128
7. Tschesche R, Schmidt W, Wulff G (1965) Reindarstellung und Strukturermittlung der Saponine des Efeus (*Hedera helix* L.) Z Naturforsch 20b:708–709
8. Kartnig T, Wegschaider O, Ri CY (1972) Ein Beitrag zur Bestimmung von Saponinen in Drogen. Planta Med 21:29–34
9. Wagner H, Reger H (1986) Folium Hederae-Extrakte. HPLC-Analyse. Dtsch Apoth Ztg 126:2613–2617
10. Mayer H, Pfandl A, Grigorieff A, Zickner I (1987) Efeu – eine alte Kult-und Heilpflanze. Pharm Ztg 132:2673–2676
11. Maffei Facino R, Carini M, Bonadeo P (1990) Efficacy of topically applied Hedera helix L. saponins for treatment of liposclerosis (so-called "cellulitis"). Acta Therap 16:337–349
12. Elias R, Diaz Lanza AM, Vidal-Ollivier E, Balansard G, Faure R, Babadjamian A (1991) Triterpenoid saponins from the leaves of *Hedera helix*. J Nat Prod 54:98–103
13. Babadjamian A, Elias R, Faure R, Vidal-Ollivier E, Balansard G (1988) Two-dimensional studies of triterpenoid glycosides. ^{1}H and ^{13}C NMR assignments

of hederasaponin C [3-O-α-L-rhamnopyranosyl-(1→2)-α-L-arabinopyranosyl-hederagenin 28-O-α-L-rhamnopyranosyl-(1→4)-β-D-glucopyranosyl-(1→6)-β-D-glucopyranosyl ester]. Spectrosc Lett 21:565–573
14. Hostettmann K (1980) Saponins with molluscicidal activity from *Hedera helix* L. Helv Chim Acta 63:606–609
15. Mahran GH, Hilal SH, El-Alfy TS (1975) The isolation and characterisation of emetine alkaloid from Hedera helix. Planta Med 27:127–132
16. Boll PM, Hansen L (1987) On the presence of falcarinol in Araliaceae. Phytochemistry 26:2955–2956
17. Bohlmann F, Arndt C, Bornowski H, Kleine K-M (1961) Über Polyine aus der Familie der Umbelliferen. Chem Ber 94:958–967
18. Bernardi R, Cardani C, Ghiringhelli D, Selva A (1970) Sull'isolamento del germacrene B, del β-elemene e di altri componenti minori dalle foglie di *Hedera helix*. Chim Ind 52:581–582
19. Tronchet J (1964) Mise en évidence d'une dorsiventralité biochimique des rameaux juvéniles de *Hedera helix* (Étude par chromatographie sur papier). C R Acad Sci 258(8):2390–2392
20. Tschesche R, Wulff G (1965) Über die antimikrobielle Wirksamkeit von Saponinen. Z Naturforsch 20b:543–546
21. Cioacá C, Margineau C, Cucu V (1978) The saponins of Hedera helix with antibacterial activity. Pharmazie 33:609–610
22. Balansard G, Timon-David P, Julien J, Bernard P, Gasquet M (1980) Douvicidal and antifungal activities of α-hederin extracted from Hedera helix leaves. Planta Med 39:234
23. Timon-David P, Julien J, Gasquet M, Balansard G, Bernard P (1980) Recherche d'une activité antifongique de plusieurs principes actifs. Extraits du Lierre grimpant: *Hedera helix* L. Ann Pharm Franc 38:545–552
24. Majester-Savornin B, Elias R, Diaz-Lanza AM, Balansard G, Gasquet M, Delmas F (1991) Saponins of the ivy plant, *Hedera helix*, and their leishmanicidic activity. Planta Med 57:260–262
25. Julien J, Gasquet M, Maillard C, Balansard G, Timon-David P (1985) Extracts of the ivy plant, *Hedera helix*, and their anthelminthic activity on liver flukes. Planta Med, pp 205–208
26. Elias R, De Méo M, Vidal-Ollivier E, Laget M, Balansard G, Dumenil G (1990) Antimutagenic activity of some saponins isolated from *Calendula officinalis* L., *C. arvensis* L. and *Hedera helix* L. Mutagenesis 5:327–331
27. El-Merzabani MM, El-Aaser AA, Attia MA, El-Duweini AK, Ghazal AM (1979) Screening system for Egyptian plants with potential anti-tumour activity. Planta Med 36:150–155
28. Agarwal SK, Rastogi RP (1974) Triterpenoid saponins and their genins. Phytochemistry 13:2623–2625
29. Jaspersen-Schib R (1990) Giftpflanzen als Weihnachtsschmuck. Dtsch Apoth Ztg 130:2766–2772
30. Vogel G, Marek M-L (1962) Zur Pharmakologie einiger Saponine. Arzneim Forsch 12:815–825
31. Turton PHJ. Poisoning by ivy. Br Med J 1925; Aug 15:294
32. Goldman L, Preston RH, Muegel HR (1956) Dermatitis venenata from English ivy (Hedera helix). Arch Dermatol 74:311–312
33. Massmanian A, Valcuende Cavero F, Ramirez Bosca A, Castells Rodellas A (1988) Contact dermatitis from variegated ivy (*Hedera helix* subsp. *canariensis* Willd.). Contact Dermatitis 18:247–248
34. Roed-Petersen J (1975) Allergic contact hypersensitivity to ivy (Hedera helix). Contact Dermatitis 1:57
35. Hambly EM, Wilkinson DS (1978) Sensitivity to variegated ivy (*Hedera canariensis*). Contact Dermatitis 4:239–240
36. Mitchell JC (1981) Allergic contact dermatitis from *Hedera helix* and *Brassaia actinophylla* (Araliaceae). Contact Dermatitis 7:158–159

37. Hansen L, Hammershøy O, Boll PM (1986) Allergic contact dermatitis from falcarinol isolated from *Schefflera arboricola*. Contact Dermatitis 14:91–93
38. Hansen L, Boll PM (1986) Polyacetylenes in Araliaceae: their chemistry, biosynthesis and biological significance. Phytochemistry 25:285–293
39. Hansen L, Boll PM (1986) The polyacetylenic falcarinol as the major allergen in *Schefflera arboricola*. Phytochemistry 25:529–530
40. Pant G, Panwar MS, Rawat MSM, Negi DS (1988) Spermicidal glycosides from Hedera nepalensis K. Koch (inflorescence). Pharmazie 43:294

Juniperus Species

D. Corrigan

Botany

The junipers constitute a genus of about 60 species of conifers of the family Cupressaceae growing in the northern hemisphere. The most significant species are *Juniperus communis* L (common juniper), *J. sabina* L. (savin), *J. oxycedrus* L. (cade) and *J. virginiana* L (cedarwood). According to the Flora Europaea, a number of species notably *J. sabina, J. virginiana, J. excelsa, J. phoenicea* and *J. thurifera* are sometimes classified as a separate genus *Sabina* Miller on morphological grounds [1].

Chemistry

The berries of *J. communis* are known to contain up to 3.4% of volatile oil. This oil consists mainly of monoterpenes such as α-pinene, myrcene, sabinene, α-thujene, β-pinene, 1,4-cineole, and the alcohol terpinen-4-ol [2]. Diterpene acids have also been reported as have sesquiterpenes such as caryophyllene and cadinene [2]. A variety of cathechin-based condensed tannins have been isolated [3]. Maarkanen et al. [4] isolated the lignan desoxypodophyllotoxin and its isomer desoxypicropodophyllotoxin from a chloroform extract of "juniper" berries but Fitzgerald et al. [5] noted that *J. communis* gave negative tests for the presence of tumour-damaging lignans (including podophyllotoxin and deoxypodophyllotoxin). These workers reported the presence of these lignans from *J. sabina* (0.25%), *J. virginiana* (0.1%), and *J. scopulorum* (0.17%) among others [6]. They found that the leaves of male plants contained podophyllotoxin while those of the female contained deoxypodophyllotoxin or podophyllotoxin depending on the species [6]. In the case of *J. sabina* var. *tamariscifolia* the leaves of the male plant yielded podophyllotoxin, while those of the female plant yielded deoxypodophyllotoxin, as did the berries of the same plant. However the wood was inactive in bioassays and yielded no lignans [5]. Serebryakova and colleagues [7] reported that *J. depressa* and *J. oxycedrus* were devoid of lignans, but that *J. foetidissima* contained deoxypodophyllotoxin [7].

Adverse Effects of Herbal Drugs, Vol. 2
(ed. by P.A.G.M. De Smet, K. Keller, R. Hänsel, R.F. Chandler)

The principle constituents of savin (*J. sabina*) essential oil are reported to include sabinene (30–40%) and sabinyl acetate (up to 53%) [8]. Fournier et al. [9] studied various commercially available samples of "savin" and "savin essential oil" and found that none of them seemed to correspond to authentic savin (*J. sabina*) but rather to various species of *J. phoenicea* L. or *J. thurifera* L, because they contained over 55% of monoterpene hydrocarbons (chiefly α-pinene) compared to 0.2% in genuine *J. sabina* oil and very little sabinyl acetate (1.1% compared to 75% in *J. sabina.*). Many ornamental juniper bushes (e.g., the varieties "aurea", "compacta", "mint julep" and "old gold") are believed to be cultivars of *J. pfitzeriana* (*Juniperus* X *media*), which is thought to have been developed as a hybrid between *J. sabina* and *J. chinensis*. All of the cultivars studied contained 15–17% of sabinyl acetate and between 2–10% of sabinene [10]. There is no indication that *J. communis* oil contains sabinyl acetate although sabinene has been recorded in samples of *J. communis* oil of Indian origin in amounts as high as 50% [11].

Juniperus oxycedrus is the source of oil of cade, which is also known as juniper tar, which may be obtained by the destructive distillation of the branches and wood of the shrub. It may be rectified by steam or vacuum distillation. It contains cadinene, cadinol, p-cresol and guaiacol [12].

Cedarwood oil is obtained from either *J. virginiana* L. (Virginia cedarwood oil) or from *J. mexicana* and/or *J. ashei* (Texas cedarwood oil) [13]. The two oils are similar in composition and contain mainly sesquiterpenes such as α and β cedrene, thujopsene (also found in *J. communis* wood oil [14]), cuparene, cedrol and widdrol. Most oils contain from 70–85% of these six components [15].

Pharmacology and Uses

Juniper berries are widely used to flavour gin, although the maximum use level in alcoholic beverages is only 0.006%, compared to the doses of 4 g of the berries, 0.3 ml of the oil and 3.7 ml of the spirit and fluid extracts used medicinally [16]. Medicinal indications include the use of the dried fruits to treat dyspepsia [17], and the fresh fruits are listed as being used to treat conditions of the urinary tract, such as acute and chronic cystitis [3]. The essential oil is formulated in capsules, tablets, inhalations, teas and bath oils which are sold as diuretics and for the treatment of rheumatic conditions [17]. Cade oil has antipruritic and keratoplastic properties and is widely used in topical preparations for psoriasis, eczema and seborrhoea [17]. Cedarwood oil is primarily used in microscopy and in perfumery although a number of creams, balsams and salves are listed in the Pharmazeutische Stoffliste for "Räucherzwecken" [17]. Savin oil and savin are similarly listed as remedies for uterine bleeding, rheumatism, gout and warts [17].

A number of Juniper species including *J. sabina* and *J. virginiana* were found to be active against the sarcoma 180 and sarcoma 37 test systems in mice [5,18]. All of the active species of juniper fall into a single subgroup (D.D.) of Bailey's taxonomic classification of the junipers [5]. *J. communis* was inactive in these tests. The active species are those which contain podophyllotoxin and deoxypodophyllotoxin [5]. These compounds were also found in *J. bermudiana*, the leaves and twigs of which were reported to inhibit the P388 lymphocytic leukaemia test system and to show cytotoxic activity toward the human nasopharyngeal epidermal carcinoma test system [19].

The deoxypodophyllotoxin in "juniper tree" is claimed by Markkanen et al. [4] to be the agent responsible for the antiherpetic (HSV-1) activity in primary human amnion cell cultures shown by chloroform extracts. Cell toxicity did not occur in the cultures at concentrations 700 times the minimum concentration required to inhibit viral growth (15 ng/ml). According to references cited by Markkanen et al. [4], juniper extract has also been found to inhibit tobacco mosaic virus and also the growth of HSV-2, influenza virus A2 and Mannheim 57 in Hela cells.

Lasheras et al. [20] investigated the pharmacological properties of a lyophilised aqueous extract of *J. communis* berries. Intravenous administration of the extract to normotensive rats produced an initial transitory rise in arterial pressure followed by a 27% reduction in blood pressure. The extract had no local anaesthetic activity and exhibited no significant depression of spontaneous motor activity. A dose of 1.2 g/kg of extract produced an analgesic response of 178% as measured by thermal stimuli in mice. These authors could not demonstrate a diuretic effect even with doses of extract as high as 1 g/kg, although Volmor and Giebel [21] had reported in 1938 that juniper berry infusion alone or in combination with ononis root increased the chloride output of the rat by 100%. Experiments on 15 mixtures of juniper berry infusion and ononis root decoction showed that the individual drugs had greater diuretic effects than combinations of the two. Combinations of large doses amplified the increased nitrogen output caused by juniper berry. Combinations of small doses were no more effective than juniper berry alone. In 1957, Janku and co-workers [22] demonstrated that 1 ml/kg of juniper berry oil injected subcutaneously into white rats produced a significant level of diuresis after 4 and 24 hours compared to controls. Terpinen-4-ol isolated from the oil was injected at a dose of 0.1 ml and this had almost twice the diuretic activity demonstrated by the oil (1 ml/kg). Further work by the same group confirmed that the diuretic activity was due to an oxygenated fraction of the oil of which 4-terpineol was the most active compound [23]. The effect was as marked as that produced by Hg diuretics but the mechanism of action was different as the 4-terpineol enhanced glomerular filtration. In addition, increased amounts of K^+, Na^+ and Cl^- were excreted. There was no effect on blood pressure in the anaesthesized cat [23].

In dogs dosed with 50 mg/kg of the essential oil of *J. macropoda*, Boiss. growing in the Himalayas, a fall in blood pressure was produced without affecting respiration [24]. Mishra and Agrawal [24] suggested that the fall in blood pressure could be due to myocardial depression, an effect which they noted with isolated frog hearts. These authors also noted a dose dependent depression of the central nervous system, similar to that induced by chlorpromazine, as well as a potentiation of pentobarbitone-induced sleep. A dose of 100 mg/kg of *J. macropoda* oil injected i.p. in rats protected the extensor tonic component in the hind limbs during seizures induced by corneal electrodes.

According to references cited by Chandler [16], juniper oil has antibacterial properties, and has been used as a genito-urinary antiseptic. Oil of cade alone or combined with olive oil (1:1) showed some *in vitro* antibacterial activity against *Micrococcus citrens, Bacillus brevis* and *M. pyogenes*, but not against *Salmonella typhosa* and *Proteus morgani* [25]. The vapour of rectified cade oil showed antibacterial activity against *Mycobacterium avium*, but not against *E. coli, Staph. aureus, B. subtilis, Strep. faecalis* or *S. typhosa* [25]. According to reports included by Opdyke [25] in his monograph, cade oil exhibited *in vitro* antifungal activity against 13 out of 15 fungi tested, while the rectified oil showed slight inhibitory activity against three wood-destroying fungi.

Fedorov [26] reported that the use of toothpastes containing CO_2 extracts of juniper berries and eucalyptus improved paradontial tissue metabolism, prevented atrophy of alveolar processes, and was anti-inflammatory on paradontial tissues when tested *in vivo* and in clinical trials.

J. sabina essential oil had a stimulatory effect on the smooth muscle fibres of the uterus and intestine [27]. It causes a strong hypertonic contraction of the uterus [28].

Adverse Reaction Profile

Juniper berry (*J. communis*) oil was given GRAS (Generally Recognised as Safe) status by the Flavouring Extract Manufacturers Association [FEMA] in 1965 and is approved by the U.S. Food and Drug Administration for food use [29]. Juniper berry was included in the Council of Europe list of substances, spices and seasonings deemed admissible for use with a possible limitation of the active principle in the final product [29]. Cade was also included in this list temporarily [25] although, according to Martindale [30], the Food Standards Committee Report on Flavouring Agents [1965] recommended that it be prohibited for use in foods as a flavouring.

In France *J. communis* berries are accepted for product registration purposes as being "traditionally used" to stimulate the appetite, to facilitate the elimination of water and as an adjuvant to diuretic remedies in benign urinary infections. If the berries are used as a tisane or as an extract in alcohol of a strength less than 30% v/v, then no toxicological dossier is required. However, if the powdered whole drug is used or a tincture or an extract prepared using alcohol stronger than 30% v/v, then a toxicological dossier must be prepared [31].

General Animal Data

The LD_{50} of a lyophilized aqueous extract of *J. communis* berries in mice was reported by Lasheras et al. [20] to be 3 g/kg injected i.p. According to von Skramlik [32], the oral LD_{50} of *J. communis* essential oil was 6.28 g/kg of body weight in the rat. Opdyke [29] refers to work by Shelanski who recorded an acute oral LD_{50} in rats for the same oil as greater than 5 g/kg. The acute dermal LD_{50} value exceeded 5 g/kg in rabbits [29].

For rectified oil of cade (*J. oxycedrus*), oral and dermal LD_{50} values greater than 5 g/kg are cited by Opdyke [25], while Jenner [33] found that cade tar (juniper tar) had an LD_{50} value of 8 g/kg. Jenner reported depression and gastrointestinal irritation as the toxic signs.

Cedarwood oil is said to have oral and dermal LD_{50} values exceeding 5 g/kg in rats and rabbits [34]. The essential oil of *J. macropoda* was reported to have an LD_{50} of 693 mg/kg in mice dosed i.p. [24].

No LD_{50} values for the oil from *J. sabina* have been recovered from the literature even though some authorities state that as little as six drops can be toxic [35]. Manceau et al. [27] report that several grammes of savin will kill a dog. They further report that 3 grammes of essence of savin per kg of body weight in guinea pigs represents the minimum lethal dose for this animal even though guinea pigs are capable of developing resistance to chronic intoxication with savin oil. The minimal lethal dose of the essential oil of *J. phoenicea* was established as 2.5 g/kg of body weight [27].

According to Manceau et al. [27] the symptoms of acute intoxication with *J. sabina* and *J. phoenicea* oils included rapid development of paralysis of the posterior limbs, profuse diarrhoea, albuminuria and hematuria. On autopsy intense congestion of the digestive and genital organs was observed. Chronic intoxication involved a rapid and significant loss of weight; at high doses animals lost a third of their weight in three days. At the same time signs of nephritis, e.g., albuminuria, were noted.

In a study of the toxicity of various preparations of juniper extract, it was found that guinea pigs gained weight even while receiving as much as 20 g of Juniper extract daily [36]. However, such large quantities cause death. On autopsy petechial hemorrhages are found in the kidneys, stomach and small intestine. Rabbits, on the other hand, could tolerate up to 40 g of extract daily and gained weight steadily. Injection of essential oil of savin (*J. sabina*) into experimental animals resulted in general congestion and lesions of all important organs [37]. Patoir et al. [38] administered commercial essential oil from *J. sabina* in doses ranging from 60–300 drops to guinea pigs and from 300–500 drops to rabbits. Seven out of thirteen treated animals succumbed to progressive toxemia characterized by pallor, dyspnea, hematuria, gastroenteritis and debility. *Juniperus thurifera* and its essential oil were studied by Revol [39] who found that the leaves and fluid extract caused intense congestion in the intestines and genito-urinary systems of guinea pigs and dogs. Inhalation of vapours from the essential oil killed mice, but toxicity in guinea pigs, cats and dogs was comparatively low.

Janku et al. [23] studied the acute toxicity of terpinen-4-ol from *J. communis* berry oil in mice. They found that the acute toxicity varied from 0.25 ml/kg after i.p. injection to 1.85 ml/kg after oral application. The LD_{50} was 0.75 ml/kg after subcutaneous injection and 0.78 ml/kg after intramuscular administration. In the rat the LD_{50} was 1.5 ml/kg i.m. They also reported that chronic administration of terpinen-4-ol from juniper berry oil caused no pathological changes in the mouse.

Dermatological Reactions

According to references cited by Opdyke [29], juniper berry (*J. communis*) oil was not irritating when applied to hairless mice and swine but was moderately irritating when applied to intact or abraded rabbit skin for 24 hours under occlusion. A patch test using full strength oil for 24 hr produced two irritation reactions in 20 subjects but a 48 hour closed patch test in humans tested with 5% oil in petrolatum produced no irritation and no sensitisation or phototoxic effects were reported [29].

According to Mitchell and Rook [40], juniper wood can produce dermatitis in woodworkers. They further noted that application of the plant to skin produces burning and slight redness and sometimes vesicles. Katz [41] reported that juniper berry oil was considered irritating to the skin.

Rectified cade oil (*J. oxycedrus*) was reported as being non-irritating in a variety of tests [25] although Mitchell and Rook [40] cite a number of reports of irritation and allergic dermatitis from application of oil of cade including acneiform eruptions. More recently Bouhlal et al. [42] extensively studied the dermatological uses of cade and reported that, of the extracts they tested, the essential oil, the concrete (the oil which remains after vacuum distillation of the hexane used as extracting solvent) and absolute (the oil which remains after removal of waxes and a further vacuum distillation of the concrete) were very weak irritants whereas extracts obtained by dry distillation, i.e., the empyreumatic oil products, were very irritating. These latter products tended to have a $pH < 5$ and the authors suggested that phenols formed during the destructive distillation were responsible for the irritant effects.

Cedarwood oil (*J. virginiana*) was moderately irritating when applied to intact or abraded rabbit skin under occlusion for 24 hrs [34]. In other references cited by Opdyke [34] it was non-irritating to hairless mice when applied undiluted, and when tested on human subjects in a 48 hour closed-patch test it also produced no irritation. Other tests showed no sensitization or phototoxic effects although there are some reports that toilet preparations containing cedarwood oils sometimes cause dermatitis if their use is followed by exposure to various rays [34]. Mitchell and Rook [40] noted that *J. virginiana* leaves were used in ointments for their irritant and rubefacient properties as was *J. sabina*. They further note that the podophyllotoxin-type lignans which have been found in both species are known irritants.

Gastrointestinal Reactions

According to the 27th edition of Martindale [43] oil of savin may cause violent gastrointestinal irritation, an effect noted also for *J. thurifera* oil by Revol [39].

Hepatic Reactions

Patoir et al. [38] studied the effect of intoxication with essential oil of savin on guinea pigs and reported liver lesions suggestive of a degenerative hepatitis without fatty infiltration.

See also the section on Fertility, Pregnancy and Lactation.

Metabolic Reactions

Manceau et al. [27], having noted that guinea pigs suffering from chronic intoxication with *J. sabina* oil, lost a third of their weight within three days, performed a quantitative study of the fatty acid, the unsaponifiable fraction as well as the free and esterified cholesterol content in lungs, kidney, liver and adrenal glands of the animals. They reported a gradual disappearance of the various lipids. This rapid weight loss was also noted by Revol [44] in his studies of the oils of *J. sabina, J. phoenicea* and *J. thurifera* in guinea pigs.

Pulmonary Reactions

Patoir et al. [38] reported that *J. sabina* essential oil caused oedema and hemorrhagic infiltration of the alveolar compartments when administered to guinea pigs and rabbits. In two human fatalities involving savin oil, Papavassilou [45] noted that the oil was concentrated in the lungs as well as in the kidneys.

According to Mitchell and Rook [40], juniper wood can give respiratory symptoms in woodworkers.

Renal Reactions

Both the British Herbal Pharmacopoeia [46] and the Kommission E. monograph [47] produced by the Bundes Gesundheits Amt (German Health Ministry) indicate that juniper berries should be avoided in renal disease. These warnings were amplified by Czygan [48] who reported that after continued use or overdosage, kidney damage arose. This included pain in the renal area associated with an increased need to pass urine as well as pain during urination. Hematuria and albuminuria could also occur. He recommended that juniper berry products should not be used without medical advice for more than 4 weeks and that these preparations were contraindicated in cases of nephritis and pyelitis. Schilcher [49] reports that juniper berry oil has a distinct kidney irritating or injuring effect because of a high percentage of monoterpene hydrocarbons. Terpinen-4-ol seems not to have any irritating effect as Janku et al. [23] reported the absence of pathological changes in a chronic toxicity study with therapeutic doses of terpinen-4-ol.

Manceau et al. [27] studied the metabolism of nitrogenous compounds in guinea pigs intoxicated with the essential oils of *J. sabina* and *J. phoenicea*. They found that the elimination of urea was increased more than ten times the normal value. Patoir et al. [38] noted hemorrhagic nephritis when *J. sabina* oil was tested in guinea pigs and rabbits. The majority of the renal tubules were congested with erythrocytes. Schilcher [49] states that long term application and/or high doses of the same essential oil can cause necrosis. Even external application of the oil could lead to intoxication with damage to the kidneys. Papavissilou [45], reporting on two cases of fatal intoxications in women by savin oil, noted that the oil was concentrated particularly in the kidneys.

Blumel [50] reported on the development of hematuria in a male who took approximately 2 g of savin tops. The symptoms included increased frequency of urination, pain in the urethra and bladder and blood in the urine.

Drug Interactions

Mice exposed to cedarwood (*J. virginiana*, and *J. ashei*) bedding exhibited reduced hypnotic effects with hexobarbitone. These effects, according to references cited by Opdyke [34], were due to the induction of microsomal enzymes. Wade et al. [51] found that cedarwood oil as well as cedrol and cedrene were effective inducers of microsomal enzymes via inhalation. Enhanced *in vivo* metabolism demonstrated that all three materials were effective inducers of aniline hydroxylase, sulfanilamide acetylase, neoprontosil azoreductase, heptachlor epoxidase and zoxazolamine hydroxylase. In rats the removal of bishydroxy coumarin from blood *in vivo* was greatly speeded up.

Fertitility, Pregnancy and Lactation

A number of publications strongly advise against the use of Juniper preparations during pregnancy [16,46,47].

Prakash [52] has reported that an acetone extract of *J. communis* seeds at a dose of 200 mg/kg had an anti-implantation activity of 60% in the rat. The extract was administered orally during the first seven days of pregnancy.

Savin (*J. sabina*) has long been used to induce abortions [45]. Prochonow [53] reported that *J. sabina* oil affected the smooth muscle of the excised uteri of cats, rabbits and guinea pigs. The initial irritation was followed by paralysis. Macht [54] also reported that savin oil had no stimulatory effect on excised uteri. On the contrary, he found that emulsions of oil in Lockes solution inhibited contractions and paralysed the uterus. The emmenagogic (i.e., abortifacient) action depended, he claimed, on general constitutional poisoning or on gastrointestinal irritation.

Support for this view comes from the already noted observation that savin oil causes violent gastrointestinal irritation, which Martindale [43] notes in the case of aloes may cause pelvic congestion, which in turn may initiate reflex stimulation of the gravid uterus [55].

In many cases the intoxication is so severe that death occurs in the mother without abortion taking place. Papavassilou [45] reported two such cases in Greek women. Revol [39] examined the effects of *J. thurifera* oil on guinea pigs and dogs and found that the leaves and fluid extract caused intense congestion in the genitourinary system and the intestines. He further noted that this oil did not cause abortions at doses at which savin oil would do so. In further work with oils and extracts of three juniper species (*J. sabina, J. phoenicea* and *J. thurifera*), Revol [44] reported that in guinea pigs death occurred due to intense congestion of the genitourinary organs in the case of *J. thurifera* and *J. sabina* while *J. phoenicea* was inactive. Rabbits, on the contrary, were resistant to the effects of high doses (15–55 ml per animal) of preparations of the three junipers.

Patoir et al. [38] reported that abortion in guinea pigs and rabbits was produced as a result of the severe general action of essential oil of savin and not as a result of a specific action. Out of nine animals treated, 6 died without aborting, while one gave birth to two dead fetuses. Two animals gave birth to live animals which died soon after birth. The livers and kidneys of the fetuses were affected like those of the mothers. It was noteworthy that the nephritic lesions were more severe than those in the mothers.

On the other hand Renaux [28] claimed that the uterine contractions produced by relatively weak doses (50 mg of aqueous extract) of savin in the isolated uterine horns of virgin guinea pigs indicated that the abortifacient effects of this plant are due to its oxytocic properties and are not just the consequence of a general intoxication.

According to Pages et al. [56], the abortive properties of *J. sabina* are generally attributed to its essential oil and more precisely to the major component of this oil, sabinyl acetate. These authors confirmed that the essential oil of *J. sabina* has abortive potential by treating mice subcutaneously with daily doses of 15–135 mg/kg body weight from gestational days 6 to 15 (i.e., during organogenesis). A significant increase in fetal resorptions or death was seen in all treatment groups without an increase in fetal malformations. All the mice that resorbed their whole litter showed a paler and smaller liver upon examination than the others, and daily doses of 45–135 mg/kg bw were associated with maternal weight loss.

Pages et al. [57] point out that sabinyl acetate is also the major component of essential oil of *Plectranthus fruticosus* L'Hérit (Labiatae). This latter oil produced not only resorptions but also malformations when administered orally at doses of 20 mg/kg bw to pregnant rats. The most frequent malformations were mono- or bilateral microphthalmia or anophthalmia [57]. As the oil gave similar results following subcutaneous treatment of mice, the different effects of *J. sabina* oil and *Plectranthus fruticosus* oil are not due to differences in animal species or route of application.

Commercially available leaves and essential oils of savin may come from the adulterants *J. phoenicea* or *J. thurifera* [9]. Pages et al. [58] have therefore also tested 135 mg/kg/day of essential oils of savin that had been obtained either commercially or by steam distillation of commercial samples of savin leaves. No treatment group of mice showed an increase in fetal resorptions or fetal malformations, so the studied materials appear to have come from a *Juniper* species other than *J. sabina*.

Mutagenicity and Carcinogenicity

Roe and Field [59] reported that cedarwood oil had neither a systemic or local effect when tested in mice during studies on tumour-promoting substances in essential oils. Fabian [60] stated that benz[α]pyrene was found in nanogram/g amounts in pic. cadi (*J. oxycedrus* tar) while Bouhlal and colleagues [42] have demonstrated that the benzopyrene content depends on the method of producing the cade. They reported that the empyreumatic oil of cade (produced by destructive distillation of *J. oxycedrus* wood) contained 8000 parts per billion (ppb) of benzopyrene, whereas the rectified oil contained less than 20 ppb.

References

1. Tutin TG, Heywood V, Burges NA, Valentine DH, Walters SM, Webb DA (1964) Flora Europaea Vol 1 Cambridge: Cambridge Univ Press pp 38–39
2. Leung AY (1980) Encyclopedia of common natural ingredients used in food, drugs and cosmetics. New York: Wiley-Interscience pp 208–209
3. Williamson EM, Evans FJ (1988) Potters new cyclopaedia of botanical drugs and preparations by Wren RC. Saffron Walden: The CW Daniel Company pp 160–161

4. Markkanen T, Makinen ML, Nikoskelainen J, Ruhonen J, Nieminen K, Jokinen P, Raunio R, Hirvonen T (1981) Antiherpetic agent from juniper tree (*Juniperus communis*), its purification, identification and testing in primary human amnion cell cultures. Drugs Exptl Clin Res 7:691–697
5. Fitzgerald DB, Hartwell JL, Leiter J (1957) Distribution of tumor-damaging lignans among conifers. J Natl Cancer Inst 18:83–99
6. Hartwell JL, Johnson JJ, Fitzgerald DB, Belkin M (1953) Podophyllotoxin from Juniperus species: Savinin. JA Chem Soc 75:235–236
7. Serebryakova AP, Filitis LN, Utkin LM (1961) Lignans of the Soviet Union Juniperus plants. Zhur Obschei Khim 31:1731–7134 [per Chem Abstr 55:26144]
8. Fournier G, Pages N, Fournier L, Callen G (1990) Contribution a l'etude des huiles essentielles de differentes especes de *Juniperus*. J Pharm Belg 45:293–298
9. Fournier G, Pages N, Baudron V, Paris M (1989) Étude d'echantillons commerciaux de sabine: rameaux feuilles et huille essentielle. Plantes Med Phytother 23:169–179
10. Fournier G, Pages N, Fournier C, Callen G (1991) Comparisons of volatile leaf essential oils of various *Juniperus pfitzeriana*. Pharm Acta Helv 66:74–75
11. Simonsen, JL (1924) Constituents of some Indian essential oils XV. Essential oil from the seeds of *J. communis*. Indian Forest Records 11:6–9 [per Chem. Abstr. 19:2723]
12. Leung AY (1980) Encyclopedia of common natural ingredients used in food, drugs and cosmetics. New York: Wiley Interscience pp 81–82
13. Leung AY (1980) Encyclopedia of common natural ingredients used in food, drugs and cosmetics. New York: Wiley-Interscience pp 105–107
14. Bredenberg JB (1961) The Chemistry of the Order Cupressales. 36. The ethereal oil of the wood of *Juniperus communis* L. Acta Chem Scand 15:961–966
15. Adams RP (1987) Investigation of *Juniperus* species of the United States for new sources of cedarwood oil. Econ Bot 41:48–54
16. Chandler RF (1986) An inconspicuous but insidious drug. Can Pharm J 119:563–566
17. Arzneiburo der Bundesvereinigung Deutscher Apothekerverbande. Pharmazeutische Stoffliste (1990) 7 Auflage. Frankfurt am Main: Werbe- und Vertriebsgesellschaft Deutscher Apotheker mbH. Io-L pp 12–19
18. Kupchan SM, Hemingway JC, Knox JR (1965) Tumour inhibitors VII. Podophyllotoxin, the active principle of *Juniperus virginiana*. J Pharm Sci 54:659–660
19. Tanimami B, Torrance SJ, Cole JR (1977) Antitumour agent from *Juniperus bermudiana* (Pinaceae): deoxypodophyllotoxin. Phytochem 16:1100–1101
20. Lasheras B, Turillas P, Cenarruzabeitia E (1986) Etude pharmacologique preliminaire de *Prunus spinosa* L, *Amelanchier ovalis* Medikus, *Juniperus communis* L. et *Urtica dioica* L. Plantes Med Phytother 20:219–226
21. Volmor H, Giebel A (1938) The diuretic action of several combinations of Juniper berry and Ononis root. Arch Exptl Path Pharmakol 190:522–534
22. Janku I, Hava M, Motl O (1957) Ein diuretisch wirksamer stoff aus wacholder (*Juniperus communis* L.). Experientia 13:255–256
23. Janku I, Hava M, Kraus R, Motl O (1960) Das diuretische prinzip des wacholders. Arch Exptl Pathol Pharmakol 238:112–113
24. Mishra P, Agrawal RK (1989) Some observations on the pharmacological activities of the essential oil of *Juniperus macropoda*. Fitoterapia 60:339–345
25. Opdyke DLJ (1975) Cade oil rectified (juniper tar). Fd Cosmet Toxicol 13:733–734
26. Fedorov Yu A, Kaliberdina NV, Todorashko VP (1977) Effect of [tooth] pastes containing biologically active ingredients on the oral cavity tissues. Maslo-Zhir prom - st 1977:22. [per Chem Abstr 89:570]
27. Manceau P, Revol L, Vernet AM (1936) Les essences de sabine du commerce. Etude d'essences authentique de *Juniperus sabina* L. et de *Juniperus phoenicea* L. Bull Soc Pharmacol 43:14–24
28. Renaux J, La Barre J (1941) Sur les effets ocytociques des essences de Rue et de Sabine. Acta Biol Belg 1:334–335

29. Opdyke DLJ (1976) Juniper Berry Oil. Fd Cosmet Toxicol 14:333
30. Reynolds JEF (ed.) (1989) Martindale. The Extra Pharmacopoeia 29th edn. London: The Pharmaceutical Press p 917
31. Ministere des Affaires Sociales et de la Solidarite (France) (1990) Medicaments a base de Plantes. Avis aux fabricants concernant les demandes d'autorisation de mise sur le marche. Bulletin Officiel No. 90/22 bis
32. Von Skramlik E (1959) Über die Giftigkeit und Vertraglichkeit von aetherischen Ölen. Pharmazie 14:435–445
33. Jenner PM, Hagan EC, Taylor JM, Cook EL, Fitzhugh OG (1964) Food flavourings and compounds of related structure 1. Acute oral toxicity. Fd Cosmet Toxicol 2:327–343
34. Opdyke DLJ (1974) Cedarwood oil virginia. Fd Cosmet Toxicol 12:845–846
35. Duke JA (1985) Handbook of Medicinal Herbs. Boca Raton: CRC Press pp 256–257
36. Rajohn CA, Wirth E (1932) The toxicity of various preparations of Extractum Juniperi. Arch Exptl Path Pharmakol 166:222–228
37. Flaminio Favero P, Veiga de Carvalho H, Novah E (1940) Experimental study of apiole, savin and rue. Anais Faculdade Med Univ S Paulo 16:499–523
38. Patoir A, Patoir G, Bedrine H (1938) Action toxique de l'essence de sabine et de l'armoise sur l'organisme. Compt Rend Soc Biol 127:1325–1326
39. Revol L (1935) *Juniperus thurifera* and its essence. Bull Sci Pharmacol 42:577–589
40. Mitchell J, Rook A (1979) Botanical Dermatology. Vancouver: Greengrass pp 242–244
41. Katz AE (1946) Dermal irritating properties of essential oils and aromatic chemicals. Spice Mill 69:46–7, 50–51 [per Chem Abstr 40:7525]
42. Bouhlal K, Meynadier J-M, Peyron J-L, Peyron L, Marion J-P, Bonetti G, Meynadier J (1988) Le Cade en dermatologie. Parfums, Cosmet Aromes 83:73–82
43. Wade A (ed) (1977) Martindale the extra Pharmacopoeia, 27th edn. London: The Pharmaceutical Press, p 1026
44. Revol L (1936) L'essence constitute t-elle l'unique principe actif des *Juniperus* de la section *Sabina*? Action physiologique d'extraits de *J. sabina, J. phoenicea, J. thurifera*. Bull Soc Pharmacol 43:139–144
45. Papavassiliou MJ (1935) Sur deux cas d'intoxication par la Sabine. La permeabilite placentaire a l'essence de sabine. Soc Med Leg 15:778–781
46. British Herbal Pharmacopoeia (1983) Bournemouth: British Herbal Medicine Association, p 124
47. Anonymous (1984) Monograph der Kommission E: Bundesanzeiger Nummer 228 vom 05-12-1984
48. Czygan F-C (1987) Warning vor unkritischem gebrauch von Wacholderbeeren. Z Phytotherapie 8:10
49. Schilcher H (1985) Effects and side-effects of essential oils. In: Essential oils and aromatic plants (ed Baerheim Svendsen A, Scheffer JJC) Dordrecht: Martinus Nijhoff, pp 226, 288, 299
50. Blumel P (1941/1943) Blutharnen bei Vergiftung mit Sadebaumspitzen. Vergiftungsfälle 12:25–28
51. Wade AE, Hall JE, Hilliard CC, Molton E, Greene FL (1968) Alteration of drug metabolism in rats and mice by an environment of cedarwood. Pharmacology 1:317–328
52. Prakash AO (1986) Potentialities of some indigenous plants for antifertility activity. Int J Crude Drug Res 24:19–24
53. Prochnow L (1912) Experimental contribution to the study of popular abortifacients. Arch Intern Pharmacodyn 21:313–319 [per Chem Abstr (1912) 6:1181]
54. Macht DI (1912) The action of so-called emmenagogue oils. J Pharmac 4:547–552 [per Chem Abstr (1913) 7:3367]
55. USP Dispensing Information (1986) Vol. 1. Drug information for the health care provider. 6th edn. United States Pharmacopoeial Convention p 928

56. Pages N, Fournier G, Chamorro G, Salazar M, Paris M, Boudene C (1989) Teratological evaluation of *Juniperus sabina* essential oil in mice. Planta Medica 55:144–146
57. Pages N, Salazar M, Chamorro G, Fournier G, Paris M, Dumitresco SM, Boudene C (1988) Teratological evaluation of *Plectranthus fruticosus* leaf essential oil. Planta Medica 54:296–298
58. Pages N, Fournier G, LeLuyer F, Marques M-C, Boudene C (1989) Les echantillons commerciaux de "Sabine" (rameaux feuilles et huile essentielle). Sont-ils teratogenes? Etude chez la souris. Plantes Med Phytother 23:186–192
59. Roe RJC, Field WEM (1965) Chronic toxicity of essential oils and certain other products of natural origin. Fd Cosmet Toxicol 3:311–324
60. Fabian F, Poliniceucu M (1985) Study on the content of aromatic polycyclic hydrocarbons of some pharmaceuticals. Farmacia (Bucharest) 33:117–122 [per Chem Abstr. 104:56487]

Larrea Tridentata

P.A.G.M. De Smet

Botany

Larrea tridentata (DC.) Coville is a zygophyllaceous shrub growing wild in the arid regions of the Southwestern United States and Mexico. It is called creosote bush, chaparral and greasewood in the United States, and gobernadora, guamis and hediondilla in Mexico [1–3].

The plant has a complex history of scientific nomenclature with many different synonyms: *Larrea divaricata* and *L. mexicana*; *Covillea tridentata* and *C. glutinosa*; *Neoschroetera tridentata*, *N. divaricata* and *N. glutinosa*; and *Zygophyllum tridentatum* [2–10]. Adding to the nomenclatural confusion is the problem that vernacular names of *Larrea tridentata* may be used to designate other botanical entities. For instance, creosote bush may also refer to South American *Larrea* species and to *Dictamnus* species of the Rutaceae, whereas greasewood may stand for *Adenostoma fasciculata* or *Sarcobatus vermiculatus* [10,11].

Chemistry

The leaves and stems of *Larrea tridentata* are covered by a thick resin, which can comprise up to 20% of the dry weight of young leaves and 10% of mature leaves. Over 80% of this resin is composed of phenolic constituents [11,12]. In one study, the total phenolics together with small amounts of lipid substances were 21% from young and vigorously growing plants and 16% from older plants [13].

The major phenolic component is a catechol lignan known as nordihydroguaiaretic acid (= NDGA) [12,14–17]. This compound has also been found in the related South American species *Larrea cuneifolia* and *L. nitida* [7]. Minor phenolics recovered from the leaves and small twigs of *L. tridentata* are norisoguaiacin, dihydroguaiaretic acid, partially demethylated dihydroguaiaretic acid and 3′-demethoxyisoguaiacin [13]. Recently, Konno et al. [18] isolated six new furanoid lignans from the leaves and stems of *L. tridentata*.

Adverse Effects of Herbal Drugs, Vol. 2
(ed. by P.A.G.M. De Smet, K. Keller, R. Hänsel, R.F. Chandler)

According to Gonzalez-Coloma et al. [12], NDGA accounts for approximately 40% of the resin content in mature leaf material of *L. tridentata*, compared to nearly 50% in young leaves. When these figures are combined with the resin contents of mature and young leaves mentioned above, they imply NDGA levels of approximately 40 mg/g in mature leaves and levels up to nearly 100 mg/g in young leaves. Gisvold [19] recovered, by means of an unspecific gravimetric procedure, levels from 0 to 65.5 mg/g of NDGA from dried samples that consisted mostly of small twigs, leaves, and flowering tops. Large twigs and stems were not included, because preliminary investigations had shown that only small amounts of NDGA could be obtained from these plant parts. Wellendorf [17] studied dried plant material from bushes of different ages by TLC analysis, and found NDGA levels between 93 and 150 mg/g. Valentine et al. [16] developed a GLC method for the determination of NDGA, and reported that 16 mg/g of this compound was present in the leaves of *L. tridentata*. This research group used boiling water to extract NDGA from the leaves, which raises a question about the completeness of the isolation procedure.

When chaparral tea is prepared by steeping the dried leaves and stems of the creosote bush in hot water, only about 40% of the available NDGA may actually pass into the tea [20]. In all probability, this incomplete passage is due to the limited solubility of NDGA in water [16]. The level of NDGA may also be reduced by leaving the tea standing for several days. In one study, the level of NDGA in an aqueous solution was stable up to 5 hours, but it declined to approximately 27% of the initial value after 14 days of keeping [16].

Alkaloids were once purported to be present in *Larrea tridentata*, but their presence has never been verified [14]. The plant contains saponins [7,11], however, and numerous flavonoids [11,12,21], such as rutin, isoquercitrin, isokaempferid, isorhamnetin, kaempferol, quercetin, quercetin-3-methylether, nicotiflorin, kumatakenin, and 5.4′-dihydroxy-3.7.3′-trimethoxyflavone [8]. Although creosote bush has a marked aromatic odour, only a very small amount of volatile oil (0.1%) is obtained upon steam distillation [14].

Pharmacology and Uses

Larrea tridentata and its phenolic constituent NDGA were at one time considered as candidate drugs for the treatment of cancer. Interest in their antitumour potential was particularly induced by a case of an elderly man with documented malignant melanoma, who apparently cured himself by drinking chaparral tea [20]. Unfortunately, an avalanche of publicity in the lay press followed, in which it was not sufficiently acknowledged that melanoma may occasionally regress spontaneously [22]. Subsequent analysis of the available animal data and preliminary testing of the chaparral tea in human cancer patients did not reveal objective evidence of a clinically relevant anticancer effect [23].

NDGA is a potent anticancer agent *in vitro*, but *in vivo* experiences have been much less impressive. Combination of NDGA with high doses of ascorbic acid was reported to inhibit Ehrlich ascites tumour in mice [20], but this evidence has been described as meager, and screening tests of NDGA in mice against other tumours have been negative [23]. In a pilot study on the effect of chaparral tea in human cancer patients, the tea appeared to stimulate the majority of malignancies, and only some malignancies went on to regress [23].

There is an Argentine report from the fifties that NDGA in intramuscular doses of e.g., 300–400 mg per day produced analgesia in cancer patients [24]. Such an effect was never reported in human users of chaparral tea, which makes it unlikely that analgesic activity is a prominent clinical effect of the tea.

Indians in the Southwestern part of the United States have used *Larrea tridentata* for many ailments. A tea from boiled leaves was drunk for venereal diseases, colds, and bowel cramps, and to stimulate urination. External preparations of the plant were used to treat rheumatism, chicken-pox, sores, and burns [14]. In Argentina, creosote bush is primarily used as firewood, but it may also serve as a household remedy, such as in baths, for moist compresses, or as a tea prepared from its leaves for painful trauma and luxations [11]. Modern herbalistic sources suggest that chaparral can be used orally for colds, influenza, diarrhoea, and urinary tract infections, and topically for dandruff [25].

NDGA has good antioxidant properties [13,26], and for this reason it was formerly added to human foods and pharmaceuticals, commonly at levels of 0.1–0.2 mg/g [20]. *In vitro* experiments have shown that the compound has antimicrobial activity [26] and that it inhibits peroxidase and catalase activity in relatively low concentrations [27]. This latter effect might have a toxicological meaning, as both enzyme systems are known to protect cellular machinery from superoxide and other reduced forms of oxygen [28]. Nowadays, NDGA is primarily used in experimental pharmacological studies as an inhibitor of the lipoxygenase pathway of arachidonic acid metabolism [28–31].

Jordan et al. [30] hypothesized that NDGA may serve as an immunosuppressive tool because of its lipoxygenase inhibiting activity. When they tested this hypothesis in a mouse model of allograft rejection, they found that NDGA (at 50 mg/kg subcutaneously per day) prevented infiltration and subsequent cytotoxicity of specifically sensitized effector cells without compromising other basic cell functions (migration).

Since lipoxygenase inhibition might have therapeutic value in psoriasis, Newton et al. [31] evaluated the usefulness of topical NDGA in humans with psoriasis, but they were unable to demonstrate a therapeutic effect.

Pharmacokinetics

A Canadian research group investigated the pharmacokinetics of NDGA in rats as part of its toxicological studies of this antioxidant (cf. the section on general animal data in the adverse reaction profile). The group determined the presence of NDGA and its metabolite *o*-quinone in tissue samples of rats, which had developed lymphatic and renal lesions after dietary exposure to 0.5 or 1.0% of NDGA for 74 weeks. No free NDGA was recovered from lymphatic or renal tissue, but *o*-quinone could be isolated from kidney tissue. The presence of this metabolite in lymphatic tissue was likely, but could not be confirmed due to the lack of sufficient material. Urine samples collected from rats fed at a level of 2% of NDGA in the diet for 36 days also yielded *o*-quinone without a detectable concentration of free NDGA [32].

When the Canadians noticed that the lymph nodes affected by the dietary feeding of NDGA were those draining the ileocaecal region of the intestine, they evaluated the formation of *o*-quinone in the ileum and caecum of rats following a single dose of 250 mg of NDGA directly into the rat intestine. A significant amount of *o*-quinone was not formed until 6 hours after administration, when the NDGA had reached the vicinity of the ileocaecal junction [32].

In a sequel study, 12–18 mg of free NDGA per day was recovered from the faeces of rats treated with 2% of NDGA for at least 6 months. The amount of *o*-quinone in the faeces could not be determined, due to contamination with bile pigments [33].

Adverse Reaction Profile

General Animal Data

The acute and chronic toxicity of NDGA in laboratory animals has been evaluated extensively in the past because of its usefulness as an antioxidant in foods for human consumption. Most chronic toxicity reports specify the tested dietary levels of NDGA without providing daily doses in mg or g per kg body weight. It should therefore be noted that, in one study, rats weighing 140–150 g ingested 0.3 g of NDGA per day, when fed ad lib with chow containing 2% of NDGA [34]. This means that each per cent of NDGA in the diet corresponded approximately to a daily dose of 1 g/kg.

Early American studies on NDGA showed approximate oral LD_{50} values of 4000 mg/kg in mice, 5500 mg/kg in rats, and 830 mg/kg in guinea pigs, and an approximate intraperitoneal LD_{50} of 550 mg/kg in mice. Dietary feeding of levels up to 1.0% did not affect the two-year mortality rate in rats, but incorporation of 1.0% into the diet for six months had an unfavourable effect on the growth rate of rats. Moreover, massive caecal hemorrhages with single and multiple cysts in the mesentery in the angle of junction between small and large intestine were sometimes observed in rats, which had been treated with dietary concentrations of 0.5% of NDGA for two years [35,36].

These findings were corroborated by a Canadian research group, which reported reduced body weight gain and cystic enlargement of the mesenteric lymph nodes at the ileocaecal junction in rats fed 0.5 or 1.0% of NDGA in the diet for 74 weeks. The overall histological picture in the lymph nodes was one of cystic reticulo-endotheliosis. In one of 33 treated animals, the nodes were invaded by a malignant reticulum cell sarcoma. Almost all treated animals showed distinctive pathological changes in the kidneys, particularly vacuolation of the cortical tubular epithelium, which involved mainly the proximal convoluted tubules. Rats treated with 2% of dietary NDGA for shorter periods of time showed widespread renal lesions, with tubular necrosis as one of the histological features [32].

In a sequel study, the dietary level of NDGA was increased from 1% during the 1st week, and 2% during the 2nd week, to 3% during the 3rd and 4th week. After the rats had been treated with this latter concentration for 15 days, the dose of NDGA had to be reduced again to 2%, as 7 of 24 animals had died [33].

The Canadian research group also gathered pharmacokinetic data to see, whether NDGA-induced toxicity should be attributed to the compound itself or its metabolite *o*-quinone (see the section on pharmacokinetics for details).

As a result of these toxicity data, the American Food and Drug Administration removed NDGA from its "Generally Recognized As Safe" (GRAS) list [2].

General Human Data

No overt toxic reactions to chaparral tea were observed in a pilot study involving 34 cancer patients. In the majority of cases, however, the tea appeared to stimulate rather than attenuate tumour growth [23].

Assuming that one liter of chaparral tea is prepared from 7–8 g of plant material containing 7–8% of NDGA, and that hot water treatment extracts 40% of the available NDGA [20], the finished tea preparation will contain 196–256 mg of NDGA per l. When 2–3 cups of this tea are consumed daily, with each cup providing 150–250 ml, the ingestion of NDGA will approximately amount to 60–190 mg per day.

Bergel [24] has reported the occurrence of hypotension, leukocytosis, eosinophilia, glucosuria, polyuria, mental confusion, nervous excitability, and insomnia in Argentine cancer patients, who received NDGA in intramuscular doses of e.g., 300–400 mg per day. The hypotension was undoubtedly a genuine side effect of the NDGA (see the section on cardiovascular reactions), and there is some evidence to suggest that the eosinophilic response may also have been related to the treatment with NDGA (see the section on hematological reactions). It is far from clear, however, whether the other effects should be attributed to NDGA or to the terminal illness and/or co-medication of the patients. For instance, the nervous excitability and insomnia observed in a patient with cerebral metastasis could have been caused or aggravated by this pathology.

Allergic Reactions

See the section on dermatological reactions.

Cardiovascular Reactions

Intravenous administration of 0.5–1 mg/kg of NDGA to cats was reported to produce a rapid fall in arterial blood pressure, which could be reversed by epinephrine and norepinephrine. When the dose was raised to 5–10 mg/kg, the hypotensive effect was accompanied by respiratory stimulation and a reduction in heart frequency. The hypotensive response was also observed in cancer patients given NDGA in intramuscular doses of e.g., 300–400 mg per day. It was treated with agents such as ephedrine and desoxycorticosterone [24].

Dermatological Reactions

There are at least sixteen cases of contact dermatitis in the literature, which are attributed either to *Larrea* plants or to the *Larrea* constituent NDGA. The capacity of *Larrea tridentata* to produce allergic contact reactions is not without practical relevance, since one of its advocated applications is that of a hair tonic [2].

Two cases of contact dermatitis from the creosote bush, both of which were confirmed by patch testing, were reported from the Southern United States [4,37]. Leonforte [11] described six cases of contact dermatitis from Argentine *Larrea* shrubs called jarilla. Three cases resulted from handling the jarilla or using it as firewood, the other three were due to taking a jarilla bath or a football with jarilla resin. Five cases were confirmed by patch tests with *Larrea* leaves and/or extracts. Patch testing in one patient showed cross sensitivity to *Zuccagnia punctata*, which plant has similarities to *Larrea*. Its Argentine name is jarilla macho, and NDGA is said to be present.

Jorgensen and Hjorth [38] recorded two cases of allergic contact sensitivity to NDGA. One case involved acute oedematous dermatitis of the face due to occupational exposure in a pharmaceutical factory. The patient showed positive patch tests to 20 mg/g of NDGA in petroleum and to hydrogenated oil of soybean containing 1.5 mg/g of NDGA. The other patient had been sensitized by a particular brand of lanolin cream containing 1 mg/g of NDGA as an antioxidant. Among 435 consecutive controls tested with 50 mg/g of NDGA in petroleum, only one (0.23%) had a weak reaction to NDGA. Roed-Petersen and Hjorth [19] patch tested 111 consecutive patients referred for eczematous dermatitis with NDGA (20 mg/g in petroleum), and found 6 positive cases (5.4%). In the three cases where the source of sensitization could still be traced, the offending preparation was the same lanolin cream with 1 mg/g of NDGA that had been incriminated earlier by Jorgensen and Hjorth [38].

A recent secondary source describes NDGA as a phototoxin [12], but this allusion is not supported by a reference to primary data.

Hematological Reactions

Tregellas and South [40] observed a positive direct antiglobulin (Coombs) test, without evidence of decreased red cell survival, in a Caucasian male who had started treatment with chaparral tablets. The reaction was shown to be due solely to IgG subclass IgG_1, and an eluate reacted with all red cells tested. After discontinuation of the herbal drug, the reaction disappeared gradually in 19 weeks, and became positive again after 5 weeks of rechallenge. Not only does this immunohematological observation demonstrate that *Larrea* preparations may interfere with compatibility procedures in the blood transfusion laboratory, it also opens up the possibility that *Larrea* products could be capable of inducing immune hemolytic anemia [41].

Bergel [24] reported the occurrence of eosinophilia in cancer patients treated intramuscularly with e.g., 300–400 mg of NDGA per day (see the section on general human data). As eosinophilia can be a sign of neoplastic diseases [42], it is difficult to attribute this effect with certainty to NDGA. A causative role of this compound is conceivable, however, as Bergel [24] also found that an intramuscular dose of 300 mg of NDGA raised the level of circulating eosinophils in normal individuals.

Hepatic Reactions[1]

The literature has not yielded animal evidence of hepatotoxicity. In one study, necrosis of the liver was occasionally noted in rats given up to 1.0% of NDGA in their diet, but this effect was also observed in control animals [35].

[1] See the note added in proof on p. 316

Katz and Saibil [25] recently described a young woman who developed subacute hepatic necrosis secondary to the use of chaparral leaf tablets. Anorexia, nausea and retrosternal pain started after three months of treatment. When the patient also began to note darkening of the urine, she reduced her daily dose from 15 tablets to one, whereupon the loss of appetite, retrosternal pain and dark urine disappeared. A few weeks later the patient unknowingly rechallenged herself by increasing the dose to seven tablets per day. The nausea and retrosternal pain returned, together with scleral icterus, fatigue, pedal edema, and increased abdominal girth. The herbal drug was subsequently stopped entirely, but the jaundice, ascites and fatigue persisted, and the patient had to be hospitalized. Serum liver tests on admission were abnormal, and a percutaneous liver biopsy showed loss of parenchymatous tissue without significant inflammatory infiltration. The patient responded to diuretic therapy and supportive care and she could be discharged after 3 weeks. One year later, her serum liver biochemistry had returned to normal values, but she still complained of fatigue.

As one of the initial symptoms in this case was loss of appetite, it is disturbing that chaparral is an ingredient in at least one over-the-counter weight loss tea [3].

Renal Reactions

The renal toxicity of NDGA in experimental animals is well-established (see the section on general animal data). NDGA-induced changes in rat kidneys include: tubular cell injury; local and focal dilation of tubules (cyst formation); tubular cell necrosis; focal proliferation of tubular epithelium; focal infiltration of interstitium and tubular lumens by polymorphonuclear leukocytes, lymphocytes, macrophages and round cells; and interstitial fibrosis [28,32–34,43]. Interestingly, NDGA is a poor or ineffective stimulus to these renal changes in germ-free rats, which indicates that they cannot be readily provoked by dietary NDGA alone [28,34].

Fertility, Pregnancy and Lactation

No data on the use of *Larrea tridentata* or its constituent NDGA during pregnancy and lactation have been recovered from the literature other than an early report that a diet providing a total dose of 0.5 g of NDGA produced slightly fewer fetal resorptions in the rat than a normal diet [44].

Mutagenicity and Carcinogenicity

The mutagenic and carcinogenic potential of *Larrea tridentata* and NDGA has not been established. There is some anecdotal evidence in the literature, however, to suggest that formal evaluation of these aspects is certainly warranted.

As was pointed out in the section on general animal data, the dietary feeding of 0.5 or 1.0% of NDGA to rats for 74 weeks produced cystic reticuloendotheliosis of paracaecal lymph nodes, and one of 33 treated animals showed invasion of the nodes by a malignant reticulum cell sarcoma [32]. As was mentioned under the heading of pharmacology and uses, chaparral tea appeared to stimulate rather than attenuate tumour growth in a pilot study on human cancer patients. If the tea would indeed have a stimulating effect on tumours, its reputation as a natural anticancer remedy would make it far from innocuous [23].

References

1. Martínez M (1979) Catálogo de Nombres Vulgares y Científicos de Plantas Mexicanas. México D.F.: Fondo de Cultura Económica, p 372 and p 1109
2. Tyler VE (1987) The New Honest Herbal. A sensible guide to herbs and related remedies. 2nd edn. Philadelphia: George F. Stickley Company, pp 18–20
3. Der Marderosian A, Liberti LE (1988) Natural product medicine. A scientific guide to foods, drugs, cosmetics. Philadelphia: George F. Stickley Company, pp 273–275
4. Smith LM (1937) Dermatitis caused by creosote bush. J Allergy 8:187–188
5. Wellendorf M (1963) Nordihydroguajaretsyre (N.D.G.A.) I. Stamplantens botanik. Dansk Tidsskr Farm 37:257–269
6. Vogel VJ (1970) American Indian Medicine. Norman: University of Oklahoma Press, pp 296–297
7. Hegnauer R (1973) Chemotaxonomie der Pflanzen. Band 6: Dicotyledoneae: Rafflesiaceae – Zygophyllaceae. Basel: Birkhäuser Verlag, pp 709–715
8. Chirikdjian JJ (1974) Isolierung von Kumatakenin und 5.4'-Dihydroxy-3.7.3.'-trimethoxyflavon aus Larrea tridentata. Pharmazie 29:292–293
9. List PH, Hörhammer L (1976) Hagers Handbuch der Pharmazeutischen Praxis. Vierte Neuausgabe. Fünfter Band. Chemikalien und Drogen (H-M). Berlin: Springer-Verlag, pp 450–451
10. Mitchell J, Rook A (1979) Botanical dermatology. Plants and plant products injurious to the skin. Greengrass: Vancouver, p 619 and p 727
11. Leonforte JF (1986) Contact dermatitis from *Larrea* (creosote bush). J Am Acad Dermatol 14:202–207
12. Gonzalez-Coloma A, Wisdom CS, Rundel PW (1988) Ozone impact on the antioxidant nordihydroguaiaretic acid content in the external leaf resin of *Larrea tridentata*. Biochem Syst Ecol 16:59–64
13. Gisvold O, Thaker E (1974) Lignans from Larrea divaricata. J Pharm Sci 63:1905–1907
14. Waller CW, Gisvold O (1945) A phytochemical investigation of *Larrea divaricata* Cav. J Am Pharm Assoc Sci Ed 34:78–81
15. Duisberg PC, Shires LB, Botkin CW (1949) Determination of nordihydroguaiaretic acid in the leaf of *Larrea divaricata* (creosote bush). Anal Chem 21:1393–1396
16. Valentine JL, McKenzie L, Kovarik F (1984) Gas chromatographic determination of nordihydroguaiaretic acid in Larrea divaricata. Anal Lett 17:1617–1626
17. Wellendorf M (1964) Nordihydroguajaretsyre (N.D.G.A.) II. Stamplantens indholdsstoffer. Dansk Tidsskr Farm 38:104–108
18. Konno C, Lu ZZ, Xue HZ, Erdelmeier CA, Meksuriyen D, Che CT, Cordell GA, Soejarto DD, Waller DP, Fong HH (1990) Furanoid lignans from Larrea tridentata. J Nat Prod 53:396–406

19. Gisvold O (1948) A preliminary survey of the occurrence of nordihydroguaiaretic acid in *Larrea divaricata*. J Am Pharm Assoc Sci Ed 37:194–196
20. Smart CR, Hogle HH, Robins RK, Broom AD, Bartholomew D (1969) An interesting observation on nordihydroguaiaretic acid (NSC-4291; NDGA) and a patient with malignant melanoma. A preliminary report. Cancer Chemother Rep 53:147–151
21. Horn GM, Gisvold O (1945) A phytochemical study of *Larrea divaricata* Cav. with special emphasis on its yellow pigments. J Am Pharm Assoc Sci Ed 34:82–86
22. Reemtsma K, Maloney Jr JV (1974) The economics of instant medical news. N Engl J Med 290:439–442
23. Anonymous (1970) Chaparral tea. CA 20:112–113
24. Bergel M (1955) Empleo del acido nordihydroguayaretico en terapeutica. La Semana Medica 2:123–131
25. Katz M, Saibil F (1990) Herbal hepatitis: subacute hepatic necrosis secondary to chaparral leaf. J Clin Gastroenterol 12:203–206
26. Oliveto EP (1972) Nordihydroguaiaretic acid. A naturally occurring antioxidant. Chem Ind 17:677–679
27. Tappel AL, Marr AG (1954) Effect of alpha-tocopherol, propyl gallate, and nordihydroguaiaretic acid on enzymatic reactions. J Agric Food Chem 2:554–558
28. Gardner KD Jr, Reed WP, Evan AP, Zedalis J, Hylarides MD, Leon AA (1987) Endotoxin provocation of experimental renal cystic disease. Kidney Int 32:329–334
29. Zedalis JM, Leon AA, Gardner KD Jr, Hylarides MD (1986) High-performance liquid chromatographic determination of nordihydroguaiaretic acid. Anal Lett 19:1443–1456
30. Jordan ML, Hoffman RA, Simmons RL (1987) Prevention of experimental allograft rejection by nordihydroguaiaretic acid. Transplant Proc 19:1307
31. Newton JA, Boodle KM, Dowd PM, Greaves MW (1988) Topical NDGA (nordihydroguaiaretic acid) in psoriasis. Br J Dermatol 119:404–406
32. Grice HC, Becking G, Goodman T (1968) Toxic properties of nordihydroguaiaretic acid. Fd Cosmet Toxicol 6:155–161
33. Goodman T, Grice HC, Becking GC, Salem FA (1970) A cystic nephropathy induced by nordihydroguaiaretic acid in the rat. Light and electron microscopic investigations. Lab Invest 23:93–107
34. Gardner Jr KD, Evan AP, Reed WP (1986) Accelerated renal cyst development in deconditioned germ-free rats. Kidney Int 29:1116–1123
35. Cranston EM, Jensen MJ, Moren A, Brey T, Bell ET, Bieter RN (1947) The acute and chronic toxicity of nordihydroguaiaretic acid. Fed Proc 6:318–319
36. Lehman AJ, Fitzhugh OG, Nelson AA, Woodard G (1951) The pharmacological evaluation of antioxidants. Adv Fd Res 3:197–208
37. Shasky DR (1986) Contact dermatitis from *Larrea tridentata* (creosote bush). J Am Acad Dermatol 15:302
38. Jorgensen G, Hjorth N (1970) Dermatitis from nordihydroguaiaretic acid, an antioxidant in fats. Contact Dermatitis Newsletter 7:151
39. Roed-Petersen J, Hjorth N (1976) Contact dermatitis from antioxidants. Hidden sensitizers in topical medications and foods. Br J Dermatol 94:233–241
40. Tregellas WM, South SF (1980) Autoimmune syndrome induced by chaparral ingestion. Transfusion 20:647–648
41. Garatty G, Petz LD (1975) Drug-induced hemolytic anemia. Am J Med 58:398–407
42. Eidson M, Philen RM, Sewell CM, Voorhees R, Kilbourne EM (1990) L-tryptophan and eosinophilia-myalgia syndrome in New Mexico. Lancet 335, 645–648
43. Evan AP, Gardner Jr KD (1979) Nephron obstruction in nordihydroguaiaretic acid-induced renal cystic disease. Kidney Int 15:7–19
44. Telford IR, Woodruff CS, Linford RH (1962) Fetal resorption in the rat as influenced by certain antioxidants. Am J Anat 110:29–36

Lithospermum Species

H. Winterhoff

Botany

Lithospermum officinale L. belongs to the Boraginaceae. Its most common vernacular name is cromwell. It is domestic nearly all over Europe and the Western parts of Asia and acclimated in China and North America.

Lithospermum ruderale Dougl. ex Lehm. is a shrub indigenous to North America, where it is widespread as a weed. The vernicular name is stone seed.

Chemistry

A complete analysis of the composition of *Lithosperumum officinale* L. has not been performed; however, various constituents were identified when searching for the active principle.

In the herb, 1.3% phosphatides were found, including phytoglucolipid, monophosphoinositide, phosphatidylethanolamine, phosphatidylcholine, a cerebroside, and β-sitosterol. Various amino acids were detected, as were 0.03% scyllitol and bornesite. A cyanogenic glycoside was isolated and identified [1]. Gallotannins and tannins of the catechin type were also found. Rutin, ellagic acid, caffeic acid, and chlorogenic acid could be identified [2]. Later on, lithospermic acid [3] and rosmarinic acid [4] were isolated.

In the root glucose, saccharose, glucofructosane, myristic acid, and fatty acids were found [5] as well as β-sitosterol, rutin and bornesit. The red pigment is probably shikonin [2]. Lithospermic acid was identified subsequently [3].

The seed contains 17–20% fatty oil, composed of neutral fats; 1.3% phosphatides and fatty acids, consisting of palmitic acid, stearic acid, hexadecadiene acid, octadecatriene acid, hydroxypentacosene acid, hydroxyeicosatriene acid [5], oleic acid, linolenic acid, tetraenic acid; and vitamin E and fructane. The ash (30%) is composed of CaO (59%), SiO_2 (27%), K_2O, MgO, P_2O_5, N_2O, and Fe_2O_3 [2].

Pyrrolizidine alkaloids have also been detected in the plant [6,7].

Adverse Effects of Herbal Drugs, Vol. 2
(ed. by P.A.G.M. De Smet, K. Keller, R. Hänsel, R.F. Chandler)

In the root of *Lithospermum ruderale* two flavonoles were identified [2] and rutin, allantoin, chlorogenic acid, and succinic acid were found [8]. The antihormonal activity of the root was attributed to its lithospermic acid content and to the presence of a very active polyphenol oxidase [9,10]. In the herb rutin, bornesite, phlobotannins, carbonic acids as well as lithospermic acid were identified [11].

Pharmacology and Uses

In former times *Lithospermum officinale* was used as a remedy in diseases of the urogenital tract and as a spasmolytic drug.

Lithospermum ruderale was used as an antidiarrhoeal drug by Indians in North America; a few tribes in Nevada used cold water extracts of the root as an oral contraceptive [12,13].

For a discussion on the effects of the plants on endocrine functions the reader is referred to the monograph on *Lycopus* species. Additional reported effects of *Lithospermum* application include a reduction of the incidence in mammary tumours in mice [14].

Adverse Reaction Profile

General Animal Data

The oral administration of 0.5 ml aqueous extract (corresponding to 1 g fresh *Lithospermum* leaves) by gavage caused no toxic signs in mice. Even when 30% of the diet were composed of dried leaves of *Lithospermum*, no toxic signs were observed in mice after a period of 14 days [15]. Correspondingly, no toxic effects were observed when rats were treated for 10 days with a suspension of 1–3 g powdered leaves daily by gavage. In contrast, repeated subcutaneous injection caused infiltrations and necroses at the injection site, and the intraperitoneal injection of high doses resulted in ascites with peritoneal irritation [15–18]. Very high doses can be lethal following severe diarrhoea [15,18]. For these findings as well as for a moderate increase in adrenal weight after repeated parenteral administration toxic constituents of the crude extracts were held responsible, not the constituents with endocrine activity [15,17].

General Human Data

Because *Lithospermum officinale* extracts have not been used in therapy in the past few decades only few observations in humans exist. Even administering 30 g extract from dried leaves of *Lithospermum officinale* for 4 days in healthy volunteers did not cause any severe side effects. A slight reduction of blood glucose was observed, but in no case were hypoglycaemic symptoms seen. The daily intake of 240 mg freeze-dried extract of *Lithospermum officinale* caused no overt adverse effects over a period of 6–8 weeks [17].

Endocrine Reactions

See the monograph on *Lycopus* species for a general discussion on endocrine effects.

Metabolic Effects

Lithospermum treatment has been associated with a moderate decrease in blood glucose in experimental animals; this effect was explained as an antiglucagon effect [17,18]. It is unclear, however, whether this finding has clinical significance (see the section on general human data).

Fertility, Pregnancy, and Lactation

The treatment of pregnant rats with aqueous *Lithospermum* extracts 8 days before conception had no influence on the duration of pregnancy, but the weight of the offspring was reduced [17].

This weight reduction was clearly more pronounced at day 10 postpartum when maternal treatment was continued, probably as a consequence of the prolactin-lowering activity of the plant extract. At present, a direct toxic action of *Lithospermum* constituents on the offspring cannot be excluded.

The pronounced antiprolactin effects as well as the possibility of direct toxic effects on the offspring suggest that use of these plants should be avoided in pregnancy and during lactation.

Mutagenicity and Carcinogenicity

No reports on mutagenic or carcinogenic effects of *Lithospermum* extracts have been found. For information on the mutagenicity and carcinogenicity of quercetin and rutin the reader is referred to the monograph on *Lycopus* species. The occurrence of pyrrolizidine alkaloids should be taken into account when the carcinogenic risk of *Lithospermum* is evaluated.

References

1. Sosa A, Winternitz F, Wylde R, Pavia AA (1977) Structure of a cyanoglycoside of Lithospermum purpureo-caeruleum. Phytochemistry 16:707
2. Hörhammer L, Wagner H, König H (1961) Zur Kenntnis der Inhaltsstoffe von Lithospermum officinale L. Arzneim Forsch 14:34–40
3. Wagner H, Wittmann D, Schäfer W (1975) Zur chemischen Struktur der Lithospermsäure aus Lithospermum officinale L. Tetrahedron Letters 8:547–550
4. Wylde R, Sosa A, Winternitz F, Gumbinger HG, Winterhoff H, Sourgens H, Kemper FH (1983) Investigations on the structure-function-relationship and the antigonadotropic activity of phenolic compounds. Naunyn-Schmiedeberg's Arch Pharmacol (Suppl 324):R58
5. Sosa A, Sosa-Bourdouil C, Hardy C (1955) Sur les constituants lipidiques de quelques espèces de "Lithospermum" (Borraginées). CR Acad Sci 240:1570
6. Anonymous (1988) Pyrrolizidine Alkaloids. Environmental Health Criteria 80:309 Geneva: World Health Organization
7. Anonymous (1988) Pyrrolizidinalkaloidhaltige Humanarzneimittel. Dtsch Apoth Ztg 128(33):62–63
8. Shaw RGA (1960) Phytochemical investigation of Lithospermum ruderale. Thesis, Indiana University
9. Gassner FX, Hopwood ML, Jöchle W, Johnson F, Sunderwirth SG (1963) Antifertility activity of an oxidized polyphenolic acid from Lithospermum ruderale. Proc Soc Exp Biol Med 114:20–25
10. Johnson G, Sunderwirth SG, Gibian H, Coulter AW, Gassner FX (1963) Lithospermum ruderale: Partial characterization of the principal polyphenol isolated from the roots. Phytochemistry 2:145–150
11. List PH, Hörhammer L (ed.) (1976) Hagers Handbuch der Pharmazeutischen Praxis. Berlin: Springer Verlag
12. Cranston EM (1945) The effect of Lithospermum ruderale on the estrous cycle of mice. J Pharmacology 83:130–142
13. Breneman WR, Carmack M, Overack DE, Creek RO, Shaw R (1960) Inhibition of anterior pituitary gonadotropins and oxytocin by extracts of Lithospermum ruderale. Endocrinology 67:583–596
14. Cranston EM, Kucera GR, Bittner JJ (1950) Lithospermum ruderale and the incidence of mammary tumors in mice. Proc Soc Exp Biol Med 75:779–781
15. Kemper F, Loeser A, Opitz K, Schwarz G (1956) Pharmakologische Eigenschaften der Steinhirse (Lithospermum officinale Linné). Arch Int Pharmacodyn 108:200–214
16. Slusher MA (1954) The influence of the pituitary-adrenal mechanism on the action of Lithospermum ruderale. Endocrinology 55:466–473
17. Kemper F (1959) Experimentelle Grundlagen für eine therapeutische Anwendung von Lithospermum officinale zur Blockierung von Hormonen des Hypophysenvorderlappens. Arzneim Forsch 9:368–375, 411–419
18. Girre L, Nettavongs M (1977) Le Lithosperme: un anticonceptionel à decouvrir. Bull Soc Pharm Ouest 19:27–48

Lycopus Species

H. Winterhoff

Botany

Lycopus europaeus L. belongs to the Lamiaceae. Its vernacular name is gipsy wort. The plant is indigenous to nearly the whole of Europe and northern parts of Russia, and it is acclimated in North America and Australia.

Another *Lycopus* species of medicinal importance is *Lycopus virginicus* Michx. Vernicular names are bugle-weed, Virginia horehound, gipsy weed, sweet bugle, American archangel, bitter bugle, gipsy wort, wood betony, and Paul's betony. The shrub is native to all of North America, from Canada to Florida.

Chemistry

A complete analysis of the chemical composition of *Lycopus europaeus* has not been performed up to now. Rather diverse constituents were identified when searching for the active principle. According to Pulatova and Sharipov [1], the herb contains 0.2% essential oil, 2.9% resin, 2.3% flavonoids, 0.12% coumarin, 0.24% alkaloids, ascorbic acid, and carotene. Hörhammer et al. [2] found amino acids, sugars, 0.15–0.17% essential oil, and a sapogenin. They identified apigenin-7-glucoside, luteolin-7-glucoside, caffeic acid, chlorogenic acid, ursolic acid, sinapinic acid, ellagic acid, and rosmarinic acid and also reported a fluorine content of 0.09%. Wagner et al. [3] detected lithospermic acid in *Lycopus europaeus* and elucidated its configuration [4]. This compound could not be isolated from *Lycopus* extracts of various other origins [5].

Systematic investigations on the chemical composition of *Lycopus virginicus* have not been performed. Only the occurrence of 0.08% essential oil, a bitter substance lycopin (chemically not defined), resin, gallic acid, and tannic acids has been described [6,7]. Hörhammer et al. [2] state that its major constituents are similar to those of *Lycopus europaeus*. Lithospermic acid was identified by Wagner et al. [3]. Caffeic acid, ferulic acid, and rosmarinic acid have also been found [5].

Adverse Effects of Herbal Drugs, Vol. 2
(ed. by P.A.G.M. De Smet, K. Keller, R. Hänsel, R.F. Chandler)

Pharmacology and Uses

Lycopus europaeus has long been used as an antipyretic, astringent, and styptic drug. Later it was given for the same indications as *Lycopus virginicus* Michx. as a specific agent against hyperthyreotic symptoms, especially in patients with tachycardia. A further therapeutic use of *Lycopus europaeus* was reported to be the therapy of irritable breast and mastopathy [8].

Lycopus virginicus Michx. was used as an astringent and in the treatment of hemorrhages. Another long-standing application of this plant is its use as a specific agent in less severe cases of hyperthyroidism, especially in patients with tachycardia.

Since it was shown in 1941 that the activity of *Lycopus europaeus* L., a plant indigenous to Europe, is nearly identical to that of *Lycopus virginicus* Michx., the latter has been more and more replaced by the former [9].

Numerous experimental studies deal with the effects of *Lycopus* species as well as with those of *Lithospermum officinale* and *Lithospermum ruderale* Dougl. ex Lehm. The spectrum of effects of these plants on the endocrine system is similar, and the same phenolic plant constituents seem to be responsible for these activities. In some cases even the same mode of action could be proven. Thus the activities of the extracts from *Lycopus* species as well as those from *Lithospermum officinale* on endocrine functions will be discussed together here. In animal experiments, antigonadotropic, antiprolactin, and antithyreotropic effects are common to all these plant extracts.

Antigonadotropic activity was found in investigations *in vitro* as well as in experiments *in vivo* in rodents [4,10–13]. The acute administration of plant extracts caused a short-term decline of LH in serum, whereas signs of peripheral gonadotropin deficiency and an increase in pituitary gonadotropin concentration were observed following repeated administration. **Antiprolactin** activity could be demonstrated by a decline of radioimmunologically determined prolactin levels [10,14].

Antithyreotropic activity was found *in vitro* as well as in experiments *in vivo* [9–11,14–22]. *In vivo* injection is followed by a rapid and distinct decline of the TSH levels in serum. Even a goitrogenic increase in thyroid weight could be reduced by repeated administration of *Lithospermum* extracts [10].

Other points of attack on the thyroid function have also been established. A direct antithyroidal TSH-independent inhibition of thyroid secretion was reported, even more pronounced that that caused by iodine [14,23]. Hints of inhibition of peripheral T_4-deiodination were obtained *in vivo* [19], and further evidence was obtained by testing the effect on isolated liver enzymes [24].

Findings about the effect of *Lycopus* extracts on iodine metabolism are contradictory. Increased iodine concentration in the thyroid gland due to reduced secretion was reported [16], whereas other authors observed only reduced iodine storage without an influence on iodine concentration

[17,25]. A direct attack at the pituitary level has also been suggested [14].

Phenolic products formed after an oxidation reaction from phenolic precursors, e.g., rosmarinic acid, caffeic acid, flavones, and flavone glucosides, are responsible for the effects of *Lithospermum* and *Lycopus* species on endocrine functions [5,12,26–28]. The concept of lithospermic acid as the only precursor of active compounds has been rejected, as caffeic acid, rosmarinic acid, chlorogenic acid, and flavonoids also represent precursors of compounds with distinct antihormonal activity. In contrast to the other endocrine effects, oxidation does not seem essential for inhibition of T_4 conversion.

The mode of inactivation of thyreotropin as well as that of the gonadotropins may be clarified as follows: a direct binding of phenolic plant constituents to the hormones accounts for a distinct loss in activity and for alterations in the secondary structure of the hormone. Following such an interaction a loss of binding to the receptor is observed [11,29–31].

Adverse Reaction Profile

General Animal Data

Pressed juice of *Lycopus europaeus* (0.75 ml corresponding to 7.5 g fresh plant) proved to be lethal in male mice [9,15]. Repeated subcutaneous injection of more than 20 mg aqueous extracts to rats caused local infiltrations and necroses, whereas higher intraperitoneal doses (100 mg freeze-dried extract) produced exudation and peritoneal irritation [14]. In addition an increase in adrenal weights was observed. Toxic constituents of the crude extracts were held responsible for these findings, not those exerting endocrine activity.

In rats an increase in thyroid weight under *Lycopus* extract treatment was reported [14]. It could be shown that the development of goiter was not an unavoidable reaction to the plant but was caused by the irregular injection intervals at which the extract was administered (8/16 h). Thus rebound phenomena seem to be responsible for this reaction. When the plant extract was given at 12-h intervals, even a reduction of thyroid weight could be observed [11,13].

Only one report deals with toxic effects of *Lycopus virginicus* extracts. Intravenous administration of 1.0 ml fresh squashed juice of the herb proved to be lethal in mice whereas even 3.0 ml of the same preparation given orally caused no toxic symptoms [9].

General Human Data

Various clinical studies deal with the treatment of patients with hyperthyreotic symptoms. Mostly preparations from *Lycopus europaeus* (Lycocyn) were used [25,32–41]. Other products used were Thyreogutt, a combination of extracts from *Lycopus* and *Leonurus cardiaca* [18,34,38–40,42–45], and extracts from *Lycopus virginicus* [46,47]. Only a few of these reports mention undesired thyroidal effects (see the section on endocrine reactions). Headache as an undesired side effect was mentioned for Thyreogutt and could be avoided by reduction of the dosage [45].

Endocrine Reactions

A few reports mention an increase in size of the thyroid gland under treatment with Lycocyn or Thyreogutt [39,40,48]. An increase in thyroid volume was repeatedly seen after treatment of patients with euthyreotic goiter [40], an indication for which *Lycopus* preparations should clearly be excluded. In one of 36 hyperthyreotic patients treated with Thyreogutt an increase in thyroid size was under discussion [48]. An initial increase of hyperthyreotic symptoms such as nervousness, tachycardia, and loss of body weight have been mentioned occasionally [9,34,49].

Drug Interactions

Interference with thyroidal radioiodine uptake during *Lycopus* treatment has been reported [49].

Fertility, Pregnancy, and Lactation

Treatment with *Lycopus* can arrest the vaginal cycle of mice and rats and reduce the number of offspring [11,13]. As a consequence of the antiprolactin activity, a decreased milk supply was observed in suckling rats [14,50].

The pronounced antiprolactin effects and the possibility of direct toxic effects on the offspring suggest that these plants should be avoided in pregnancy and during lactation.

Mutagenicity and Carcinogenicity

Mutagenic or carcinogenic effects of *Lycopus* extracts have not been reported. Such effects have only been reported for the widespread constituents rutin and quercetin [e.g., 51,52]. These findings started a broad and controversial discussion [53]. Several *in vivo* investigations have now disproved the *in vitro* findings, as long-term studies have shown no increase in the incidence of carcinoma [54–57]. In addition, both compounds are common in vegetables as well as in medicinal plants. Thus a small additional supply through a herbal medicine will not be of great importance. Moreover, ellagic acid, another constituent of this plant, may perhaps counteract carcinogenic effects [58].

References

1. Pulatova TP, Sharipov SHN (1969) Pharmacognostic study of Lycopus europaeus grown in Uzbekistan. Chem Abstracts 70:230
2. Hörhammer L, Wagner H, Schilcher H (1962) Zur Kenntnis der Inhaltsstoffe von Lycopus europaeus. Arzneim Forsch 12:1–7
3. Wagner H, Hörhammer L, Frank U (1970) Lithospermsäure, das antihormonale Wirkprinzip von Lycopus europaeus L. (Wolfsfuß) und Symphytum officinale L. (Beinwell). Arzneim Forsch 20:705–713
4. Wagner H, Wittmann D, Schäfer W (1975) Zur chemischen Struktur der Lithospermsäure aus Lithospermum officinale L. Tetrahedron Letters 8:547–550
5. Wylde R, Sosa A, Winternitz F, Winterhoff H, Kemper FH (1980) Sur l'isolement des principes responsables de l'activité antigonadotropique a partir de diverses espèces de Lithospermum et Lycopus. Planta Med 39:35
6. Schindler H (1955) Die Inhaltsstoffe von Heilpflanzen und Prüfungsmethoden für pflanzliche Tinkturen: Lycopus virginicus. Arzneim Forsch 5:99–102
7. List PH, Hörhammer L (1976) Hagers Handbuch der Pharmazeutischen Praxis. Berlin: Springer Verlag
8. Mohr, H (1969) Behandlung mit einem Thyreoregulans bei Mastodynie und Mastopathie. Ärztliche Praxis 21:3613
9. Madaus G, Koch FrE, Albus G (1941) Tierexperimentelle Untersuchungen über die antithyreoide Wirksamkeit von Lycopus europaeus und Lycopus virginicus (Wolfsfuß). Z Ges Exp Med 109:411–424
10. Sourgens H, Winterhoff H, Gumbinger HG, Kemper FH (1982) Antihormonal effects of plant extracts: TSH- and prolactin-suppressing properties of Lithospermum officinale and other plants. Planta Med 45:78–86
11. Winterhoff H (1988) Pharmakologische Charakterisierung von Arzneipflanzen-Inhaltsstoffen mit Wirkungen auf das Endokrinium. Habilitationsschrift, Münster
12. Winterhoff H, Gumbinger HG, Sourgens H (1988) On the antigonadotropic activity of Lithospermum and Lycopus species and some of their phenolic constituents. Planta Med 55:101–106
13. Schaffstein W (1989) Untersuchungen zum Einfluß pflanzlicher Extrakte und ihrer Inhaltsstoffe auf endokrine Parameter und Organgewichte der weiblichen Ratte unter Beachtung des Östruszyklus. Thesis, Münster
14. Sourgens H (1984) Pharmakologische Grundlagen einer Beeinflussung endokriner Systeme, insbesondere der Schilddrüse, durch Pflanzeninhaltsstoffe. Habilitationsschrift, Münster
15. Koch FrE (1952) Weitere Untersuchungen über die antithyreoide Wirkung von Lycopus europaeus (Wolfsfuß). Madaus Jahresberichte 6:107–112
16. Hiller E, Girod E (1954) Experimentelle Untersuchungen über die Beeinflußbarkeit der Schilddrüse durch Konzentrate aus Lycopus europaeus unter Berücksichtigung der Histologie und des Jodstoffwechsels. Arzneim Forsch 4:380–388
17. Hartenstein H, Müller WA (1961) Untersuchungen über die Wirkung von Lycopus europaeus und Lithospermum officinale auf den Schilddrüsenstoffwechsel der Ratte. Hippokrates 32:284–288
18. Kemper F, Loeser A, Richter A (1961) Antihormonale Wirksamkeit von Lycopus (Wolfsfuß). Arzneim Forsch 11:92–94

19. Winterhoff H, Sourgens H, Gumbinger HG, Kemper FH (1979) Effects of acute and chronical application of antihormonal plant extracts. Acta Endocrinol (Kbh.) 225 (Suppl):43
20. Mendes R, Sourgens H, Kemper FH (1980) Interaction of different plant ingredients with hypothalamic-hypophyseal hormones in the rat. Naunyn Schmiedeberg's Arch Pharmacol 311 (Suppl):209
21. Sourgens H, Winterhoff H, Kemper FH (1980) Phytotherapie bei Schilddrüsenerkrankungen. Phys Med Rehabil 21:100–102
22. Sourgens H, Winterhoff H, Gumbinger HG, Kemper FH (1986) Effects of Lithospermum officinale and related plants on hypophyseal and thyroid hormones in the rat. Int J Crude Drug Res 24:53–63
23. Frömbling-Borges A (1987) Intrathyreoidale Wirkung von Lycopus europaeus, Pflanzensäuren, Tyrosinen, Thyroninen und Lithium-chlorid. Darstellung einer Schilddrüsensekretionsblockade. Thesis, Münster
24. AufmKolk M, Koehrle J, Gumbinger H, Winterhoff H, Hesch RD (1984) Antihormonal effects of plant extracts: iodothyronine deiodinase of rat liver is inhibited by extracts and secondary metabolites of plants. Horm Metab Res 16:188–192
25. Schach H (1955) Beeinflussung der Schilddrüsenfunktion durch Lycopus vulgaris. Münch Med Wschr 25:824–826
26. Gumbinger HG, Winterhoff H (1980) Characterisation of antihormonal active substances from Lithospermum officinale and Lycopus virginicus. Naunyn Schmiedeberg's Arch Pharmacol 311 (Suppl):208
27. Gumbinger HG, Winterhoff H, Sourgens H, Kemper FH, Wylde R (1981) Formation of compounds with antigonadotropic activity from inactive phenolic precursors. Contraception 23:661–666
28. Wylde R, Sosa A, Winternitz F, Gumbinger HG, Winterhoff H, Sourgens H, Kemper FH (1983) Investigations on the structure-function-relationship and the antigonadotropic activity of phenolic compounds. Naunyn-Schmiedeberg's Arch Pharmacol 324 (Suppl):R58
29. Gumbinger HG (1983) Isolation of TSH-inhibitor-complexes and investigations on their secondary structure by circular dichroism spectroscopy. Naunyn-Schmiedeberg's Arch Pharmacol 322 (Suppl):R59
30. AufmKolk M, Ingbar J, Amir S, Winterhoff H, Sourgens H, Hesch RD, Ingbar SH (1984) Inhibition by certain plant extracts of the binding and adenylate cyclase stimulatory effect of bovine thyrotropin in human thyroid membranes. Endocrinology 115:527–534
31. AufmKolk M, Ingbar J, Kubota K, Amir SM, Ingbar SH (1985) Extracts and autooxidized constituents of certain plants inhibit the receptor-binding and the biological activity of Graves' immunoglobulins. Endocrinology 116:1687–1693
32. Mattausch F (1943) Aus der Praxis-für die Praxis. Hippokrates 14:168–171
33. Assmann E (1950) Lycopus europaeus. Allg Hom Ztg 2:55–67
34. Falk E (1950) Ein neuer Weg der Behandlung von Thyreotoxikosen für den praktischen Arzt. Hippokrates 21:718–720
35. Leppert H (1951/52) Zur konservativen Therapie der Thyreotoxikosen. Therapiewoche 2:571–572
36. Hiller E, Deglmann H (1955) Der Einfluß von Extrakten aus Lycopus europaeus auf die Jodverteilung im menschlichen Serum. Arzneim Forsch 5:465–470
37. Frank J (1959) Gefahrlose Hyperthyreose-Behandlung in der Allgemeinpraxis. Münch Med Wschr 101:203–204
38. Klein E (1964) Die Indikationen zu den verschiedenen Behandlungsverfahren der Hyperthyreose. Therapiewoche 14:1183–1189
39. Freyschmidt P (1967) Langzeittherapie der Strumen. Therapiewoche 17:623–628
40. Freyschmidt P (1968) Schilddrüsenerkrankungen. Georg Thieme Verlag, Stuttgart
41. Karl HJ (1974) Schilddrüsenhormone und Thyreostatica. Dtsch Apoth-Ztg 114:187–188
42. Pleimes (1951/52) Therapie der Thyreotoxikose. Therapiewoche 2:361–362

43. Keil A, Dworacek A (1952) Neuere Erfahrungen bei der Behandlung von Hyperthyreosen und vegetativen Dystonien. Die Medizinische 26:891–893
44. Lobenhofer G (1953) Klinische Erfahrungen mit Thyreogutt. Münch Med Wschr 51:1375
45. Sittig H (1955) Über Operationsvorbereitung der Thyreotoxikosen und des Morbus Basedow mit pflanzlichen Wirkstoffen. Münch Med Wschr 97:826–832
46. Volk G (1930) Einige Beobachtungen und Bemerkungen zur homöpathischen Behandlung von Kreislaufkranken. Hippokrates 2:293–309
47. Braun H (1978) Mehrjährige Erfahrungen mit Lycoaktin. Arch Arzneither 3:15–54
48. Wolf G (1954) Über Hyperthyreosebehandlung in der freien Praxis. Landarzt 30:756–763
49. Samec V (1962) Diagnostische und therapeutische Möglichkeiten bei Störungen der Schilddrüsenfunktion. Mitteilungen aus Forschung und Praxis (Dr. Willmar Schwabe GmbH Karlsruhe) 3:207–215
50. Kolodziej C, Sourgens H, Gumbinger HG, Kemper FH (1984) Beeinflussung des Hypophysenvorderlappenhormons Prolaktin durch Lycopus europaeus. Farm Tijdschr Belg 61:312
51. Alvi NK, Rizvi RY, Hadi SM (1986) Interaction of quercetin with DNA. Bioscience Rep 6(10):861–868
52. De Smet PAGM, Vulto AG (1988) Drugs used in non-orthodox medicine. In: Dukes MMG, Beeley L (ed) Side effects of Drugs Annual 12, Amsterdam: Elsevier Science Publishers, pp 402–415
53. World Health Organization (1982) Quercetin. IARC Monographs on the evaluation of the carcinogenic risk of chemicals to humans 31:213–223
54. Saito D, Shirai A, Matsushima T, Sugimura T, Hirono I (1980) Test of carcinogenicity of quercetin, a widely distributed mutagen in food. Teratogen Carcinogen Mutagen 1:213–221
55. Aeschbacher HU, Meier H, Ruch E (1982) Nonmutagenicity *in vivo* of the food flavonol quercetin. Nutr Cancer 4(2):90–98
56. Morino K, Matsukura N, Kawachi T, Ohgaki H, Sugimura T, Hirono I (1982) Carcinogenicity test of quercetin and rutin in golden hamsters by oral administration. Carcinogenesis 3:93–97
57. Bertram B (1989) Flavonoide: Eine Klasse von Pflanzeninhaltsstoffen mit viefältigen biologischen Wirkungen, auch mit karzinogener Wirkung? Dtsch Apoth Ztg 47:2561–2571
58. Sayer JM, Yagi H, Wood AW, Conney AH, Jerina DM (1982) Extremely facile reaction between the ultimate carcinogen benzo(a)pyrene-7,8-diol 9,10-epoxide and ellagic acid. J Am Chem Soc 104:5562–5564

Phytolacca Americana

P.A.G.M. De Smet

Botany

Phytolacca americana L. (syn. *P. decandra* L.) belongs to the Phytolaccaceae [1]. English vernacular names include poke, pokeweed, pokeroot, pokeberry, inkberry, pigeon berry, American nightshade, scoke, pocan, red ink, and garget [2–5]. The plant is known as Kermes in German and as phytolaque in French [2].

Chemistry

In the 19th century, the roots of *P. americana* were believed to contain an alkaloidal substance named "phytolaccine", together with phytolaccic acid, tannin, resin, gum and fixed oil [6]. However, later researchers were unable to confirm the presence of any alkaloid [7–9]. Although this makes "phytolaccine" a confusing concept, the term still is occasionally encountered in modern toxicological literature [10,11].

After the presence of alkaloids had been disproved, phytochemical research on the roots of *P. americana* focused primarily on the presence of saponins. Ahmed et al. [8] reported the isolation of a toxic acidic steroidal saponin. Stout et al. [12] designated this material as phytolaccatoxin, and obtained from it, by acid hydrolysis, a triterpene aglycone named phytolaccagenin. Woo and co-workers [13–15] subsequently demonstrated that the roots also yielded the closely related aglycone phytolaccagenic acid. They isolated seven different triterpene saponins, which were designated as phytolaccosides A, B, D, E, G, F and D_2. In addition, several sterols were identified [16].

Johnson and Shimizu [17] obtained, from the fresh berry juice of *P. americana*, 0.6% of a crude saponin mixture. This fraction afforded, on acid hydrolysis, the triterpene aglycones phytolaccagenin (the major aglycone), desmethylphytolaccagenin (= jaligonic acid), and phytolaccinic acid (= phytolaccagenic acid). Oleanolic acid, the major aglycone in berries of *P. dodecandra*, was detected only in a trace amount. The presence of

Adverse Effects of Herbal Drugs, Vol. 2
(ed. by P.A.G.M. De Smet, K. Keller, R. Hänsel, R.F. Chandler)

phytolaccagenin, jaligonic acid, and phytolaccagenic acid in the hydrolysate was confirmed by Kang and Woo [18]. These researchers also detected the structurally related pokeberrygenin and esculentic acid, together with a trace of acinosolic acid [18]. The berries of *P. americana* contain a considerable amount of red pigment, phytolaccanin, which is identical to the betanin pigment of beetroot (*Beta vulgaris*) [19,20].

The leaves and seeds of *P. americana* yield proteins which have been designated as pokeweed antiviral proteins (PAPs) because of their antiviral activity [21–24]. A pokeweed antiviral protein also occurs in the seeds of the related *P. acinosa* [25]. The seeds of *P. americana* also contain lignans that are known as americanin A, americanin B, and americanin D [26].

Pharmacology and Uses

The root of *P. americana* was at one time described as an alterative, cathartic, emetic, a narcotic, and a gargle, as well as a remedy for conjunctivitis, cancer, dyspepsia, glandular swelling, chronic rheumatism, ringworm, scabies, and ulcers. There is no satisfactory evidence, however, that it has any therapeutical usefulness [2,11,27,28].

Poke root has also been used in non-western folk medicine for treating edema and rheumatism, and it is alleged that its saponins have anti-inflammatory activity [14]. A Chinese text book recommends the roots of *P. americana* and *P. acinosa* internally for oliguria, edema and ascites, and externally for trauma, hemorrhage, carbuncle, and pyogenic skin infections [29].

Poke berries have also been employed in folk medicine for the treatment of rheumatism and arthritis [28], and their purple juice has reputedly been used to color food and wine [19,27]. Similar to the fruit of *P. dodecandra*, which yields a potent molluscicidal substance known as "endod", the fruit of *P. americana* has been shown to contain one or more molluscicidal principles [17,30].

The sprouts of the young poke plant are sometimes eaten as potherbs after being boiled in two changes of water [3].

The pokeweed antiviral proteins occurring in the leaves and seeds of *P. americana* exhibit antiviral activity and inhibit protein synthesis in cell-free systems [21,22,25,31]. The seed protein was shown to have immunomodulatory activity in experimental animals [23].

Adverse Reaction Profile

The toxicity of *P. americana* is generally believed to reside in its triterpene saponins and its mitogenic proteins [8,28,32,33]. The toxicology of the related *P. dodecandra* has been reviewed by Duncan [34]. According to an early source, death has occurred following the administration of 10 to 15 g of the juice of raw fresh leaves of *P. dodecandra* [35].

General Animal Data

Macht [27] studied the toxicity of fluid alcoholic extracts of poke root and poke berries in experimental animals. The extracts were administered as such or in the form of saline suspensions obtained by evaporating the alcohol and replacing it by physiological saline. The saline suspensions proved to be very irritating, and their intraperitoneal lethality for mice, rats, and guinea pigs was found to be quite high. Intravenous injection into anesthesized cats markedly depressed respiratory and circulatory functions. Administration of diluted poke root extract by stomach tube to cats produced violent vomiting. Large oral doses of fluid extracts did not impair the kidney function of rabbits, but liver function was markedly impaired by this treatment.

Goldstein et al. [7] observed the following sequence of symptoms in cats following intraperitoneal administration of a hydroalcoholic extract, corresponding to 1.0 g of poke root per kg body weight: discomfort, retching and sometimes emesis; gradual loss of the use of hind and front legs; stupor, somnolence and diminished perception of pain; profound narcosis; slower and weaker heart beat and shallower respiration; and ultimately death from respiratory failure.

Ahmed et al. [8] tested the toxicity of an acidic steroidal saponin obtained from the root of *P. americana* in mice. Its intraperitoneal LD_{50} was computed as 0.065 mg/kg. With lethal doses, the substance showed marked depressant activity, especially on circulation and respiration, and it acted as a potent convulsant in relatively larger doses.

Experimental studies of the toxicity of poke berries in poultry have produced conflicting results. In one feeding study, they were harmless to some chickens and a duck [36], whereas in another study the administration of berries to turkey poults produced a reduction of growth rate, ataxia, inability to walk and death [37].

Accidental poisoning in animals is rare, partly because the root (which is generally considered to be the most toxic part of the plant) is underground, and partly because the plant is not particularly palatable [38].

General Human Data

Human intoxication by *P. americana* commonly involves an initial burning sensation in the mouth and throat, followed within a few hours by nausea, protracted vomiting, sometimes with hematesis, salivation, profuse diaphoresis, severe abdominal cramps and pain, watery or bloody diarrhoea, generalized weakness, headache, dizziness, hypotension and tachycardia [5,33,38–42]. Urinary incontinence, confusion, unconsciousness, and gross tremors of the hands may also occur [5], and sometimes melena, visual disturbances, weakened respiration, lethargy, stupor, and convulsions have been observed [10,38,42]. All recently described patients recovered within 24–48 hours, often with the aid of supportive care [5,33,40–42], but fatalities have occurred in the 19th century [33,42].

Several case reports specified that the plant had been used inappropriately, viz. by chewing the root without boiling it prior to consumption [42], by eating the raw leaves [40], or by drinking a herbal tea prepared by extracting the leaves and stems [5] or the powdered root [33] with boiling water. These comments can be retraced to a widespread belief that the young green shoots or leaves can be consumed safely as vegetables after boiling them in water, discarding the cooking water and then reboiling them [3,10,28,38,40,43]. Moreover, a Chinese text states that the toxicity of Shanglu (the root of *P. acinosa* or *P. americana*) may be greatly reduced by boiling the drug for two hours [29]. It should be noted, however, that an outbreak of 21 cases of pokeweed poisoning occurred in a group of campers, who had taken a pokeweed salad prepared by boiling, draining, and reboiling the young leaves. Contrary to claims that this preparation ensures harmlessness, the campers experienced the typical symptoms of pokeweed intoxication, and four of them required hospitalization because of protracted vomiting and dehydration. The camp counselor had been preparing pokeweed salad for many years without apparent ill effects, and it remained unexplained, why his latest salad resulted in an outbreak of gastrointestinal illness [41]. So long as the factors which govern the toxicity of pokeweed preparations remain unknown, abstinence from any preparation seems the only course of action which is guaranteed to be absolutely safe.

Secondary sources generally agree that the root is the most toxic part and that toxicity increases with plant maturity, the only exception being that green berries are considered to be more toxic than mature red berries [10,28,41,42]. Unfortunately, such secondary statements are not supported by primary references, and controversy exists about the relative toxicity of poke berries [28]. It is sometimes alleged that ten berries, if eaten uncooked by a preschool child, are very toxic [10], whereas other sources feel that references to the poisoning of children by the berries are not conclusive [38]. A two-year-old child died after eating berries that were undisputedly pokeweed berries. An original report about this case has never been presented in the literature, however, because the hospital staff members involved disagreed over etiology and the autopsy findings. The hospital pathologist was convinced that the child died from a viral infection, but he noted enlarged lymphocytes, apparently showing mitotic activity, in the brain sections, which eventually led to the discovery of the mitotic capacity (see the section on hematological reactions) [43]. It is sometimes claimed that the berries are edible if cooked [10], but primary information on this subject is quite limited. There is a recent report about a group of boy scouts and their leader, who ate pokeberry pancakes (prepared by stirring mashed pokeberries into pancake batter and frying the mixture over wood fire). No apparent side effects occurred other than mild or moderate diarrhoea [11].

In 1979, the American Herb Trade Association issued a policy statement that pokeroot should not be sold as a herbal beverage or food because of its toxicity. The Association recommended that no part of the mature plant should be sold for ingestion and that all poke products, except immature leaves, should be withdrawn from sale in the United States [33].

Cardiovascular Reactions

Tachycardia and hypotension are commonly noted in intoxications by *P. americana* (see the section on general human data). In one case, ECG-abnormalities suggestive of ischemia were observed [42].

Dermatological Reactions

The green plant and root often produce inflammation of the skin, and topical preparations derived from these parts can result in smarting and burning [44]. Early researchers claimed that this irritant action of poke root is not due to its toxic alcohol-soluble principle, but to one or more water-soluble principles [7].

According to a preamble of a Directive of the European Communities regarding cosmetic products, it is necessary to prohibit the use of *Phytolacca* spp. to protect public health [45].

Gastrointestinal Reactions

Poisoning by *P. americana* is characterized by nausea, vomiting, abdominal cramps and pain, and diarrhoea (see the section on general human data). The latter effect explains, why pokeweed is reputed to be a cathartic (see the section on pharmacology and uses). It should be added, however, that saline suspensions, obtained by evaporating the alcohol from fluid alcoholic extracts of *P. americana* and replacing it by physiological saline, were shown to paralyze *in vitro* intestinal loops from cats and rabbits [27].

Hematological Reactions

The roots of *P. americana* yield five physiochemically distinct proteins with mitogenic properties [46], whereas two mitogenic proteins have been found in the root of the related *P. octandra* [47,48].

In vitro, extracts of *P. americana* have mitogenic effects on human peripheral blood cells in dilutions up to 1:1000000 [49,50]. *In vivo*, large immature basophilic lymphocytes and typical plasma cells appeared in the peripheral blood of two adults shortly after accidental exposure to a root extract (one through the conjunctiva and the other through a subcutaneous puncture wound). An extensive search revealed no mitotic cells, and all other hematological findings were within normal limits [51]. Barker et al. [50] reported a significant increase in the number of plasmacytoid lymphocytes in the peripheral blood of children, who had either ingested the berries of *P. americana* or handled the berries with freshly cut or abrased hands. No distinctive clinical features were seen in association with this peripheral blood plasmacytosis.

The peripheral plasmacytosis may persist for two or more months [4,42].

Ocular Reactions

Since pokeroot has been described as a remedy for conjunctivitis (see the section on pharmacology and uses), it should be noted that the dust of dried poke root is irritant to the eye and that occupational exposure to the fresh plant may result in serious inflammation of the eye lids [7]. Instillation of saline suspensions (obtained by evaporating the alcohol from fluid alcoholic extracts of *P. americana* and replacing it by physiological saline) into rabbit eyes resulted in marked reddening and irritation of the conjunctivae [27].

Respiratory Reactions

Ahmed et al. [8] studied the effect of an acidic steroidal saponin obtained from the root of *P. americana* on the respiratory tract. Inhalation of the substance caused an extreme sternutatory effect, followed by rhinitis, pharyngitis, sore throat, cough with pains in the chest, and persistent headache.

Due to the potent irritant action of poke root, occupational exposure to its dust may cause severe complications. Two subjects, who were engaged in the milling of poke root and accidentally inhaled the dust, developed respiratory irritation and gastroenteritis, which were so severe that one subject required hospitalization. Several other occupants of the same building were also forced to discontinue their work because of rhinitis and gastroenteritis [7].

Fertility, Pregnancy and Lactation

According to secondary sources, abortion in cows has been described as a result of pokeberry toxicity [18,37]. Yeung et al. [52] reported that acetone-precipitated powders obtained from the related *P. acinosa* showed mid-term abortifacient activity in mice, when given in intraperitoneal doses corresponding to 4.76 g of the fresh leaves, 4.35 g of the fresh roots, or 0.55 g of the fresh seeds per kg body weight. As the abortifacient activity could be destroyed by heat and by the proteolytic enzyme pepsin, the suggestion was raised that the active principle was most likely a protein. Stolzenberg et al. [53] observed antifertility activity of a butanolic extract from the related *P. dodecandra*, when given by intrauterine injection to the rat. In contrast, oral treatment of mice with an aqueous extract of *P. dodecandra* had no significant effects on reproduction [54], and subcutaneous treatment with an aqueous extract of *P. esculenta* for 5 days did not affect the fertility of female mice [55].

Saponins from *P. americana* [56], *P. dodecandra* [57,58], and *Phytolacca* plants used in Chinese medicine [29] have all been shown to possess spermicidal properties.

No data have been recovered from the literature about the teratogenicity of *P. americana* or about its effects on the suckling child, when used by a breast-feeding mother.

Mutagenicity and Carcinogenicity

Butanol extracts from the seeds or fruit of *P. americana* did not demonstrate mutagenic activity in *Salmonella typhimurium* strain TM677 either in the presence or absence of a metabolic activating system [30].

Data about the carcinogenicity of *P. americana* have not been recovered from the literature.

References

1. Penso G (1983) Index Plantarum Medicinalium Totius Mundi Eorumque Synonymorum. Milano: Organizzazione Editoriale Medico Farmaceutica, p 735
2. Osol A, Farrar GE (1955) The Dispensatory of the United States of America. 25th edn. Philadelphia: J.B. Lippincott Company, 1806–1807
3. Lust J (1974) The Herb Book. Toronto: Bantam Books, p 317
4. Kell SO (1982) Pokeweed. Vet Hum Toxicol 24 (Suppl):138
5. Jaeckle KA, Freemon FR (1982) Pokewood poisoning. South Med J 74:639–640
6. Millspaugh CF (1974) American Medicinal Plants. New York: Dover Publications, pp 557–560
7. Goldstein SW, Jenkins GL, Thompson MR (1973) A chemical and pharmacological study of *Phytolacca americana*. J Am Pharm Assoc 26:306–312
8. Ahmed ZF, Zufall CJ, Jenkins GL (1949) A contribution to the chemistry and toxicology of the root of *Phytolacca americana* L. J Am Pharm Assoc 38:443–448
9. Lascombes S, Bastide A (1976) Recherche d'alcaloides dans *Phytolacca decandra* L. (*Phytolacca americana* L.). Plant Med Phytothér 10:182–187
10. Mack RB (1982) Toxic encounters of the dangerous kind. No Carolina Med J 43:365
11. Edwards N, Rodgers GC (1982) Pokeberry pancake breakfast – or – it's gonna be a great day! Vet Hum Toxicol 24 (Suppl):135–137

12. Stout GH, Malofsky BM, Stout VF (1964) Phytolaccagenin. A light atom x-ray structure proof using chemical information. J Am Chem Soc 86:957–958
13. Woo WS, Kang SS (1976) Phytolaccoside B: triterpene glucoside from *Phytolacca americana*. Phytochemistry 15:1315–1317
14. Woo WS, Kang SS, Wagner H, Seligmann O, Chari VM (1978) Triterpenoid saponins from the roots of Phytolacca americana. Planta Med 34:87–92
15. Kang SS, Woo WS (1987) Two new saponins from *Phytolacca americana*. Planta Med pp 338–340
16. Woo WS (1974) Steroids and pentacyclic triterpenoids from *Phytolacca americana*. Phytochemistry 13:2887–2889
17. Johnson A, Shimizu Y (1974) Phytolaccinic acid, a new triterpene from *Phytolacca americana*. Tetrahedron 30:2033–2036
18. Kang SS, Woo WS (1980) Triterpenes from the berries of *Phytolacca americana*. J Nat Prod 43:510–513
19. Driver MG, Francis FJ (1979) Purification of phytolaccanin (betanin) by removal of phytolaccatoxin from *Phytolacca americana*. J Food Sci 44:521–523
20. Forni E, A Trifilò, Polesello A (1983) Researches on the utilisation of the pigment from *Phytolacca decandra* L. as a food colorant: Part 1 – preparation of an extract free from toxic substances. Food Chem 10:35–46
21. Irvin JD, Kelly T, Robertus JD (1980) Purification and properties of a second antiviral protein from *Phytolacca americana* which inactivates eukaryotic ribosomes. Arch Biochem Biophys 200:418–425
22. Barbieri L, Aron GM, Irvin JD, Stirpe F (1982) Purification and partial characterization of another form of the antiviral protein from the seeds of *Phytolacca americana* L. (pokeweed). Biochem J 203:55–59
23. Spreafico F, Malfiore C, Moras ML et al (1983) The immunomodulatory activity of the plant proteins *Momordica charantia* inhibitor and pokeweed antiviral protein. Int J Immunopharmacol 5:335–343
24. Bjorn MJ, Larrick J, Piatak M, Wilson KJ (1984) Characterization of translational inhibitors from *Phytolacca americana*. Amino-terminal sequence determination and antibody-inhibitor conjugates. Biochim Biophys Acta 790:154–163
25. Xiamei Z, Zhong H (1989) Preparation of the antiviral protein from pokeweed seeds and assay of its toxicity. Acta Botan Yunnanica 11:440–448
26. Woo WS, Kang SS, Seligmann O, Chari M, Wagner H (1980) The structure of new lignans from the seeds of Phytolacca americana. Tetrahedron Lett 21:4255–4258
27. Macht DI (1937) A pharmacological study of Phytolacca. J Am Pharm Assoc Sci Ed 26:594–599
28. Tyler VE (1987) The New Honest Herbal. A sensible guide to herbs and related remedies. 2nd edn. Philadelphia: George F. Stickley Company, pp 182–183
29. Shiying G (1987) Shanglu. In: Chang H-M, But PP-H, ed. Pharmacology and Applications of Chinese Materia Medica. Vol. 2. Singapore: World Scientific Publishing, pp 1131–1134
30. Pezzuto JM, Swanson SM, Farnsworth NR (1984) Evaluation of the mutagenic potential of endod (*Phytolacca dodecandra*), a molluscicide of potential value for the control of schistosomiasis. Toxicol Lett 22:15–20
31. Aron GM, Irvin JD (1988) Cytotoxicity of pokeweed antiviral protein. Cytobios 55:105–111
32. Lampe KF (1974) Systemic plant poisoning in children. Pediatrics for the Clinician 54:347–351
33. Lewis WH, Smith PR (1979) Poke root herbal tea poisoning. JAMA 242:2759–2760
34. Duncan J (1985) The toxicology of plant molluscicides. Pharmacol Ther 27:243–264
35. Holland JH (1922) The useful plants of Nigeria. Part IV. Royal Botanical Gardens, Kew. Bulletin of Miscellaneous Information. Additional Series IX. p 549
36. Hendrickson JM, Hilbert KF (1931) Pokeweed berries not poisonous for chickens. J Am Vet Med Assoc 78:556–558
37. Barnett BD (1975) Toxicity of pokeberries (fruit of *Phytolacca americana* Large) for turkey poults. Poultry Sci 54:1215–1217

38. Kingsbury JM (1964) Poisonous Plants of the United States and Canada. Englewood Cliffs: Prentice-Hall, Inc, p 227
39. Guthrie A (1887) Poisoning by poke root. JAMA 9:125
40. Stein ZLG (1979) Pokeweed-induced gastroenteritis. Am J Hosp Pharm 36:1303
41. Anonymous (1981) Plant poisonings – New Jersey. MMWR 30:65–67
42. Roberge R, Brader E, Martin ML et al (1986) The root of evil – pokeweed intoxication. Ann Emerg Med 15:470–473
43. Kingsbury JM (1980) One man's poison. BioScience 30:171–176
44. Mitchell J, Rook A (1979) Botanical Dermatology. Plants and plant products injurious to the skin. Vancouver: Greengrass, 1979, p 513
45. Anonymous (1988) European communities. Int Dig Health Legislation 39:683
46. Basham TY, Waxdal MJ (1974) Mitogenic activity of 5 lectins from *Phytolacca americana*. Fed Proc 33:793
47. Bodger MP, McGiven AR, Fitzgerald PH (1979) Mitogenic proteins of pokeweed. I. Purification, characterization and mitogenic activity of two proteins from pokeweed (*Phytolacca octandra*). Immunology 37:785–792
48. Bodger MP, McGiven AR, Fitzgerald PH (1979) Mitogenic proteins of pokeweed. II. The differentiation of human peripheral blood B lymphocytes stimulated with purified pokeweed mitogens (Po-2 and Po-3) from pokeweed, *Phytolacca octandra*. Immunology 37:793–799
49. Farnes P, Barker BE, Brownhill LE, Fanger H (1964) Mitogenic activity in Phytolacca americana (pokeweed). Lancet 2:1100–1101
50. Barker BE, Farnes P, LaMarche PH (1966) Peripheral blood plasmacytosis following systemic exposure to *Phytolacca americana* (pokeweed). Pediatrics 38:490–493
51. Barker BE, Farnes P, Fanger H (1965) Mitogenic activity in Phytolacca americana (pokeweed). Lancet 1:170
52. Yeung HW, Feng Z, Li WW, Cheung WK, Ng TB (1987) Abortifacient activity in leaves, roots and seeds of *Phytolacca acinosa*. J Ethnopharmacol 21:31–35
53. Stolzenberg SJ, Parkhurst RM, Reist EJ (1976) Blastocidal and contraceptive actions by an extract and compounds from endod (*Phytolacca dodecandra*). Contraception 14:39–51
54. Mamo E, Worku M (1987) Oral administration of a water extract of *Phytolacca dodecandra* l'Herit in mice – effects on reproduction. Contraception 35:155–161
55. Matsui AS, Rogers J, Woo YK, Cutting WC (1967) Effects of some natural products on fertility in mice. Med Pharmacol Exp Int J Exp Med 16:414–424
56. Ismail SI, Hammouda FM, Hassan NM, Ciliana SP (1985) Isolation of the spermicidal principle from *Phytolacca americana* and determination of its mutagenic capacity. Acta Agronom Acad Sci Hung 34 (Suppl):92
57. Stolzenberg SJ, Parkhurst RM (1974) Spermicidal actions of extracts and compounds from *Phytolacca dodecandra*. Contraception 10:135–143
58. Dorsaz A-C, Hostettmann K (1986) Further saponins from Phytolacca dodecandra: their molluscicidal and spermicidal properties. Planta Med p 557

Podophyllum Species

I.H. Bowen and I.J. Cubbin

Botany

Podophyllum (family Berberidaceae) is a medicinally important genus in which there are two principal species, *P. peltatum* L., which is indigenous to the eastern parts of North America and Canada, and *P. emodi* Wallich, which is found in northern India and on the slopes of the Himalayas. In both areas it is a drug of commerce [1].

American podophyllum, *P. peltatum*, is a perennial herb with a rhizome growing up to 1 m in length with many roots arising from it. It is the rhizome and the roots which are used in medicine. Most of the synonyms for podophyllum derive from its structure, namely may-apple, hog-apple, wild or ground lemon, ducks-foot, devils-apple and racoonberry; the other name by which it is frequently termed in commerce is American mandrake [2,3]. This should never be confused with mandrake root (*Mandragora officinarum*) or English mandrake (*Bryonia dioca*), both of which exert very different pharmacological effects [4].

Indian podophyllum, *P. emodi* Wallich, is the *P. hexandrum* of Royle [5] and is very similar in botanical character to the American species. It is known in India as papri or bukra, and its fruit has a scarlet-red colour. It has also been referred to as vegetable calomel [6].

Malaysian folk-medicine has employed the underground part of *P. difforme* and related species [7].

Chemistry

The constituents of Podophyllum can be considered in two groups, those which form the resin, which has long been known as podophyllin [8], and those which do not. The medicinal action is entirely attributable to the resin, which is prepared by alcoholic percolation of the rhizomes and roots. The percolate is then concentrated and added to acidulated water and the resulting precipitate is collected and dried. The yield of resin from American podophyllum is 3.5–6% and approximately twice that amount (up to 12%) is obtained from *P. emodi* [3,9].

Adverse Effects of Herbal Drugs, Vol. 2
(ed. by P.A.G.M. De Smet, K. Keller, R. Hänsel, R.F. Chandler)

The chief constituents of the American drug are the C_{18} lignans, of which podophyllotoxin forms 20% in the resin obtained from *P. peltatum*. The peltatins, α- and β-, form respectively 5 and 10%, although the exact proportion is variable depending on seasonal changes. Other lignans which have been isolated include demethylpodophyllotoxin, deoxypodophyllotoxin and podophyllotoxone. All these compounds occur in the free form and as the glycosides – however the glycosides being water-soluble are almost invariably lost to the resin due to the method of preparation [3,10].

The Indian resin contains approximately 40% podophyllotoxin, and the other lignans in much the same proportions as the American resin, with the exception of the peltatins which are absent. Since it is believed that these are responsible for the purgative action of the drug, this must raise questions about the purgative efficacy of the Indian product, or at least prompt further investigations. Since the resins are not identical it is possible to distinguish them by simple chemical tests [11,12].

Several flavonoids have also been isolated from the resin including astragalin, isorhamnetin, kaempferol and quercetin. This latter is ubiquitous throughout the plant and also occurs as a variety of glycosides in aqueous fractions.

Those constituents which have been isolated external to the resin include albumen, calcium oxalate, gallic acid, starch, quercetin and both volatile and fixed oils [13].

Epimerisation at C-4 is the first stage in the production of the semi-synthetic compounds etoposide and teniposide which exert a quite different pharmacological action. Etoposide (VP-16) has ethylidene-β-D-glucopyranose substituted at the C-4 position of the C ring, is demethylated at the C-4′ position of the E ring, and is currently marketed in Britain as Vepesid (Bristol-Myers); while teniposide (VM-26, Sandoz), which is a sulphur containing derivative is registered in The Netherlands as Vumon [14–16].

Pharmacology and Uses

The activity of the drug is due to the presence of a lactone ring in the *trans* configuration. In weakly alkaline medium the podophyllotoxin readily epimerises to give the less strained *cis* isomer picropodophyllotoxin which is physiologically inactive.

Podophyllum resin, the isolated podophyllin and podophyllotoxins have been used at various times and in varying formulations for a number of clinical applications including purgative, emetic, anthelmintic and the treatment of various growths on the skin [17–19]. The resin is a powerful and irritant purgative and is nowadays much less employed for this purpose. Since the early 1800's podophyllum preparations have been employed for the treatment of plantar, anal and urogenital warts, including condyloma acuminatum, which is now the principal use of podophyllum products

[20,21]. It is, perhaps, less efficacious in the treatment of common and plantar warts since it does not easily penetrate the thicker horny layers which these warts produce [22]. Oily formulations are an improvement in this respect [22,23] and have also produced encouraging results in the treatment of skin carcinomas [24–28]. Podophyllotoxin in similar formulations has an even better cure rate and, in a study of the cutaneous cytodestructive potency of podophyllum lignans, it was shown that podophyllotoxin was the most potent, followed by the peltatins and 4′-demethylpodophyllotoxin [29]. It was concluded that 0.1–0.5% podophyllotoxin may be an appropriate concentration range for achieving "notable cutaneous injury" from repeated applications of ethanolic podophyllum preparations to human anogenital areas. Comparisons between podophyllin treatment and surgical removal of warts have been carried out [30]. Irrigation of the bladder with podophyllin solution has been used to treat papillomas [31] although in many cases severe pain and accompanying infection lead to discontinuation of treatment [32]. Similarly, early reports of podophyllum treatment of laryngeal papillomatosis [33] do not seem to have been substantiated [34] perhaps because of disappointing long-term effects [35]. German patents exist for the use of oral, anal and parenteral formulations, incorporating podophyllum, for treating obstruction of the lymph system [36].

Podophyllum is a mitotic poison, arresting cells in the metaphase of the mitotic cycle, subsequently leading to epithelial cell death. Nucleoside transport into cells is also inhibited and this property, but not the same mitotic toxicity, is also shared with the semi-synthetic podophyllotoxin derivative etoposide [37].

A study of the cutaneous cytodestructive potency of podophyllum lignans, assessed by induced changes in skinfold thickness in the albino rabbit, suggested that podophyllotoxin had twice the potency of α-peltatin and both were more potent than 4′-demethylpodophyllotoxin and β-peltatin which were not significantly more active than controls. If visual irritation indices (assessed erythema) are used as the criterion then the order of potency remains as above but all four lignans show more activity than controls [29]. The authors draw comparisons between the permeability of rabbit skin and of occluded human skin and suggest a concentration range of 0.1–0.5% podophyllotoxin for clinical use. Lassus [38] draws attention to the variability of podophyllin preparations and appears to suggest that, though generally more expensive, podophyllotoxin preparations have a more predictable effect.

Pharmacokinetics

Pharmacokinetic data for podophyllum resin or its constituents have not been recovered from the literature, but in a detailed study of a case of fatal poisoning by podophyllum, Cassidy [39] reported blood analyses before and after hemoperfusion. In his discussion he stated that podophyllotoxin is eliminated in the bile with a half life of 48 h.

Adverse Reaction Profile

General Animal Data

In studies of the effects of podophyllum lignans on guinea pig, skin reactions including erythema, oedema and erosion were examined [40]. The reactions were judged to be non-allergic toxic responses due to the cutaneous destructive action of the lignans, the most potent of which was podophyllotoxin. Philips et al. [41] quoted the following LD_{50} values for podophyllotoxin in toxicity studies on several animal species: rat 8.7 mg/kg, cat 1.7 mg/kg, rabbit 5 mg/kg (intravenous); mouse 33 mg/kg, rat 15 mg/kg (intraperitoneal); cat 4 mg/kg, rat 3 mg/kg (intramuscular). Cats and dogs receiving seven or more intravenous doses of 0.5 mg/kg survived without alarming consequences, and mice tolerated 8 mg/kg per day by intraperitoneal injection [42]. Animals receiving fatal doses succumbed within 24 hours, the initial signs being emesis and respiratory stimulation, with dogs occasionally displaying bradycardia and ventricular systole. Terminal stages were associated with slow respiration, falling blood pressure and respiratory failure. In cats and rats, but not dogs, fatal doses also led to severe pulmonary damage. Other toxic symptoms included gastrointestinal, hepatic or renal damage and disturbances of hematopoiesis. Toxic doses promoted granulocytopenia from which recovery was rapid following withdrawal.

General Human Data

The fruit, which resembles a yellow rose hip, being up to 6 cm in length, is the only edible part of the plant; fatalities have occurred using the roots and foliage for culinary purposes [2].

Toxicity due to podophyllum may occur from ingestion or by absorption through the skin. Dudley [43] has reported the death of an elderly female following ingestion of only 300 mg of podophyllum resin and Petersen et al. [44] described a similar case which followed ingestion of 350 mg. In both cases toxic symptoms included lethargy, hyperpnoea and coma. Accidental ingestion of approximately 4 g of podophyllum in tincture of benzoin was reported to lead to hypotension, lethargy and hypocalcemia accompanied by severe CNS disturbance and some GI ulceration. Following intensive therapy the patient recovered but peripheral neuropathy with walking difficulties and reduced touch sensation in the fingers persisted even after 10 months [45]. Cooper [46] has similarly suggested 300 mg as the toxic dose. Balucani and Zellers [47] reported complete recovery of a patient following ingestion of 1 g of podophyllum resin, whereas Clarke and Parsonage [48] recorded survival after a dose of 2.8 g.

Similar symptoms follow poisoning after topical application of podophyllum preparations, Slater [49] reporting recovery of a patient after charcoal hemoperfusion but noting residual signs of peripheral neuropathy after some 4 months. Similar reports are listed in Martindale [50] but many cases include additional effects such as foetal death, teratogenicity and carcinogenicity which are dealt with under the relevant headings below.

Cassidy et al. [39] have noted a pronounced lactic acidosis in a fatal case of podophyllum poisoning but did not consider the degree of acidosis to be sufficient to explain the depth of the patient's coma.

The presence of podophyllum in some herbal preparations for use as laxatives or slimming preparations can lead to accidental poisoning [51,52]. The average user is often unaware of the potential toxicity of the preparation.

Fatalities have also been reported following topical application [3]. When used carefully, with the patient confining application to the affected area and taking care to wash the site 4–8 hours after application, podophyllum and its preparations seem only rarely to cause major problems. The majority of the adverse reactions reported above are due to inappropriate use or to accidental poisoning.

Allergic Reactions

No allergic reactions to podophyllum have been recovered from the literature. The skin reactions to podophyllum applications have in fact been shown to be non-allergic [40].

Cardiovascular Reactions

Whilst no specific effects on the heart have been noted, systolic murmur [45] and tachycardia [53] have been recorded among the symptoms of podophyllum toxicity. Hypotension is one of the commonest symptoms of podophyllum poisoning (see general human data).

Dermatological Reactions

Common dermatological reactions to the use of podophyllum preparations (cf general animal data) include erythema, oedema and erosion. Contact dermatitis in workers handling podophyllum resin has been reported [54]. Histological changes to the genital skin and mucosa of young adults of both sexes have been recorded [55]. The changes are indistinguishable from squamous cell carcinoma in situ (Bowen's disease and related conditions) but there seems to be some uncertainty whether these are true or pseudo malignancies (see also under mutagenicity and carcinogenicity). It has been suggested that the condition be described as genital keratinocytic displasia. In one recorded case the condition has led to amputation of the penis [56]. Sullivan and King [57] named these bizarre forms of epithelial cells "podophyllin cells", and Wade and Ackerman [56] suggest that they can in fact be distinguished from squamous cell carcinoma. Skin sensitization may also develop from the incorporation of allergenic materials not arising from podophyllum into the product formulation [56,58].

Gastrointestinal Reactions

The symptoms of systemic toxicity due to podophyllum products include nausea and vomiting [53]. Geffroy et al. [59] report a case of cathartic colon induced by pills containing podophyllin, and a case of paralytic ileus following topical application of 25% podophyllin solution has been described by Grabbe [60]. The mechanism of action on the gastrointestinal tract is unclear but the cathartic action of podophyllum is postulated to be secondary to irritation [39].

Hematological Reactions

Toxic effects of podophyllum include leukopenia, anemia and thrombocytopenia [53]. Granulocytopenia in animal studies, reversible on discontinuation of the drug, has been noted [41]. Chronic use has been associated with hypokalemia due to increased stool potassium loss, and morphological changes in circulating lymphocytes have been observed following overdosage [39].

Hepatic Reactions

No specific references to liver damage have been recovered from the literature for podophyllum, its constituents or their semi-synthetic derivatives. Elevation of liver enzymes following topical use of podophyllin resin may, however, suggest some hepatotoxicity [53].

Nervous System Reactions

Among the symptoms of podophyllum poisoning are confusion, peripheral neuropathy and paresthesia [45,54,61,62], and there may be a delay in onset of symptoms of 10–13 hours after ingestion [39]. Peripheral neuropathy progressively worsens and may not appear until two weeks after application [3]. True psychotic effects have only been reported by Stoudemire [63], who additionally mentions a case of visual hallucinations in a child who was overdosed with a cathartic that included podophyllum in its formulation [64]. The patient exhibited vagueness of speech, disorientation, poor memory and seizures, deteriorating into a stupour. During recovery she continued to have hallucinations. Paresthesia generally leads to a lack of touch sensations in fingers, hands and feet, which may persist for several weeks. Peripheral neuropathy is often much longer-lasting [45] and causes gait problems, often associated with difficulties in hand and arm movements. During recovery mechanical supports are often needed to aid walking [52,54], and there is a risk of residual symptoms such as sensory impairment in the hands and feet [52].

Ocular Reactions

Direct contact with the eyes should be avoided; corneal damage has resulted from application of podophyllum preparations to verrucae near the eyes [3,17].

Renal Reactions

Although direct effects on the kidney have not been recovered from the literature, renal damage is seen in animals following fatal doses of podophyllum [41].

Respiratory Tract Reactions

Stoehr et al. [53] report both stimulation and depression of respiration in cases of podophyllum poisoning.

Fertility, Pregnancy and Lactation

Toxicity studies in animals have indicated that podophyllum and its preparations are more toxic to the fetus than to the pregnant mother and instances of fetal death and abortion have occurred [65,66]. Graber [67] suggests that this is due to vascular spasm of the vessels of the decidua basalis with resulting embarrassment of the fetal ciculation and oxygenation. Chamberlain et al. [62] described intrauterine death in the 34th week of pregnancy following topical application of 25% solution of podophyllum resin for the treatment of vulvar warts, and podophyllum has been used in attempts to cause termination of pregnancy [68]. Congenital deformities following use of slimming pills containing podophyllum, indicative of possible teratogenicity, have been reported. These included skin tags on the ear and cheek, heart defects, limb abnormalities and polyneuritis [51]. A simian crease of the left hand and a preauricular skin tag were noted in a child born to a mother who had been treated topically with podophyllum resin from the 23rd to 29th weeks of pregnancy [69]. The authors advise against the use of podophyllum preparations during pregnancy because of their teratogenic potential. Similar sentiments are expressed by Chamberlain et al. [62] who also doubt that the toxic nature of podophyllum is sufficiently appreciated. Jelinek [70] did not see evidence of intrauterine death which could be attributed to podophyllum, despite long use of the drug in his practice. He comments on the need to wash off the applied preparation three hours after application to avoid local reaction and absorption. American text books, however, caution against the topical use of podophyllum in pregnancy because of the known incidence of teratogenic effects and fetal death [71,72]. In addition, although there are no documented problems in breast-fed infants, the ease with which topical podophyllum is systemically absorbed suggests caution in administration of podophyllum to nursing mothers [71].

Mutagenicity and Carcinogenicity

The production of atypical cells during podophyllum treatment has already been mentioned (see dermatological reactions), and pseudo or true malignancies similar to squamous cell carcinoma may present as a result of the treatment itself. Ridley [73] also notes that podophyllum might produce epidermal atypia but, quoting from other sources, comments that it is probably not frankly carcinogenic in vulval warts and the cervix. A confirmed case of cancer (epithelioma) of the penis following treatment of condyloma acuminata with podophyllin has been reported by Boneff [74] and the preparations obviously need to be administred with care, particularly in occluded sites.

References

1. Wren RC (1956) Potter's New Cyclopaedia of Botanical Drugs and Preparations. 7th edn. (enlarged by Wren RW). London: Potter and Clark Ltd, pp 196–197
2. Grieve M (1974) A Modern Herbal. London: Jonathan Cape, pp 512–513
3. Graham NA, Chandler FR (1990) Herbal Medicine, Podophyllum. Can Pharm J 123:330–333
4. Kraemer H (1920) Scientific and Applied Pharmacognosy. London: Chapman and Hall, pp 231–233

5. Chopra RN, Nayar SL, Chopra IC (1956) Glossary of Indian Medicinal Plants. New Delhi: Council of Scientific and Industrial Research, p 198
6. Dey KL (1896) The Indigenous Drugs of India. 2nd edn. Calcutta: Thacker, Spink and Co, pp 251–254
7. Perry LM, Mertzger J (1980) Medicinal Drugs of East and Southeast Asia. London: MIT Press, p 56
8. Hanbury D, Fluckiger FA (1879) Pharmacographia. 2nd edn. London: Macmillan, pp 35–37
9. Tyler V, Brady LR, Robbers JE (1988) Pharmacognosy. 9th edn. Philadelphia: Lea and Febiger, pp 141–142
10. Trease GE, Evans WC (1983) Pharmacognosy. 12th edn. Eastbourne: Bailliere Tindall, pp 643–647
11. Denston TC (1951) A Textbook of Pharmacognosy. 5th edn. London: Pitmans, pp 299–304
12. Wallis TE, Goldberg S (1931) Podophyllum rhizome, American and Indian. Q J Pharm Pharmacol 4:28
13. Duke JA (1985) CRC Handbook of Medicinal Herbs. Florida: CRC Press Ltd, pp 387–388
14. Stahelin H (1970) 4-Demethylepipodophyllotoxin thenylidene glucoside (VM26). A podophyllotoxin compound with a new mechanism of action. Eur J Cancer 6:303–311
15. Pullockaran AJ, Kingston DGI (1989) Synthesis of stereospecifically deuterated desoxypodophyllotoxins and ^{1}H-NMR assignment of desoxypodophyllotoxin. J Nat Prod 52:1290–1295
16. Walker G (Compiler) (1989–90) ABPI Data Sheet Compendium. London: Datapharm Public Ltd, pp 261–262
17. Miller RA (1985) Podophyllin. Int J Dermatol 24:491–498
18. Steinmetz EF (1954) Materia Medica Vegetabilis. Amsterdam: Steinmetz, pp 353–354
19. Hartwell JL (1968) Plants used against cancer. A survey II. J Nat Prod 31:71–170
20. Scutt R (1954) Treatment of ano-genital warts with podophyllin. Br Med J 2: 397–398
21. Singh KG, Bajaj AK, Sharma R (1988) Perianal condyloma acuminata in an infant. Int J Dermatol 27:181–182
22. Bettley FR (1971) The treatment of skin carcinoma with podophyllum derivatives. Br J Dermatol 84:74–82
23. Carslaw RW, Neill J, Thom JA (1963) Linseed oil in the treatment of plantar warts. Br J Dermatol 75:280
24. Nelson LM (1953) Use of Podophyllin (Podophyllum resin) in dermatology. Arch Derm 67:488–495
25. Nelson LM (1966) Podophyllin-salicylic acid solution in treatment of basal cell carcinomas. Arch Derm 93:457–459
26. Hall AF (1950) Treatment of senile keratoses with podophyllin. Arch Derm 62: 362–369
27. Shanon J, Sagher F (1955) Podophyllin treatment in various skin diseases. Dermatologica 111:319–327
28. Smith LM, Garrett HD (1950) Resin of podophyllum in treatment of cancerous and precancerous conditions of skin. Effect on basal cell epithelioma and seborrhoeic, senile and radiation keratoses. Arch Derm 61:946–956
29. Von Krogh G, Maibach HI (1983) Cutaneous cytodestructive potency of lignans. A comparative evaluation of macroscopic-toxic influence on rabbit skin subsequent to repeated 10-day applications. Dermatologica 167:70–77
30. Jenson SJ (1985) Comparison of podophyllin application with simple surgical excision in clearance and recurrence of perianal condylomata acuminata. Lancet 2:1146–1148
31. Richardson EJ (1959) The use of podophyllin in the treatment of papillomas of the bladder. J Urol 82:234–235

32. Gibson GR (1969) Chemotherapy in the management of bladder tumours. Aust NZ J Surg 38:281–283
33. Hollingsworth JB, Kohlmoos HW, McNaught RC (1950) Treatment of juvenile papilloma of the larynx with resin of podophyllum. Arch Otolaryngol 52:82–85
34. Robbins KT, Woodson GE (1984) Current concepts in the management of laryngeal papillomatosis. Head Neck Surg 6:861–866
35. Szunapar J (1967) Laryngeal papillomatosis. Acta Otolaryngol 63:74–86
36. Sichert R (1971) Medicinal extracts for treating obstruction of the lymphatic system. Ger Offen DE1963706; 24 Jun, 14pp. Addn to Ger Offen 1931467
37. Loike JD, Horowitz SB (1976) Effects of podophyllotoxin and VP16–213 on microtubule assembly and nucleoside transport in HeLa cells. Biochemistry 15: 5435–5442
38. Lassus A (1987) Podophyllin/podophyllotoxin. Lancet 2:1395
39. Cassidy DE, Drewry J, Fanning JP (1982) Podophyllum toxicity: a report of a fatal case. J Toxicol Clin Toxicol 19:35–44
40. Von Krogh G, Maibach HI (1983) Guinea pig maximisation test: Podophyllum lignans. Contact Dermatitis 9:95–98
41. Philips FS, Chenoweth, Hunt CC (1948) Studies on the toxicology of podophyllotoxin and related substances. Fed Proc 7:249
42. Greenspan EM, Leiter J (1949) Toxicity and haematologic changes produced by alpha-peltatin, beta-peltatin and podophyllotoxin. Cancer Res 9:626
43. Dudley WH (1980) Fatal podophyllum poisoning. Med Rec 37:409
44. Petersen F, Haines WS, Webster RW (1923) Legal Medicine and Toxicology. Vol 2. 2nd edn. Philadelphia: WB Saunders [reported in ref 45]
45. McFarland MF, McFarland J (1981) Accidental ingestion of podophyllum. Clin Toxicol 18:973–977
46. Cooper P (1974) Poisoning by drugs and chemicals, plants and animals – an index of toxic effects and their treatment. London: Alchemist, p 179
47. Balucani M, Zellers DD (1964) Podophyllum resin poisoning with complete recovery. J Am Med Assoc 189:639–640
48. Clark ANG, Parsonage MJ (1957) A case of podophyllum poisoning with involvement of the nervous system. Br Med J 2:1155–1157
49. Slater GE, Rumack BH, Peterson RG (1978) Podophyllum popisoning, systemic toxicity following cutaneous application. Obstet Gynecol 52:94–96
50. Reynolds JEF (ed) (1982) Martindale: The Extra Pharmacopoeia. 28th edn. London: The Pharmaceutical Press, pp 1366–1367
51. Cullis JE (1962) Congenital deformities and herbal "slimming tablets". Lancet 2:511–512
52. Dobb GJ, Edis RH (1984) Coma and neuropathy after ingestion of herbal laxative containing podophyllin. Med J Aust 140:495–496
53. Stoehr GP, Peterson AL, Taylor WJ (1978) Systemic complications of local podophyllin therapy. Ann Intern Med 89:362–363
54. O'Donovan WJ (1935) Dermatitis due to podophyllin resin. Br J Dermatol 47:13–21
55. Kwitten J (1982) Genital keratinocytic displasia. Mt Sinai J Med 49:289–296
56. Fisher AA (1981) Severe systemic and local reactions to topical podophyllum resin. Cutis 28:233, 236, 242
57. Sullivan M, King L (1947) Effects of resin of podophyllum on normal skin, condyloma acuminatum and verrucae vulgares. Arch Dermatol Syphilol 56:30–47
58. Mitchell J, Rook A (1979) Botanical dermatology: Plants and plant products injurious to the skin. Vancouver: Greengrass, p 720
59. Geffroy Y, Hecketsweiler P, Colin R (1973) Aetiology of ulcerative colitis. Lancet 1:1451
60. Grabbe W (1951) Gefahren bei der Behandlung spitzer Kondylome mit Podophyllin bei gleichzeitiger Neosalvarsan-Therapie. Hautzart 2:325–326
61. Moher LM, Maurer SA (1979) Podophyllum toxicity: Case report and literature review. J Fam Pract 9:237–240

62. Chamberlain MJ, Reynolds AL, Yeoman WB (1972) Toxic effect of podophyllum application in pregnancy. Br Med J 3:391–392
63. Stoudemire A, Baker N, Thompson TL (1981) Delirium induced by topical application of podophyllin: a case report. Am J Psychiatry 138:1505–1506
64. Coruh M, Argun G (1965) Podophyllin poisoning: a case report. Turk J Paediatr 7:100–103
65. Didcock KA, Picard CW, Robson JM (1952) The action of podophyllotoxin on pregnancy. J Physiol 117:65–66
66. Thiersch JB (1963) Effect of podophyllin and podophyllotoxin on the rat litter in utero. Proc Soc Exp Biol Med 113:124–127
67. Graber EA, Barber HRK, O'Rourke MD (1967) Simple surgical treatment for condyloma acuminatum of the vulva. Obstet Gynecol 29:247–250
68. Kelsey FO (1963) Drug Embryopathy. Md State Med J 12:594–597
69. Karol MD, Conner CS, Murphrey KJ (1980) Podophyllum: suspected teratogenicity from topical application. Clin Toxicol 16:283–286
70. Jelinek G (1972) Toxicity of podophyllum. Br Med J 3:699
71. Anonymous (1990) USP Dispensing Information. Vol 1B. Rockville: The United States Pharmacopeial Convention, p 2270
72. McEvoy GK (ed) (1990) AHFS Drug Information. Bethesda: American Society of Hospital Pharmacists, pp 2056–2057
73. Ridley CM (1972) Toxicity of podophyllum. Br Med J 3:698
74. Boneff A (1969) Cancer de la verge apres traitment des condylome acumines a la podophylline. Arch Belg Dermatol Syphiligr 25:455–457

Polygala Species

P.A.G.M. De Smet

Botany

More than thirty species of the genus *Polygala* (Polygalaceae) are or have been used as medicinal plants [1]. The most well-known medicinal species is undoubtedly *P. senega* L., which serves as the source of senega root. Synonyms of this crude drug include rattlesnake root, seneca snake root, seneca root, snake root (E); Klapperschlangenwurzel, Virginische Schlangenwurzel (G); racine de sénéga, racine de Polygala [2–4]. The vernacular term snakeroot is confusing, as it has also been applied to a wide range of other plants including *Eupatorium urticaefolium*, *Aristolochia serpentaria* and *Senecio aureus* [5]. Another medically important *Polygala* species is *P. tenuifolia* Willd. (syn. *P. sibirica* L.) [1,6]. The root bark of this plant is used in traditional Chinese medicine under the name of Yuanzhi for a variety of disorders [7].

Data about the medical botany of some other *Polygala* species are listed in Table 1.

Chemistry

The roots of *P. senega* contain 6–16% of crude saponin, depending on the source of the sample [3,47,48]. Brieskorn and Renke [10] found eight saponins in the root of *P. senega* var. *typica*, and showed that all of them had presenegenin as the aglycone. Shoji and co-workers [49–51] isolated three different saponins from the roots of *P. senega* var. *latifolia* and identified them as glycosides of presenegenin. The oligosaccharides and cinnamic acid derivatives obtained from the roots of this variety have been studied in detail [52–54]. Other constituents of *P. senega* include phenolic glycosides [49], 0.1–0.3% of methylsalicylate [2,55,56], and traces of essential oil [3].

The roots of *P. tenuifolia* yield seven triterpenoid saponins, known as onjisaponins. The structure of five of these saponins has been determined [57,58]. Upon basic hydrolysis, the crude saponin of *P. tenuifolia* yields

Adverse Effects of Herbal Drugs, Vol. 2
(ed. by P.A.G.M. De Smet, K. Keller, R. Hänsel, R.F. Chandler)

Table 1. The medical botany (B), chemistry (C) and pharmacology (P) of some other *Polygala* species than *P. senega* and *P. tenuifolia*

Polygala acicularis Oliv.
B: Leaves and roots used in Africa [8].
C: 0.22% of saponin in the roots with presenegenin as aglycone [8].

Polygala alba Nutt.
B: Used in East Asia [1]. The root is considered a substitute or adulterant of *P. senega* [6,9].
C: Saponin in the roots with presenegenin as aglycone [10].

Polygala alpestris Rchb.
C: Complex mixture of saponins yielding tenuifolin as prosapogenin [11].

Polygala amara L. (syn. *P. amarella* Cr.)
B: Used in Europe and the former Soviet Union [1]. The medicinal plant part is the herb [6,9].
C: 1–2% of saponins in the roots [6]. The aerial parts of *P. amarella* yield the bitter principle amarelloside, together with flavonoids and a hydroxycinnamoyl ester [12].

Polygala arillata Benth. & Ham.
B: Used in Asia [13].
C: Xanthones in stems and roots [13].

Polygala brasiliensis L.
B: Whole plant used medicinally [6].
C: Saponin [6].

Polygala chamaebuxus L.
B: Herb used medicinally [6,9].
C: Saponins [14], the prosapogenin tenuifolin [14], and phenolic glycosides [11,15] in aerial parts.

Polygala chinensis L.
B: Used in India and East Asia [1,16].
C: Saponins in the roots with presenegenin as aglycone of the major saponin [17]; lactonic lignan glycosides and flavonol glycosides in roots [18]; 0.23–0.35% of lignans in whole plant [16,19,20].
A herbal Chinese tablet available on the Dutch market purportedly contained an analgesic and hypnotic alkaloid from *P. chinensis*. Chemical analysis revealed the presence of *l*-tetrahydropalmatine [21]. Analgesic tablets containing this alkaloid are indeed used in Chinese medicine but come from *Stephania* spp. [22].

Polygala comosa Schkuhr.
C: Complex mixture of saponins yielding, on basic hydrolysis, tenuifolin as prosapogenin [11].

Polygala erioptera DC.
C: 0.47% of saponin in the roots with presenegenin as aglycone [23].
P: Molluscicidal activity [24].

Polygala exelliana Troupin
C: 0.64% of saponin in the roots with presenegenin as aglycone [25].

Polygala fruticosa Berg. (syn. *P. oppositifolia* L.)
B: Roots used in South Africa [26].
C: Chromonocoumarins in leaves and root bark [26].
P: The chromonocoumarin, frutinone A, in the leaves has antifungal activity against the plant pathogenic fungus *Cladosporium cucumerinum* [26].

Polygala japonica Houtt.
B: Used in East Asia [1]. The medicinal plant part is the leaf [9].
C: Triterpene saponins in aerial parts [27,28].

Table 1. *Continued*

Polygala klotzchii Chod.
P: The plant is toxic to lifestock [29,30].

Polygala macradenia Gray
C: The lignan 4'-demethyldeoxypodohyllotoxin [31], xanthones [32,33].
P: Cytotoxic and tumor inhibitory activities of 4'-demethyldeoxypodophyllotoxin [31].

Polygala macrostigma Chod.
C: 0.53% of saponin in the roots with presenegenin as aglycone [34].

Polygala microphylla L.
C: Saponins and essential oil in roots and rhizomes [35,36].
P: Sedative activity of infusion prepared from roots and rhizomes and administered intraperitoneally to mice [36].

Polygala nitida T.S. Brandegee
B: Roots used in Middle America [37].
C: Xanthones in roots [37].

Polygala paniculata L.
B: Used in South America [1,9]. The medicinal plant parts are the leaf and the root [9].
C: Coumarin derivatives in dried plant [38,39].
P: Petrol ether and chloroform extracts show molluscicidal properties and antifungal activity against the plant pathogenic fungus *Cladosporium cucumerinum* [39].

Polygala persicariifolia DC.
B: Used in Africa [1].
C: 0.38% of saponin in the roots with presenegenin as aglycone [40].

Polygala paenea L.
C: The lignan 4'-demethyldeoxypodophyllotoxin [31].
P: Cytotoxic and tumor inhibitory activities of 4'-demethyldeoxypodophyllotoxin [31].

Polygala polygama Walt. (syn. *P. rubella* Willd.)
B: Used in East Asia and North America [1].
C: Podophyllotoxin and other lignans [41,42].
P: Antitumor and cytotoxic activities [41,42].

Polygala pruinosa Boiss.
C: A saponin in the roots of ssp. *pruinosa* with presenegenin as aglycone [43].

Polygala rarifolia DC. (syn. *P. rehmannii* Chod.)
B: Used in Africa [1].
C: Saponins and the prosapogenin presenegin glucoside [6].

Polygala spectabilis DC.
B: Used in South America [44].
C: Stigmasterol and xanthone derivatives in branches [44].

Polygala vayredae Costa
B: The root is considered a substitute for *P. senega* [6].
C: Complex mixture of saponins yielding tenuifolin as prosapogenin [11].

Polygala virgata
C: 74% of monoacetotriglycerides in seed oil [45].

Polygala vulgaris L.
B: Used in Europe [1]. The medicinal plant part is the herb [6,9].
C: Saponins, flavonoids, tannins, phenolic acids and alkaloids in aerial parts [46].
P: Saponins show antifungal activity [46].

tenuifolin (= presenegenin 3β-O-glucoside) [59]. According to a Chinese text book, the root core of *P. tenuifolia* contains much less saponins than the root bark [7]. Other compounds recovered from the roots or rhizomes of *P. tenuifolia* are xanthones [60,61], 3,4,5-trimethoxycinnamic acid [60], and β-carboline alkaloids [62].

Data about the chemistry of some other *Polygala* species are listed in Table 1.

Pharmacology and Uses

The root of *P. senega* is employed primarily as an expectorant [3,4]. Diaphoretic, sialogogue and emetic effects are also among its reputed virtues [48,56]. Intraperitoneal administration of a crude saponin preparation extracted from senega root was reported to increase the plasma levels of ACTH, corticosterone and glucose in the rat [63].

The root bark of *P. tenuifolia* is prescribed in traditional Chinese medicine for a variety of disorders, including cough, common cold, neurasthenia, amnesia, and insomnia [7]. Decoctions of the herb and root of *P. tenuifolia* have anthelmintic activity [64], and root saponins of this plant are inhibitors of cAMP phosphodiesterase [65].

Data about the pharmacology of some other *Polygala* species are listed in Table 1.

Pharmacokinetics

According to Briggs [48], senega saponins are poorly absorbed from the intestine.

Adverse Reaction Profile

General Animal Data

Tschesche and Wulff [66] reported a parenteral LD_{50} of 3 mg/kg in rats for a mixture of senega saponins.

Intragastric administration of the root bark of *Polygala tenuifolia* yielded an LD_{50} of 10 g/kg in mice compared to approximately 17 g/kg for the whole root. The root core was not lethal in doses up to 75 g/kg [7]. This difference in the LD_{50} values of root bark and root core suggests that there are chemical differences between these plant parts (cf. the section on chemistry).

General Human Data

Senega root is officially recognized as a crude herbal drug in Germany [3] and France [67]. Literature data about adverse reactions appear to be limited to statements about irritating effects on the gastrointestinal tract (see below).

Dermatological Reactions

An authoritative text book on botanical dermatology lists *P. senega* as an irritant plant without reproducing original reports [68].

Gastrointestinal Reactions

Overdosage with senega root preparations results in nausea, vomiting and diarrhoea due to gastrointestinal irritation. In sensitive individuals gastrointestinal effects may already occur at the therapeutic dose level [3,48].

Fertility, Pregnancy and Lactation

Data concerning the effects of *P. senega* or *P. tenuifolia* on fertility or concerning their effects during pregnancy and lactation have not been recovered from the literature.

Mutagenicity and Carcinogenicity

Morimoto et al. [69] did not observe mutagenic effects of aqueous or methanolic extracts from roots of *P. senega* or *P. tenuifolia* in the *Bacillus subtilis* rec-assay or in *Salmonella typhimurium* strains TA98 and TA100.

Data about the carcinogenicity of *P. senega* or *P. tenuifolia* are not available.

References

1. Penso G (1983) Index Plantarum Medicinalium Totius Mundi Eorumque Synonymorum. Milano: Organizzazione Editoriale Medico Farmaceutica, pp 761–762
2. Osol A, Farrar GE (1955) The Dispensatory of the United States of America. 25th edn. Philadelphia: J.B. Lippincott Company, pp 1225–1226
3. Wichtl M (1989) Senegawurzel. In: Wichtl M (ed) Teedrogen. Ein Handbuch für die Praxis auf wissenschaftlicher Grundlage. 2. Auflage. Stuttgart: Wissenschaftliche Verlagsgesellschaft, pp 447–448

4. Reynolds JEF (ed) (1989) Martindale The Extra Pharmacopoeia. 29th edn. London: The Pharmaceutical Press, pp 913–914
5. Vogel VJ (1970) American Indian medicine. Norman: University of Oklahoma Press, pp 368–369
6. List PH, Hörhammer L (1977) Hagers Handbuch der Pharmazeutischen Praxis. Vierte Neuausgabe. Sechster Band. Chemikalien und Drogen, Teil A: N-Q. Berlin: Springer-Verlag, pp 802–811
7. Zhigui C (1986) Yuanzhi. In: Chang H-M, But PP-H (eds) Pharmacology and Applications of Chinese Materia Medica. Singapore: World Scientific Publishing, pp 551–553
8. Delaude C (1971) Étude comparative des saponines extraites de deux Polygalacées africaines. Le *Securidaca longependunculata* Fres. var. *parvifolia* et le *Polygala acicularis* Oliv. Bull Soc R Sci Liège 40:397–405
9. Hoppe HA (1975) Drogenkunde. Band 1. Angiospermen. 8. Auflage. Berlin: Walter de Gruyter, pp 859–862
10. Brieskorn CH, Renke F (1968) Chemischer Aufbau, physikalische Eigenschaften und Unterscheidungsmerkmale einiger Polygala-Saponine. Dtsch Apoth Ztg 108:1601–1605
11. Hamburger M, Hostettmann K (1986) Glycosidic constituents of some European Polygala species. J Nat Prod (Lloydia) 49:557
12. Dubois M-A, Neszmelyi A, Heubl G, Fiebig M, Wagner H (1989) Amarelloside, a bitter tri-*O*-acetyl tri-*O*-benzoyl tetrasaccharide from *Polygala amarella*. Phytochemistry 28:3355–3359
13. Ghosal S, Banerjee S, Chauhan RBPS, Srivastava RS (1977) Extractives of *Polygala*. Part 5. New trioxygenated xanthones of *P. arillata*. J Chem Soc Perkin Trans 1:740–743
14. Hamburger M, Hostettmann K (1986) New saponins and a prosapogenin from *Polygala chamaebuxus*. Helv Chim Acta 69:221–227
15. Hamburger M, Hostettmann K (1985) Hydroxycinnamic acid esters from *Polygala chamaebuxus*. Phytochemistry 24:1793–1797
16. Ghosal S, Kumarswamy C, Chauhan RPS, Srivastava RS (1973) Lactonic lignans of *Polygala chinensis*. Phytochemistry 12:2550–2551
17. Brieskorn CH, Kilbinger W (1975) Struktur eines Saponin aus *Polygala chinensis* L. Arch Pharm (Weinheim) 308:824–832
18. Ghosal S, Chauhan RPS, Srivastava R (1974) Lignan and flavonol glycosides of *Polygala chinensis*. Plant Biochem J 1:64–72
19. Ghosal S, Chauhan RPS, Srivastava RS (1974) Structure of chinensin: a new lignan lactone from *Polygala chinensis*. Phytochemistry 13:2281–2284
20. Ghosal S, Chauhan RPS, Srivastava RS (1974) Two new aryl naphthalide lignans from *Polygala chinensis*. Phytochemistry 13:1933–1936
21. De Smet PAGM, Elferink F, Verpoorte R (1989) Linksdraaiend tetrahydropalmatine in chinese tablet. Ned T Geneesk 133:308
22. Quansheng C (1986) Yanhusuo. In: Chang H-M, But PP-H (eds) Pharmacology and Applications of Chinese Materia Medica. Singapore: World Scientific Publishing, pp 515–524
23. Delaude C, Davreux M (1972) Contribution a l'étude chimique des saponines des Polygalacées. Identification de la saponine extraite de *Polygala erioptera* DC. Bull Soc R Sci Liège 41:576–578
24. Ahmed EHM, Bashir AK, El Kheir YM (1984) Investigations of molluscicidal activity of certain Sudanese plants used in folk medicine. Part IV. Planta Med pp 74–77
25. Delaude C (1973) Contribution a l'étude des saponines que contiennent les Polygalacées. Identification de la saponine extraite du *Polygala exelliana* Troupin. Bull Soc R Sci Liège 42:631–634
26. Di Paolo ER, Hamburger M, Stoeckli-Evans H, Rogers C, Hostettmann K (1989) New chromonocoumarin (= 6*H*, 7*H*-[1]benzopyrano[4,3-*b*[1]-benzopyran-6,7-dione) derivatives from *Polygala fruticosa* Berg. Helv Chim Acta 72:1455–1462

27. Fang Z-P, Vin G-J (1986) Study on the structure of a new triterpene saponin B from *Polygala japonica* Houtt. Acta Bot Sin 28:196–200
28. Fang Z-P, Vin G-J (1989) Studies on the structures of two new triterpene saponins C and D from *Polygala japonica* Houtt. Acta Bot Sin 31:708–712
29. Temperini JA, Retz L, Andrade SO (1976) Correlaçao entre atividade biológica e compostos químicos em plantas do gênero *Polygala* (Polygalaceae). Arq Inst Biol Sao Paulo 43:15–23
30. Habermehl GG, Busam L, Itakura Y, Martz W, Krebs HCh (1988) Progress in plant toxin research. Toxicon 26:23–24
31. Hoffmann JJ, Wiedhopf RM, Cole JR (1977) Cytotoxic and tumor inhibitory agent from *Polygala macradenia* Gray (Polygalaceae): 4′-demethyldeoxypodophyllotoxin. J Pharm Sci 66:586–587
32. Dreyer DL (1969) Extractives of *Polygala macradenia* Gray (Polygalaceae). Tetrahedron 25:4415–4420
33. Stout GH, Fries JL (1969) Polygalaxanthone A – a revised structure. Tetrahedron 25:5295–5299
34. Delaude C (1974) Contribution a l'étude des saponines contenues dans les Polygalacées. Identification de la saponine extraite du *Polygala macrostigma* Chod. Bull Soc R Sci Liège 43:249–252
35. Carretero Accame ME, Pardo Garcia MP (1984) Contribución al estudio de la esencia de la *Polygala microphylla* (L.) (Poligalaceae). An Real Acad Farm 50:211–214
36. Carretero ME, Benedi J, Pardo MP (1986) Études pharmacodynamiques préliminaires de *Polygala microphylla* (L.), sur le système nerveux central. Plant Méd Phytother 20:148–154
37. Domínguez XA, Sosa MG, Ortiz C, Jakupovic J (1990) Xanthone derivatives from *Polygala nitida*. Planta Med 56:126–127
38. Hamburger M, Stoeckli-Evans H, Hostettmann K (1984) A new pyranocoumarin diester from *Polygala paniculata* L. Helv Chim Acta 67:1729–1733
39. Hamburger M, Gupta M, Hostettmann K (1985) Coumarins from *Polygala paniculata*. Planta Med pp 215–217
40. Delaude C (1973) Contribution a l'étude des saponines contenues dans les Polygalacées. Identification de la saponine extraite du *Polygala persicariifolia* DC. Bull Soc R Sci Liège 42:635–638
41. Hokanson GC (1978) Podophyllotoxin and 4′-demethylpodophyllotoxin from *Polygala polygama* (Polygalaceae). Lloydia 41:497–498
42. Hokanson GC (1979) The lignans of *Polygala polygama* (Polygalaceae): deoxypodophyllotoxin and three new lignan lactones. J Nat Prod 42:378–384
43. Sezik E, Yesilada E (1985) A new saponin from the roots of *Polygala pruinosa*. Fitoterapia 56:159–163
44. Andrade CHS, Fo RB, Gottlieb OR, Silveira ER (1977) The chemistry of Brazilian Polygalaceae. I. Xanthones from *Polygala spectabilis*. Lloydia 40:344–346
45. Smith Jr CR, Madrigal RV, Weisleder D, Plattner RD (1977) *Polygala virgata* seed oil – a new source of acetotriglycerides. Lipids 12:736–740
46. Chesne C, Amoros M, Girre L (1983) Étude de l'activité antifongique de plantes supérieures: III. – Étude comparative de techniques d'isolement d'un saponoside antifongique des parties aériennes du *Polygala vulgaris* L. Plant Méd Phytothér 17:191–201
47. Kita F, Aikawa H, Takido M, Kimura Y (1969) Studies on the standardization of crude crugs. XVIII. Studies on the analytic method of Senega saponins. Yakugaku Zasshi 89:1111–1114
48. Briggs CJ (1988) Senega snakeroot – a traditional Canadian herbal medicine. Can Pharm J 121:199–201
49. Shoji J, Kawanishi S, Tsukitani Y (1971) Studies on the constituents of Senegae radix. I. Isolation and quantitative analysis of the glycosides. Yakugaku Zasshi 91:198–202

50. Tsukitani Y, Shoji J (1973) Studies on the constituents of Senegae Radix. III. The structures of senegin-III and senegin-IV, saponins from *Polygala senega* Linne var. *latifolia* Torry et Gray. Chem Pharm Bull (Tokyo) 21:1564–1574
51. Tsukitani Y, Kawanishi S, Shoji J (1973) Studies on the constituents of Senegae Radix. II. The structure of senegin-II, a saponin from *Polygala senega* Linne var. *latifolia* Torry et Gray. Chem Pharm Bull (Tokyo) 21:791–799
52. Akada Y, Yuki H, Takiura K (1972) Studies on glycone moiety of senega saponins. II. Composition of cinnamic acid derivatives and monosaccharides of purified saponins, and oligosaccharides obtained by partial hydrolysis of crude saponin. Yakugaku Zasshi 92:232–237
53. Takiura K, Yamamoto M, Murata H, Takai H, Honda S, Yuki H (1974) Studies on oligosaccharides. XIII. Oligoccharides in *Polygala senega* and structures of glycosyl-1,5-anhydro-D-glucitols. Yakugaku Zasshi 94:998–1003
54. Takiura K, Yamamoto M, Murata H, Takai H, Honda S, Yuki H (1975) Studies on oligosaccharides. XVI. New trisaccharides found in Senega radix. Yakugaku Zasshi 95:166–169
55. Hashimoto Y, Kawanishi K, Tomita H, Moriyasu M, Uhara Y, Kato A (1983) Enfleurage chromatography. A new technique for identifying volatile components in a small amount of samples from natural occurrence. Anal Lett 16:317–322
56. Tyler VE (1987) The New Honest Herbal. A sensible guide to herbs and related remedies. 2nd edn. Philadelphia: George F. Stickley Company, pp 218–219
57. Sakuma S, Shoji J (1982) Studies on the constituents of the root of *Polygala tenuifolia* Willdenow. I. Isolation of saponins and the structures of onjisaponins G and F. Chem Pharm Bull (Tokyo) 29:2431–2441
58. Sakuma S, Shoji J (1982) Studies on the constituents of the root of *Polygala tenuifolia* Willdenow. II. On the structures of onjisaponins A, B and E. Chem Pharm Bull (Tokyo) 30:810–821
59. Pelletier SW, Nakamura S, Soman R (1971) Constituents of *Polygala* species. The structure of tenuifolin, a prosapogenin from *P. senega* and *P. tenuifolia*. Tetrahedron 27:4417–4427
60. Ito H, Taniguchi H, Kita T, Matsuki Y, Tachikawa E, Fujita T (1977) Xanthones and a cinnamic acid derivative from *Polygala tenuifolia*. Phytochemistry 16:1614–1616
61. Ikeya Y, Sugama K, Okada M, Mitsusashi H (1991) Two xanthones from *Polygala tenuifolia*. Phytochemistry 30:2061–2065
62. Han BH, Park JH, Park MH, Han YN (1985) Beta-carboline alkaloids of *Polygala tenuifolia*. Arch Pharmacol Res (Seoul) 8:243–248
63. Yokoyama H, Hiai S, Oura H, Hayashi T (1982) Effects of total saponins extracted from several crude drugs on rat adrenocortical secretion. Yakugaku Zasshi 102:555–559
64. Rhee JK, Woo KJ, Baek BK, Ahn BJ (1981) Screening of the wormicidal Chinese raw drugs on *Clonorchis sinensis*. Am J Chin Med 9:277–284
65. Nikaido T, Ohmoto T, Saitoh H, Sankawa U, Sakuma S, Shoji J (1982) Inhibitors of cyclic adenosine monophosphate phosphodiesterase in *Polygala tenuifolia*. Chem Pharm Bull (Tokyo) 30:2020–2024
66. Tschesche R, Wulff G (1973) Chemie und Biologie der Saponine. In: Zechmeister L, Herz W, Grisebach H, Kirby GW (eds) Fortschritte der Chemie organischer Naturstoffe. Wien: Springer Verlag, pp 461–606
67. Anonymous (1990) Avis aux fabricants concernant les demandes d'autorisation de mise sur le marché des médicaments à base de plantes. Bulletin Officiel no. 90/22 bis. Paris: Ministère des Affairs Sociales et de la Solidarité
68. Mitchell J, Rook A (1979) Botanical dermatology. Plants and plant products injurious to the skin. Greengrass: Vancouver, pp 533
69. Morimoto I, Watanabe F, Osawa T, Okitsu T (1982) Mutagenicity screening of crude drugs with *Bacillus subtilis* rec-assay and Salmonella/microsome reversion assay. Mutat Res 1982;97:81–102

Quillaja Saponaria

P.A.G.M. De Smet

Botany

Quillaia bark is the dried inner part of the bark of *Quillaja saponaria* Molina and of other species of *Quillaja* (Rosaceae). The bark is also known as quillaja bark, soap tree bark, soap bark, Panama bark, China bark or Murillo bark (E); Seifenrinde, Waschrinde, Panamarinde (G); écorce de quillaya, écorce de Panama, écorce de saponaire (F) [1–4].

Chemistry

Quillaia bark contains about 9–10% of a triterpenoid saponin mixture. Acid hydrolysis yields two sapogenins, quillaic acid (= hydroxygypsogenin) and gypsogenin [1,4–6]. Treatment with weak alkali produces two desacylsaponins that have been identified as quillaic acid 3,28-*O*-bisglycosides. The structures of these desacylsaponins and of the eliminated acyl groups have been elucidated [7,8]. Other constituents of quillaia bark include calcium oxalate and about 10–15% of tannins [4].

Pharmacology and Uses

Quillaia bark has been used as emulsifying or frothing agent in foods, beverages and pharmaceuticals. It has been employed as an expectorant but this use has become obsolete. It may also be included in external preparations because of its detergent effects [1–4, 6]. The French health authorities permit topical medicinal use as a softening agent [9].

Recent pharmacological studies of quillaia saponins focus on the lipid-lowering activity of dietary feeding to laboratory animals [10–12] and on the enhancement of the immune response to vaccines [13–20].

Adverse Effects of Herbal Drugs, Vol. 2
(ed. by P.A.G.M. De Smet, K. Keller, R. Hänsel, R.F. Chandler)

Pharmacokinetics

Concrete information about the pharmacokinetic fate of quillaia saponins appears to be limited to some early reports that are not particularly informative [21]. One researcher described the excretion of two sapogenins in the feces following oral dosing in dogs [21]. Other experimenters found no or low urinary excretion of sapogenins following oral administration of quillaia saponin to dogs [22].

Recently, immunopotentiating effects were shown following oral administration of quillaia saponins. These observations do not prove, however, that the saponins enter the general circulation because the underlying mechanism may be initial activation of the mucosal immune system leading to further immunological events [14–16,18].

Adverse Reaction Profile

General Animal Data

A Russian research group obtained the following LD_{50}-values for quillaia bark saponins in the mouse: 1625 mg/kg p.o., 650 mg/kg s.c., 275 mg/kg i.p. and 275 mg/kg i.v. [23]. According to Osol and Farrar [1], 0.4 mg/kg of quillaic acid injected intravenously in a cat was sufficient to cause death, whereas 2 g administered by mouth was not fatal.

The acute toxicity of different saponin fractions of quillaia bark was recently assessed by Kensil and co-workers [19] who determined mortality after intradermal injection in mice. A commercially purchased crude saponin mixture known as Quil-A was lethal in the dose range of 100–125 μg. Purified saponins (isolated from quillaia bark by silica and reverse phase chromatography and designated as QS-7, QS-18 and QS-21) varied considerably in their toxicity. QS-7 was nonlethal in doses up to 500 μg and QS-21 killed one of five mice at 500 μg, whereas QS-18 (the predominant saponin in quillaia bark and Quil-A) was lethal at 25 μg. There was no correlation between lethality and hemolytic activity.

Speijers et al. [24] investigated local reactions and hematological changes following intramuscular administration of Quil-A to rats. A concentration of 600 μg/ml caused inflammatory reactions in all animals, but at a concentration of 50 μg/ml an inflammatory reaction occurred in only one of six animals. It was concluded that there are no objections against the incorporation of Quil-A in vaccines at a concentration of 50 μg/ml.

Coulson and Evans [25] studied the effects of dietary feeding of quillaia saponins in rats. They observed a dose-related reduction in the rate of body weight gain at levels of 0.5–2.0% and high mortality at a level of 3.0%. Oser [26] did not find an adverse effect on weight gain following the dietary administration of 0.05% of quillaia extract to rats for 12 weeks. Rao and Kendall [11] found no adverse effects on food consumption, body weight and gross autopsy findings in rats after treatment with 0.75% of quillaia saponins in the diet for 8 or 24 weeks.

The most extensive studies on the toxicity of quillaia bark were conducted by a group of the British Industrial Biological Research Association which investigated short-term and long-term effects of a spray-dried aqueous extract of quillaia bark in rodents [21,27,28]. Short-term toxicity was assessed by feeding rats with diets containing 0.0, 0.6, 2.0 or 4.0% of the extract. Treatment for 13 weeks produced a transitory reduction in the rate of body weight gain with parallel changes in the intakes of food and water. Dietary feeding of 2.0 and 4.0% was associated with changes in the relative weights of some body organs (most notably lower liver weights and higher stomach weights) but these changes were not accompanied by histopathological abnormalities. Effects on hematological parameters (including erythrocyte fragility in hypotonic saline) were not observed at any dose level [21].

The long-term toxicity of quillaia bark extract was tested in mice [27] and in rats [28]. In the first study, mice were given dietary levels up to 1.5% for 84 weeks. No level of treatment had a significant effect on death rate or histopathological features, including incidences of malignant and benign tumours. A lower rate of body weight gain was seen only at the level of 1.5% (corresponding to a daily intake of approximately 2.2 g/kg) [27]. In the second study, quillaia bark extract was fed to rats at dietary levels up to 3% (approximately equivalent to an intake of 1.5 g/kg/day) for 2 years. This treatment had no adverse effects on death rate, serum chemistry or hematological parameters, or on the incidence of histopathological findings, including tumours. Male rats fed the highest dietary level had lower body weights than did control animals, consequent to a decreased food intake [28].

General Human Data

Secondary sources claim that the ingestion of large amounts of quillaia may result in systemic poisoning with liver damage, respiratory failure, convulsions and coma [3,23], but such statements are not supported by a primary reference.

In 1986, the FAO/WHO Expert Committee on Food Additives established, on the basis of the available toxicological data (see the section on general animal data), an acceptable daily intake for quillaia extract of 0–5 mg/kg body weight [29].

Allergic Reactions

One well-documented case has been reported, where occupational exposure to the dust of raw quillaia bark resulted in allergic asthmatic symptoms that persisted even despite the use of a protective mask [30].

Gastrointestinal Reactions

Ingestion of quillaia bark preparations can produce gastrointestinal irritation leading to vomiting and diarrhoea [1,4,30].

Respiratory Reactions

Powdered quillaia bark is very sternutatory due to its local irritant properties [1].

Leroy and Marbarger [31] exposed hamsters for 1 hour per day to nebulized solutions containing 0.5–1.0% of quillaia saponin. After 60–90 days of treatment there was hyperplasia of the bronchiolar epithelium and focal lesions consisting of giant cells and histiocytes containing lipid droplets and hemosiderin pigment.

See also the section on allergic reactions.

Drug Interactions

The capacity of quillaia bark saponins to form insoluble, poorly absorbed complexes with nutrients has been studied *in vitro* by West and colleagues [32,33]. They observed a 39% binding of provitamin D_3 but no complexation of vitamin A, vitamin D_3, vitamin E, zinc, iron or magnesium. Coulson and Evans [25] found no influence of quillaia saponin on the absorption of ergocalciferol (= vitamin D_2) or its curative effect upon rickets in rats.

Fertility, Pregnancy and Lactation

A pure saponin isolated from quillaia bark named quillinin-A was found active against rat sperm at a concentration of 0.05% but it was inactive against human spermatozoa at a level of 0.5% [5].

Other data about the effects of quillaia bark on fertility or about its use during pregnancy and lactation have not been recovered from the literature.

Mutagenicity and Carcinogenicity

Data about the mutagenicity of quillaia bark have not been recovered from the literature.

Long-term toxicity studies in mice and in rats (see the section on general animal data) have not yielded evidence for carcinogenic activity of quillaia bark extract at dietary levels up to 1.5% in mice [27] or up to 3% in rats [28].

References

1. Osol A, Farrar GE (1955) The Dispensatory of the United States of America. 25th edn. Philadelphia: J.B. Lippincott Company, pp 1153–1154
2. Madaus G (1979) Lehrbuch der biologischen Heilmittel. Band III. Hildesheim: Georg Olms Verlag, pp 2278–2280
3. Reynolds JEF (ed) (1989) Martindale The Extra Pharmacopoeia. 29th edn. London: The Pharmaceutical Press, p 1248
4. Wichtl M (1989) Seifenrinde. In: Wichtl M, red. Teedrogen. Ein Handbuch für die Praxis auf Wissenschaftlicher Grundlage. 2. Auflage. Stuttgart: Wissenschaftliche Verlagsgesellschaft, pp 440–441
5. Varshney IP, Beg MFA, Sankaram AVB (1985) Saponins and sapogenins from *Quillaia saponaria*. Fitoterapia 56:254–256
6. Price KR, Johnson IT, Fenwick GR (1987) The chemistry and biological significance of saponins in foods and feeding stuffs. CRC Crit Rev Food Sci Nutr 26:27–135
7. Higuchi R, Tokimitsu Y, Fujioka T, Komori T, Kawasaki T, Oakenful DG (1987) Structure of desacylsaponins obtained from the bark of *Quillaja saponaria*. Phytochemistry 26:229–235
8. Higuchi R, Komori T (1987) Structures of compounds derived from the acyl moieties of quillajasaponin. Phytochemistry 26:2357–2360
9. Anonymous (1990) Avis aux fabricants concernant les demandes d'autorisation de mise sur le marché des médicaments à base de plantes. Bulletin Officiel no. 90/22 bis. Paris: Ministère des Affairs Sociales et de la Solidarité
10. Oakenfull DG, Topping DL, Illman RJ, Fenwick DE (1984) Prevention of dietary hypercholesterolaemia in the rat by soya bean and quillaja saponins. Nutr Rep Int 29:1039–1046
11. Rao AV, Kendall CW (1986) Dietary saponins and serum lipids. Food Cosmet Toxicol 24:441
12. Sidhu GS, Oakenfull DG (1986) A mechanism for the hypocholesterolaemic activity of saponins. Br J Nutr 55:643–649
13. Dalsgaard K (1978) A study of the isolation and characterization of the saponin Quil A. Evaluation of its adjuvant activity, with a special reference to the application in the vaccination of cattle against foot-and-mouth disease. Acta Vet Scand 69 (Suppl) pp 1–40
14. Maharaj I, Froh KJ, Campbell JB (1986) Immune responses of mice to inactivated rabies vaccine administered orally: potentiation by *Quillaja* saponin. Can J Microbiol 32:414–420
15. Chavali SR, Francis T, Campbell JB (1987) An *in vitro* study of immunomodulatory effects of some saponins. Int J Immunopharmacol 9:675–683
16. Chavali SR, Campbell JB (1987) Adjuvant effects of orally administered saponins on humoral and cellular immune responses in mice. Immunobiol 174:347–359
17. Chavali SR, Campbell JB (1987) Immunomodulatory effects of orally-administered saponins and nonspecific resistance against rabies infection. Int Arch Allergy Appl Immunol 84:129–134
18. Chavali SR, Barton LD, Campbell JB (1988) Immunopotentiation by orally-administered *Quillaja* saponins: effects in mice vaccinated intraperitoneally against rabies. Clin Exp Immunol 74:339–343
19. Kensil CR, Patel U, Lennick M, Marciani D (1991) Separation and characterization of saponins with adjuvant activity from *Quillaja saponaria* Molina cortex. J Immunol 146:431–437
20. Wu JY, Gardner BH, Murphy CI, Seals JR, Kensil CR, Recchia J, Beltz GA, Newman GW, Newman MJ (1992) Saponin adjuvant enhancement of antigen-specific immune responses to an experimental HIV-1 vaccine. J Immunol 148:1519–1525
21. Gaunt IF, Grasso P, Gangolli SD (1974) Short-term toxicity study of quillaia extract in rats. Food Cosmet Toxicol 12:641–650

22. Fieger J (1918) Über die Ausscheidung von Saponinen durch den Harn und ihre Wirkung auf das Blut nach innerlicher Darreichung. Biochem Z 86:243–297
23. Anonymous (1982) Quillaia extracts. In: Toxicological evaluation of certain food additives. WHO Food Additives Series no. 17, pp 180–184
24. Speijers GJA, Danse LHJC, Beuvery EC, Strik JJTWA, Vos JG (1988) Local reactions of the saponin Quil A and a Quil A containing iscom measles vaccine after intramuscular injection of rats: a comparison with the effect of DPT-polio vaccine. Fundam Appl Toxicol 10:425–430
25. Coulson CB, Evans RA (1960) The effect of saponin, sterols and linoleic acid on the weight increase of growing rats. Br J Nutr 14:121–134
26. Oser BL (1966) An evaluation of *Yucca mohavensis* as a source of food grade saponin. Food Cosmet Toxicol 4:57–61
27. Phillips JC, Butterworth KR, Gaunt IF, Evans JG, Grasso P (1979) Long-term toxicity study of quillaia extract in mice. Food Cosmet Toxicol 17:23–27
28. Drake JJ-P, Butterworth KR, Gaunt IF, Hooson J, Evans JG, Gangolli SD (1982) Long-term toxicity study of quillaia extract in rats. Food Chem Toxicol 20:15–23
29. Anonymous (1986) Evaluation of certain food additives and contaminants. 29th Report of the Joint FAO/WHO Expert Committee on Food Additives. Technical Report Series 733. Geneva: World Health Organization, p 43
30. Raghuprasad PK, Brooks SM, Litwin A, Edwards JJ, Bernstein IL, Gallagher J (1980) Quillaja bark (soapbark)-induced asthma. J Allergy Clin Immunol 65:285–287
31. Leroy EP, Marbarger JP (1969) Evolution of lesions in hamster's lung caused by inhaled aerosols of triterpenoid saponins from Quillaja saponaria. Am J Pathol 55:41a–42a
32. West LG, Greger JL, White A, Nonnamaker BJ (1978) *In vitro* studies on saponin-mineral complexation. J Food Sci 43:1342–1343
33. West LG, Greger JL (1978) *In vitro* studies on saponin-vitamin complexation. J Food Sci 43:1340–1343

Scutellaria Species

P.A.G.M. De Smet

Botany

Species of *Scutellaria* (skullcap), which belong to the family Labiatae, have been employed as herbal remedies in various parts of the world.

Scutellaria baicalensis Georgi (Baikal skullcap) is the species most commonly utilized in Europe [1]. It should be noted, however, that an investigation of herbal preparations in the United Kingdom showed that skullcap herb available from some wholesale suppliers was not in fact a *Scutellaria* species but was a *Teucrium* species [2]. In traditional Oriental medicine, the root of *Scutellaria baicalensis* (Scutellariae Radix) is used under the names of Huangqin in China [3,4] and Ogon or Wogon in Japan [5,6]. *Scutellaria amoena* C.H. Wright, *S. hypericifolia* Levl., *S. ikonnikovii* Juz., *S. likiangensis* Diels, *S. rehderiana* Diels, and *S. viscidula* Bge. may all serve as alternative sources of Huangqin [3,7]. Another skullcap valued in Chinese medicine is the dried whole plant of *S. barbata* D. Don (barbat skullcap) [4].

In the United States, the dried overground plant of *S. lateriflora* L. (mad dog skullcap) was formerly official in the Pharmacopeia and National Formulary. This species as well as *S. parvula* Michx. (small skullcap) and *S. galericulata* L. = *S. epilobifolia* Hamilton (marsh skullcap) used to be source plants of American Indian medicines [8].

Other *Scutellaria* species that are or have been used as herbal medicines, primarily in Asian regions, include *S. canescens* Nutt. = *S. incana* Spreng. (Western skullcap), *S. discolor* Colebr., *S. indica* L., *S. luzonica* Rolfe = *S. marivelensis* Elm., *S. macrantha* Fisch and *S. scordifolia* L. [9,10].

Chemistry

The root of *Scutellaria baicalensis* contains sterols [5] and more than 30 different flavonoids, such as baicalein (= scutellarein), baicalin (= baicalein 7-glucuronide), baicalein 7-*O*-β-D-glycopyranoside, wogonin, wogonin-7-*O*-glucuronide, oroxylin A, oroxylin A 7-*O*-glucuronide, dihydrooroxylin A,

Adverse Effects of Herbal Drugs, Vol. 2
(ed. by P.A.G.M. De Smet, K. Keller, R. Hänsel, R.F. Chandler)

skullcapflavone I, skullcapflavone II, and chrysin [3,5,6,11–17]. Tani et al. [18] identified baicalin and wogonin 7-*O*-glucuronide as the two major root flavonoids. Both glucuronides were distributed in the cortex, phloem and xylem at high concentrations, whereas their aglycones, baicalein and wogonin, were localized in the outermost periderm and inner slightly decayed xylem and pith. As a consequence, the usual preparation of Scutellariae Radix (by removing of the outer peel from the fresh root) may result in appreciable loss of bioactive constituents [18]. Analytical studies of commercial samples of Scutellariae Radix have shown variable concentrations of 0.1–20.6% of baicalin, <0.1–5.4% of wogonin 7-*O*-glucuronide, <0.1–5.2% of baicalein, 0.1–2.1% of wogonin, and <0.1–4.1% of oroxylin A 7-*O*-glucuronide [6,17,18].

The major root flavonoids of *S. baicalensis* are not found in the flower or leaf, but low amounts occur in the upper stem (0.58% of baicalin and 0.07% of wogonin 7-*O*-glucuronide), and higher amounts in the lower stem (4.3% of baicalin and 3.3% of wogonin 7-*O*-glucuronide) [18]. However, the leaves of *S. baicalensis* do contain the flavonoids carthamidin, isocarthamidin, and isoscutellarein-8-*O*-glucuronide [19,20].

The herb of *S. barbata* contains alkaloids, flavonoids, phenols, and steroids [4].

Pharmacology and Uses

Skullcap has been utilized primarily for its reputed tonic, tranquilizing and antispasmodic effects [1,8].

The roots of *Scutellaria baicalensis* and/or their flavonoid components have been associated with a variety of pharmacological actions, such as antibacterial effects [7,21], anti-inflammatory activity [22–24], antiallergic effects [3,25], decreased blood urea nitrogen [26], decreased lipid levels in serum and liver [27,28], and increased blood viscosity in betamethasone-treated rats [29]. Also reported were inhibitory effects on blood platelet aggregation [30], mouse liver sialidase [31], complement-mediated cytotoxicity in cultured mouse hepatocytes [32], lipid peroxidation in rat liver [33–35], rat hepatic aryl hydrocarbon hydroxylase [36], beef heart mitochondrial NADH-oxidase activity [37] and cAMP phosphodiesterase from beef heart [38]. There is also evidence of increased DNA recombination activity *in vitro* [39] and decreased mutagenicity of benzo[*a*]pyrene in *Salmonella typhimurium* strains TA 98 and TA 100 [40].

Pharmacokinetics

After oral administration of baicalin to rats, approximately 50% of the dose was excreted in the bile in the form of metabolites. The two major metabolites were 6-O-β-glucopyranuronosylbaicalein 7-O-sulfate and baicalein 6,7-di-O-β-glucopyranuronoside. These metabolites could also be recovered from the bile of rats treated with the aglycone baicalein. Since biliary excretion was slower in the case of baicalin, it may be that this glucuronide undergoes hydrolysis in the gastrointestinal tract to baicalein before it is absorbed [41].

Adverse Reaction Profile

General Animal Data

Chinese studies of the acute toxicity of various preparations from the root of *Scutellaria baicalensis* have been reviewed by Wenqing [3], who concluded that such preparations have very low toxicity when given orally.

Kiwaki et al. [42,43] studied the subacute oral toxicity of Sairei-tô (dried decoction of Scutellariae Radix and 11 other herbs) and Saiboku-tô (dried decoction of Scutellariae Radix and 9 other herbs) in rats. Their results suggested maximum no-effect dose levels of >2 g/kg/day in the case of Sairei-tô [42] and of 1 g/kg/day for male rats or >2 g/kg/day for female rats in the case of Saiboku-tô [43].

Baicalin was reported to have an intraperitoneal LD_{50} of 3 g/kg in mice [21].

General Human Data

In traditional Chinese medicine, neither oral administration of root preparations of *Scutellaria baicalensis* nor injection of baicalin and baicalein have been associated with ill effects other than rare gastric discomfort and diarrhoea [3].

Hepatic Reactions[1]

There is an increasing number of case reports to suggest that the ingestion of skullcap-containing preparations can induce hepatotoxic reactions [44–46].

A recent report from the United Kingdom described four women with hepatitis or jaundice after the use of stress-relieving herbal tablets [45]. Three patients presented with jaundice after taking Kalms tablets in dosages from one tablet daily for 3 days to two tablets daily for 2 months. Liver biopsies disclosed severe acute hepatitis with centrilobular and bridging necrosis in one patient and moderately acute hepatitis in another. Liver function test results of these two patients returned to normal 2–3 months after stopping the herbal medicine. In the third patient liver biopsy was

[1] See the note added in proof on p. 317

unsuccessful, but it took her liver function tests 19 months to return to normal values. The fourth patient showed jaundice after using Neurelax tablets for three weeks (about 30 tablets). Her clinical condition deteriorated and she developed ascites and encephalopathy. A liver biopsy performed three months later revealed chronic aggressive hepatitis with advanced fibrosis. The patient could not return to work until ten months later, when the results of her liver function tests had almost returned to normal. The authors pointed out that the Welsh Drug Information Centre had received inquiries about jaundice following the use of Kalms and Neurelax, and also after the intake of Box's nerve tablets, which have an identical formulation to Neurelax. They suggested that, out of several ingredients common to Neurelax and Kalms tablets, skullcap and valerian would seem to be the most likely offenders, even though there were no reports to show that these ingredients can actually produce liver damage.

There is another British case report on the induction of hepatitis by a herbal drug product that seemingly contained skullcap without the addition of valerian [44]. A 49-year-old woman presented with similar symptoms (nausea, general malaise, and a dull ache in the right hypochondrium) on two different occasions. Both episodes coincided with the ingestion of herbal tablets for several weeks. The tablets were taken for nervous tension and were reported to contain mistletoe, motherwort, kelp, wild lettuce and skullcap. After the settling of symptoms and the return of liver function tests to normal, a formal challenge test with the tablets was arranged. The nausea and general malaise returned after 10 days of continuous ingestion, and a liver biopsy taken 4 days later showed extensive inflammatory-cell infiltration, considerable focal necrosis, and distortion of liver architecture. Complement concentrations were normal, and screening for autoimmune antibodies was negative, but there was polyclonal increase in serum IgG concentration. Liver histology and liver function tests gradually returned to normal. The authors suggested that the hepatitis was probably due to mistletoe, because this was the only constituent known to contain potential toxins. However, this view was challenged by others [47,48], and the mistletoe component was later reported to be absent in the herbal product in question [49].

The development of hepatitis following the use of skullcap in combination with other botanical drugs was also reported recently from Australia [46]. A 56-year-old woman presented to hospital with weight loss, jaundice, and hepatomegaly. Serology testing proved negative for viral causes, but several liver function tests gave abnormal results. Liver biopsy confirmed a diagnosis of chronic active hepatitis of unclear etiology. The patient had taken three different herbal remedies in addition to her conventional medicines (verapamil, chlordiazepoxide, thyroxine). The first herbal preparation reportedly contained mistletoe, the second one celery fruit, guaiacum, burdock root and sarsaparilla, and the third valerian, skullcap and passion flower. After stopping all medications with exception of the thyroxine, the patient started to improve, and she could be discharged after two weeks on a regimen of thyroxine and temazepam.

Additional cases of liver damage, even with fatal consequences, were recently observed in Norwegian patients. Some patients had been taking several herbal remedies, including skullcap, whereas others had used a herbal remedy, in which skullcap was the only ingredient [50–52].

Drug Interactions

The flavonoid glucuronide baicalin occurring in *Scutellaria baicalensis* forms complexes with the alkaloid berberine [53]. These complexes might have an absorption profile other than their separate components due to altered physicochemical properties.

Fertility, Pregnancy and Lactation

Matsui et al. [54] did not observe decreased fertility in female mice which were treated subcutaneously with an aqueous extract of *Scutellaria baicalensis* for 5 days.

Kiwaki et al. [55] tested the teratogenic potential of Sairei-tô (dried decoction of a mixture of Scutellariae Radix and 11 other traditional Chinese herbs). Oral treatment of female rats with doses up to 2 g/kg/day from day 7 to day 17 of the pregnancy did not produce increased fetal mortality, inhibited fetal growth or teratogenicity, and the growth, development and reproductive capacity of the offspring were not affected.

Kim et al. [56] treated female rats with aqueous extract concentrates of Scutellariae Radix at oral dose levels of 0.25, 12.5 and 25 g/kg/day from day 7 to 17 of gestation, and observed dose-dependent increases in the incidence of lumbar rib and abnormal urinary system (mainly dilatation of the ureter).

Mutagenicity and Carcinogenicity

Although the mutagenicity testing of *Scutellaria* root extracts in bacteria can be hampered by a killing effect [57–59], Lee et al. [59] demonstrated mutagenic effects of aqueous extracts in *Salmonella typhimurium* strains TA 98 and TA 100 with and without S9 activation. Morimoto et al. [57] only found a positive response to an aqueous extract in TA 100 + S9 mix and also showed mutagenicity of a methanolic extract in the *Bacillus subtilis* rec-assay. Nagao et al. [60] obtained negative results with baicalein in *S. typhimurium* TA 98 and TA 100, whereas wogonin was positive in TA 100 in the presence of S9 mix.

As far as is known, *Scutellaria* extracts have not been submitted to formal carcinogenicity testing.

References

1. Tyler VE (1987) The New Honest Herbal. A sensible guide to herbs and related remedies. 2nd edn. Philadelphia: George F. Stickley Company, pp 216–217
2. Phillipson JD, Anderson LA (1984) Herbal remedies used in sedative and anti-rheumatic preparations: Part 1. Pharm J 233:80–82
3. Wenqing L (1987) Huangqin. In: Chang H-M, But PP-H, ed. Pharmacology and Applications of Chinese Materia Medica. Vol II. World Scientific Publishing Co, Singapore, pp 1022–1028
4. National Institute for the Control of Pharmaceutical and Biological Products (1987) Colour atlas of Chinese traditional drugs. Vol 1. Beijing: Science Press, pp 239–240
5. Takido M, Aimi M, Takahashi S, Yamanouchi S, Torii H, Dohi S (1975) Constituents of aqueous extracts of crude drugs. I. Root of *Scutellaria baicalensis* Georgi (Wogon) (I). Yakugaku Zasshi 95:108–113
6. Takino Y, Miyahara T, Arichi E, Arichi S, Hayashi T, Karikura M (1987) Determination of some flavonoids in Scutellariae Radix by high-performance liquid chromatography. Chem Pharm Bull (Tokyo) 35:3494–3497
7. Franzblau SG, Cross C (1986) Comparative *in vitro* antimicrobial activity of Chinese medicinal herbs. J Ethnopharmacol 15:279–288
8. Vogel VJ (1970) American Indian medicine. Norman: University of Oklahoma Press, pp 366–367
9. Hoppe HA (1975) Drogenkunde. Band 1. Angiospermen. 8. Auflage. Berlin: Walter de Gruyter, pp 984–985
10. Penso G (1983) Index Plantarum Medicinalium Totius Mundi Eorumque Synonymorum. Milano: Organizzazione Editoriale Medico Farmaceutica, pp 866–867
11. Takido M, Yasukawa K, Matsuura S, Iinuma M (1979) On the revised structure of skullcapflavone I, a flavone compound in the roots of *Scutellaria baicalensis* Georgi (Wogon). J Pharm Soc Japan 99:443–444
12. Takagi S, Yamaki M, Inoue K (1980) Studies on the water-soluble constituents of the roots of *Scutellaria baicalensis* Georgi (Wogon). Yakugaku Zasshi 100:1220–1224
13. Takagi S, Yamaki M, Inoue K (1981) On the minor constituents of the roots of *Scutellaria baicalensis* Georgi (Wogon). Yakugaku Zasshi 101:899–903
14. Tomimori T, Miyaichi Y, Kizu H (1982) On the flavonoid constituents from the roots of *Scutellaria baicalensis* Georgi. I. Yakugaku Zasshi 102:388–391
15. Tomimori T, Miyaichi Y, Imoto Y, Kizu H, Suzuki C (1984) Studies on the constituents of *Scutellaria* species. IV. On the flavonoid constituents of the root of *Scutellaria baicalensis* Georgi (4). Yakugaku Zasshi 104:529–534
16. Tomimori T, Miyaichi Y, Imoto Y, Kizu H, Tanabe Y (1984) Studies on the constituents of *Scutellaria* species. III. On the flavonoid constituents of the root of *Scutellaria baicalensis* Georgi (3). Yakugaku Zasshi 104:524–528
17. Tomimori T, Jin H, Miyaichi Y, Toyofuku S, Namba T (1985) Studies on the constituents of *Scutellaria* species. VI. On the flavonoid constituents of the root of *Scutellaria baicalensis* Georgi (5). Quantitative analysis of flavonoids in Scutellaria roots by high-performance liquid chromatography. Yakugaku Zasshi 105:148–155
18. Tani T, Katsuki T, Kubo M, Arichi S (1985) Histochemistry. VII. Flavones in Scutellariae radix. Chem Pharm Bull (Tokyo) 33:4894–4900
19. Takido M, Aimi M, Yamanouchi S, Yasukawa K, Torii H, Takahashi S (1976) Studies on the constituents in the water extracts of crude drugs. II. On the leaves of *Scutellaria baicalensis* Georgi (1). Yakugaku Zasshi 96:381–383
20. Nagai T, Miyaichi Y, Tomimori T, Yamada H (1989) Inhibition of mouse liver sialidase by plant flavonoids. Biochem Biophys Res Commun 3:25–31
21. Tsao T-F, Newman MG, Kwok Y-Y, Horikoshi AK (1982) Effect of Chinese and western antimicrobial agents on selected oral bacteria. J Dent Res 61:1103–1106
22. Kato M, Marumoto M, Hayashi M, Maeda T, Hayashi E (1984) Pharmacological studies on Saiko-prescriptions. IV. Effect of Shosaiko-to on swelling of rat hind paws induced by carrageenin. Yakugaku Zasshi 104:509–515

23. Kato M, Marumoto M, Hayashi M, Maeda T, Hayashi E (1984) Pharmacological studies on Saiko-prescriptions. V. Mechanisms of actions of Shosaiko-to on swelling of rat hind paws induced by carrageenin. Yakugaku Zasshi 104:516–523
24. Kubo M, Matsuda H, Tanaka M, et al. (1984) Studies on Scutellariae radix. VII. Anti-arthritic and anti-inflammatory actions of methanolic extract and flavonoid components from Scutellariae radix. Chem Pharm Bull (Tokyo) 32:2724–2729
25. Koda A, Nishiyori T, Nagai H, Matsuura N, Tsuchiya H (1982) Anti-allergic actions of crude drugs and blended Chinese traditional medicines. Effects of type I and type IV allergic reactions. Folia Pharmacol Jpn 80:41
26. Nagasawa T, Shibutani S, Oura H (1979) Effect of crude drugs on rat serum constituents after the administration. II. Yakugaku Zasshi 99:71–77
27. Kimura Y, Kubo M, Tani T, Arichi S, Ohminami H, Okuda H (1981) Studies on Scutellariae radix. III. Effects on lipid metabolism in serum, liver and fat cells of rats. Chem Pharm Bull (Tokyo) 29:2308–2312
28. Kimura Y, Kubo M, Kusaka K, Tani T, Higashino M, Arichi S, Okuda H (1982) Studies on Scutellariae radix. V. Effects on ethanol-induced hyperlipemia and lipolysis in isolated fat cells. Chem Pharm Bull (Tokyo) 30:219–222
29. Tani T, Ohno T, Inoue K, Katsuki T, Arichi S (1986) Effect of crude drugs and their prescriptions on the blood rheology affected by glucocorticoid treatment. IV. Effect of Sho-saiko-to Dai-saiko-to and their constituent crude drugs on adverse reactions in betamethasone treated rat. Yakugaku Zasshi 106:808–817
30. Kubo M, Matsuda H, Tani T, Arichi S, Kimura Y, Okuda H (1985) Studies on Scutellariae radix. XII. Anti-thrombotic actions of various flavonoids from Scutellariae radix. Chem Pharm Bull (Tokyo) 33:2411–2415
31. Nagai T, Yamada H, Otsuka Y (1989) Inhibition of mouse liver sialidase by the root of *Scutellaria baicalensis*. Planta Med 55:27–29
32. Kiso Y, Suzuki M, Yasuda M, Watanabe H, Minegishi T, Hikino H, Yang L-L, Yen K-Y (1990) Antihepatotoxic actions of traditional Chinese medicines. 2. The pharmacological interaction of components of Dai-saiko-tô employing complement-mediated cytotoxicity in primary cultured mouse hepatocytes. Phytother Res 4:36–38
33. Kimura Y, Kubo M, Tani T, Arichi S, Okuda H (1981) Studies on Scutellariae radix. IV. Effects on lipid peroxidation in rat liver. Chem Pharm Bull (Tokyo) 29:2610–2617
34. Kimura Y, Okuda H, Tani T, Arichi S (1982) Studies on Scutellariae radix. VI. Effects of flavanone compounds on lipid peroxidation in rat liver. Chem Pharm Bull (Tokyo) 30:1792–1795
35. Kimura Y, Okuda H, Taira Z, Shoji N, Takemoto T, Arichi S (1984) Studies on Scutellariae radix. IX. New component inhibiting lipid peroxidation in rat liver. Planta Med 50:290–295
36. Friedman FK, West D, Sugimura T, Gelboin HV (1985) Flavone modulators of rat hepatic aryl hydrocarbon hydroxylase. Pharmacology 31:203–207
37. Duval D, Hodnick WF, Pardini RS (1988) Inhibition of mitochondrial respiration, auto-oxidation and cyanide mediated oxygen consumption by selected flavonoids. Fed Am Soc Exp Biol J 2(4):A773
38. Nikaido T, Ohmoto T, Kinoshita T, et al. (1989) Inhibition of adenosine 3′,5′-cyclic monophosphate phosphodiesterase by flavonoids. III. Chem Pharm Bull (Tokyo) 37:1392–1395
39. Higashitani A, Tabata S, Hayashi T, Hotta Y (1989) Plant saponins can affect DNA recombination in cultured mammalian cells. Cell Struct Funct 14:617–624
40. Sakai Y, Nagase H, Ose Y, Sato T, Kawai M, Mizuno M (1988) Effects of medicinal plant extracts from Chinese herbal medicines on the mutagenic activity of benzo[*a*]pyrene. Mutat Res 206:327–334
41. Abe K, Inoue O, Yumioka E (1990) Biliary excretion of metabolites of baicalin and baicalein in rats. Chem Pharm Bull (Tokyo) 38:208–211
42. Kiwaki S, Ono C, Sakai K, Tada H, Oketani Y (1989) Ninety-day toxicity study of a Chinese herb medicine, *Sairei-tô* extract in rats. Pharmacometrics 38:241–254

43. Kiwaki S, Yamashita Y, Yamamae H, Nakamura T, Oketani Y (1989) Ninety-day toxicity study of a Chinese herb medicine Saiboku-to extract in rats. Pharmacometrics 38:495–510
44. Harvey J, Colin-Jones DG (1981) Mistletoe hepatitis. Br Med J 282:186–187
45. MacGregor FB, Abernethy VE, Dahabra S, Cobden I, Hayes PC (1989) Hepatotoxicity of herbal remedies. Br Med J 299:1156–1157
46. Weeks GR, Proper JS (1989) Herbal medicines – Gaps in our knowledge. Aust J Hosp Pharm 19:155–157
47. Fletcher Hyde F (1981) Mistletoe hepatitis. Br Med J 282:739
48. Farnsworth NR, Loub WD (1981) Mistletoe hepatitis. Br Med J 282:1058
49. McIntyre M (1984) Exposed: the inaccurate reporting behind the herbal medicine "scare". J Altern Med, January, pp 2–3
50. Myhr K. Department of Pharmacy, University Hospital of Trondheim. Personal communications, September and November 1991
51. Leander S, Skogstrøm L. Naturmedisin kan gi leverskade. Aflenposten November 6, 1991
52. Moum B, Aukrust P, Schrumpf E, Mørk T, Mathisen Ø, Elgjo K (1992) Naturmidler kan forårsake helseskader. Tidsskr Nor Laegeforen 112:1308–1311
53. Nolan JE, Brain KR (1985) Component interaction in Chinese herbal medicines. Acta Agronom 34 (Suppl):113
54. Matsui AS, Rogers J, Woo YK, Cutting WC (1967) Effects of some natural products on fertility in mice. Med Pharmacol Exp Int J Exp Med 16:414–424
55. Kiwaki S, Ono C, Sakai K, Nakamura T, Oketani Y (1989) A teratological evaluation of orally administered *Sairei-tô* extract in rats. Pharmacometrics 38:255–270
56. Kim SH, Kim Y-H, Han S-S, Roh JK (1988) Reproduction (Seg. II) study of Scutellaria radix in rat. J Toxicol Sci 13:340
57. Morimoto I, Watanabe F, Osawa T, Okitsu T (1982) Mutagenicity screening of crude drugs with *Bacillus subtilis* rec-assay and Salmonella/microsome reversion assay. Mutat Res 97:81–102
58. Yamamoto H, Mizutani T, Nomura H (1982) Studies on the mutagenicity of crude drug extracts. I. Yakugaku Zasshi 102:596–601
59. Lee HK, Kim YK, Kim Y-H, Roh JK (1987) Effect of bacterial growth-inhibiting ingredients on the Ames mutagenicity of medicinal herbs. Mutat Res 192:99–104
60. Nagao M, Morita N, Yahagi T, et al. (1981) Mutagenicities of 61 flavonoids and 11 related compounds. Environ Mut 3:401–419

Taraxacum Officinale

P.A.G.M. De Smet

Botany

Taraxacum officinale Weber (syn. *T. officinale* Wiggers, *T. dens leonis* Desr., *Leontodon taraxacum* L.) belongs to the family Asteraceae. Common vernacular names are dandelion (E), Löwenzahn (G), dent de lion and pissenlit (F) [1,2]. The vernacular term dandelion may also refer to another asteraceous plant, however, namely *Arctotheca calendula* [3]. The parts used medicinally are the root and the root with herb [1,2].

Chemistry

From the roots of dandelion, Hänsel et al. [4] isolated four different sesquiterpene lactones, namely 4α.15.11β.13-tetrahydroridentin B, taraxacolide-1′-O-β-D-glucopyranoside, taraxinic acid-1′-O-β-D-glucopyranoside and its 11,13-dihydroderivative. Rauwald and Huang [5] later found the γ-butyrolactone glucoside taraxacoside in the roots. Chemical studies of dandelion root or its milk sap have also yielded a number of triterpenes (taraxasterol, PSI-taraxasterol, its acetate, taraxole, taraxerole, b-amyrin) and steroles (b-sitosterol, its b-D-glucopyranoside, stigmasterol [4,6,7]. Other root constituents are inulin, organic acids [1,8], b-D-fructofuranosides and b-fructofuranosidases [9,10]. The reputed presence of lactucopicrin [1] has not been verified [4].

The sesquiterpene lactones taraxinic acid-1′-O-β-D-glucopyranoside and its 11,13-dihydroderivative have also been obtained from aerial parts of dandelion [4,11]. Other leaf constituents include *p*-hydroxyphenylacetic acid [11], amino acids [1], apigenin-7-glucoside and luteolin-7-glucoside [1], β-sitosterole [11], furan fatty acids [12], and vitamins such as vitamin A [1,8,13].

The flowers contain triterpenes (arnidiol, faradiol, β-amyrin), β-sitosterol, and carotinoids [1,8,14,15].

Adverse Effects of Herbal Drugs, Vol. 2
(ed. by P.A.G.M. De Smet, K. Keller, R. Hänsel, R.F. Chandler)

Pharmacology and Uses

Dandelion is primarily employed as a cholagogue, as a diuretic and as a bitter principle to stimulate appetite. It is also used in folk medicine as a laxative and blood purifier as well as in diabetes [2,8]. Some positive evidence for choleretic and diuretic effects has been obtained in rat experiments [16,17]. Animal studies on the hypoglycemic activity of dandelion have produced equivocal results. In one study, oral doses of 1–2 g/kg of the whole dried and powdered plant produced a hypoglycemic response in normal rabbits without giving significant results in alloxan-treated animals [18]. In another study, oral treatment with dried roots and leaves (as such incorporated in the diet and as a decoction replacing drinking water) did not affect glucose homeostasis in either non-diabetic or streptozotocin-diabetic mice [19].

A hot water extract from *Taraxacum officinale* was reported to show antitumor activity following intraperitoneal administration to mice [20].

The roasted root of dandelion may serve as a coffee surrogate, while the young leaves are sometimes eaten as a salad [1,2,8]. The plant is also collected to serve as an animal fodder [7,21,22].

Adverse Reaction Profile

A general discussion on the adverse reaction profile of medicinal plants containing sesquiterpene lactones was presented in the first volume of this book series [23].

General Animal Data

Rácz-Kotilla et al. [17] determined the acute toxicity of fluid extracts from dandelion root and dandelion herb in mice, and obtained intraperitoneal LD_{50} values of 36.6 g/kg and 28.8 g/kg, respectively. Akhtar et al. [18] treated rabbits orally with 3–6 g/kg of the whole dried and powdered dandelion plant without observing visible signs of acute toxicity.

General Human Data

According to a German text book [24], dandelion may produce poisoning especially when children suck the milk sap from the flower stems. Toxic symptoms are nausea, vomiting, diarrhea, and cardiac arrhythmias.

The consumption of dandelion as a green salad can result in human fascioliasis, when the plant is contaminated by the sheep liver fluke *Fasciola hepatica* [25,26]. This disease is characterized by liver enlargement and peripheral eosinophilia.

Allergic Reactions

Dandelion can produce allergic contact dermatitis due to the presence of the sesquiterpene lactone taraxinic acid-1'-O-β-D-glucopyranoside (see the section on dermatological reactions).

Dandelion pollen are among the plant pollens that can act as an allergen [27–29]. Cohen et al. [30] described three patients who experienced an immediate allergic reaction after their first ingestion of bee pollen as a health food. All three patients had a history of seasonally exacerbating rhinitis. Immunological evaluation revealed that they were sensitive to bee pollen, dandelion and to another member of the Asteraceae, short ragweed. The incriminated bee pollen products were found to contain the pollen of dandelion or a close relative.

The Russian literature describes a case of anaphylactic shock following the use of aspirin and a gargle containing *Calendula*. Five years before, the patient had experienced a similar reaction after smelling at dandelion [31]. Another report about a systemic reaction to dandelion that may have had an allergic basis appeared in the 19th century in The Lancet. Ingestion of a decoction of the dandelion plant produced itching and tingling erythema, papules and wheals followed by desquamation [32].

Dermatological Reactions

Dandelion juice is not irritant [22] but topical exposure to dandelion can produce an allergic response [3,7,21,22,33–37]. There are several well-documented cases in the literature where collection of dandelions as an animal fodder resulted in allergic dermatitis [7,21,22,33,34]. Hausen [38] demonstrated that the sesquiterpene lactone taraxinic acid-1'-O-β-D-glucopyranoside is responsible for these reactions. This compound is the only sesquiterpene lactone in *Taraxacum officinale* which has the α-methylene group exocyclic to the γ-lactone that is needed for contact allergenic properties.

Experiments in guinea pigs have shown that dandelion is a weak sensitizer [39]. This is also evident from a human study on Asteraceae-sensitive patients. Patch testing of 17 patients to dandelion gave only one strong and two weak to moderate reactions. The latter two patients showed cross-reactions to chamomile and yarrow, while the former also reacted to arnica. One patient who did not react to dandelion showed a positive response to the autumnal hawkbit (*Leontodon autumnalis*) [35]. This latter plant may serve as an adulterant of *T. officinale* [2].

Cross-sensitivity to other allergenic plant sources of sesquiterpene lactones (e.g., chamomile, laurel oil) has also been observed by other authors [7,33]. Lovell and Rowan [37] recently produced evidence, however, that patch testing with a sequiterpene lactone mix is not a reliable screening test for dandelion allergy. When seven subjects with a history suggestive of dandelion dermatitis were patch tested with extracts of dandelion and with a sesquiterpene lactone mix, all were positive to dandelion extracts, but only 2 reacted to the mix.

Gastrointestinal Reactions

Gastrointestinal side effects from normal therapeutic use have not been documented but since dandelion acts as a bitter principle, hyperacidic gastric complaints cannot be excluded [2].

There is one case report in the literature about a dandelion green bezoar following antrectomy and vagotomy [40].

Metabolic Reactions

See the section on pharmacology and uses for details on hypoglycemic potential.

Fertility, Pregnancy and Lactation

Data about *T. officinale* have not been recovered from the literature. Matsui et al. [41] reported that subcutaneous treatment with an aqueous extract of the related *T. mongolicum* for 5 days did not affect the fertility of female mice.

Mutagenicity and Carcinogenicity

Hirono et al. [42] tested the carcinogenicity of *Taraxacum platycarpum* Dahlst. in rats. The rhizomes of this dandelion have been used as a stomachic or lactagogue in Chinese medicine. Incorporation of 32% of the rhizomes in the diet for 209 days did not produce evidence of carcinogenicity.

References

1. List PH, Hörhammer L (1979) Hagers Handbuch der Pharmazeutischen Praxis. Vierte Neuausgabe. Sechster Band. Chemikalien und Drogen. Teil C: T-Z. Berlin: Springer-Verlag, pp 16–21

2. Willuhn G (1989) Löwenzahnkraut-, wurzel. In: Wichtl M, ed. Teedrogen. Ein Handbuch für die Praxis auf wissenschaftlicher Grundlage. 2. Auflage. Stuttgart: Wissenschaftliche Verlagsgesellschaft, pp 315–318
3. Burry JN, Kuchel R, Reid JD, Kirk J (1973) Australian bush dermatitis. Compositae dermatitis in South Australia. Med J Aust 1:110–116
4. Hänsel R, Kartarahardja M, Huang J-T, Bohlmann F (1980) Sesquiterpenlacton-β-glucopyranoside sowie ein neues Eudesmanolid aus *Taraxacum officinale*. Phytochemistry 19:857–861
5. Rauwald HW, Huang J-T (1985) Taraxacoside, a type of acylated γ-butyrolactone glycoside from *Taraxacum officinale*. Phytochemistry 24:1557–1559
6. Burrow S, Simpson JCE (1938) The triterpene group. Part IV. The triterpene alcohols of *Taraxacum* root. J Chem Soc 141:2042–2047
7. Larrègue M, Rat J-P, Gallet P, Bressieux J-M, Pousset J-L (1978) Eczéma de contact au pissenlit, a l'huile de laurier noble et au frullania par allergie croisée. Ann Dermatol Venereol (Paris) 105:547–548
8. Faber K (1958) Der Löwenzahn – *Taraxacum officinale* Weber. Pharmazie 13:423–436
9. Rutherford PP, Deacon AC (1972) β-Fructofuranosidases from roots of dandelion (*Taraxacum officinale* Weber). Biochem J 126:569–573
10. Rutherford PP, Deacon AC (1972) The mode of action of dandelion root β-fructofuranosidases on inulin. Biochem J 129:511–512
11. Kuusi T, Pyysalo H, Autio K (1985) The bitterness properties of dandelion. II. Chemical investigations. Lebensm Wiss Technol 18:347–349
12. Hannemann K, Puchta V, Simon E, Ziegler H, Ziegler G, Spiteller G (1989) The common occurrence of furan fatty acids in plants. Lipids 24:296–298
13. Tyler VE (1987) The New Honest Herbal. A sensible guide to herbs and related remedies. 2nd edn. Philadelphia: George F. Stickley Company, pp 83–84
14. Kleinig H, Nietsche H (1968) Carotinoid-Muster in gelben Blütenblättern. Phytochemistry 7:1171–1175
15. Cadosch H, Vögeli V, Rüedi P, Eugster CH (1978) Über die Carotinoide Flavoxanthin und Chrysanthemaxanthin: ^{1}H-NMR.-, ^{13}C-NMR.- und Massen-Spektren und absolute Konfiguration. Helv Chim Acta 61:783–794
16. Büssemaker J (1936) Über die choleretische Wirkung des Löwenzahns. Arch Exp Pathol Pharmakol 181:512–513
17. Rácz-Kotilla E, Rácz G, Solomon A (1974) The action of Taraxacum officinale extracts on the body weight and diuresis of laboratory animals. Planta Med 26:212–217
18. Akhtar MS, Khan QM, Khaliq T (1985) Effects of Portulaca oleracae (Kulfa) and Taraxacum officinale (Dhudhal) in normoglycaemic and alloxan-treated hyperglycaemic rabbits. JPMA 35:207–210
19. Swanston-Flatt SK, Day C, Flatt PR, Gould BJ, Bailey CJ (1989) Glycaemic effects of traditional European plant treatments for diabetes. Studies in normal and streptozotocin diabetic mice. Diabetes Res 10:69–73
20. Baba K, Abe S, Mizuno D (1981) Antitumor activity of hot water extract of dandelion, *Taraxacum officinale* – Correlation between antitumor activity and timing of administration. Yakugaku Zasshi 101:538–543
21. Hausen BM, Schulz KH (1978) Allergische Kontaktdermatitis durch Löwenzahn (Taraxacum officinale Wiggers). Dermatosen 26:198
22. Davies MG, Kersey PJW (1986) Contact allergy to yarrow and dandelion. Contact Dermatitis 14:256–257
23. Hausen BM (1992) Sesquiterpene lactones – general discussion. In: De Smet PAGM, Keller K, Hänsel R, Chandler RF (eds) Adverse Effects of Herbal Drugs. Volume 1. Heidelberg: Springer-Verlag, pp 227–236
24. Gessner O, Orzechowski G (1974) Gift- und Arzneipflanzen von Mitteleuropa. 3. Auflage. Heidelberg: Carl Winter Universitätsverlag, p 383

25. Rondelaud D (1980) Données épidémiologiques surs la distomatose humaine à *Fasciola hepatica* L. dans la région du Limousin, France. Les plantes consommées et les limnées vectrices. Ann Parasitol (Paris) 55:393–405
26. Rondelaud D, Amat-Frut E, Pestre-Alexandre M (1982) La distomatose humaine à *Fasciola hepatica* L. Étude épidémioloqique de 121 cas survenus sur une période de 25 ans. Bull Soc Pathol Exot Filiales 75:291–300
27. Eriksson NE (1977) Diagnosis of reaginic allergy with house dust, animal dander and pollen allergens in adult patients. IV. An evaluation of the clinical value of skin test, radioallergosorbent test, case history and combinations of these methods. Int Arch Allergy Appl Immunol 53:450–458
28. Déchamp C, Michel J, Deviller P, Perrin LF (1984) Choc anaphylactique au céleri et sensibilisation à l'ambroisie et à l'armoise. Allergie croisée ou allergie concomitante? Presse Méd 13:871–874
29. Birnbaum J, Tafforeau M, Vervloet D, Charpin J, Charpin D (1989) Allergy to sunflower honey associated with allergy to celery. Clin Exp Allergy 19:229–230
30. Cohen SH, Yunginger JW, Rosenberg N, Fink JN (1979) Acute allergic reaction after composite pollen ingestion. J Allergy Clin Immunol 64:270–274
31. Gol'dman II (1974) Anafilakticheskii shok posle poloskaniia nastoki kalenduly. Klin Med (Mosk) 52:142–143
32. Mitchell J, Rook A (1979) Botanical dermatology. Plants and plant products injurious to the skin. Greengrass: Vancouver, pp 219–220
33. Janke D (1950) Durch Löwenzahn (Taraxacum officinale) verursachtes Ekzem. Ein Beitrag zur Kenntnis phytogener Dermatosen. Hautartz 1:177–181
34. Janson P (1953) Citrusfrüchte und Hauterkrankungen. Ztschr Haut Geslechtskrankh 14:144–147
35. Hausen BM (1979) The sensitizing capacity of Compositae plants. III. Test results and cross-reactions in Compositae-sensitive patients. Dermatologica 159:1–11
36. Guin JD, Skidmore G (1987) Compositae dermatitis in childhood. Arch Dermatol 123:500–502
37. Lovell CR, Rowan M (1991) Dandelion dermatitis. Contact Dermatitis 25:185–188
38. Hausen BM (1982) Taraxinsäure-1′-O-β-D-glucopyranosid, das Kontaktallergen des Löwenzahns (Taraxacum officinale Wiggers). Dermatosen 30:51–53
39. Zeller W, De Gols M, Hausen BM (1985) The sensitizing capacity of *Compositae* plants. VI. Guinea pig sensitization experiments with ornamental plants and weeds using different methods. Arch Dermatol Res 277: 28–35
40. Collins JM, Miller DR (1966) Dandelion green bezoar following antrectomy and vagotomy. Case report. J Kans Med Soc 67:303–304
41. Matsui AS, Rogers J, Woo YK, Cutting WC (1967) Effects of some natural products on fertility in mice. Med Pharmacol Exp Int J Exp Med 16:414–424
42. Hirono I, Mori H, Kato K, Ushimaru Y, Kato T, Haga M (1977) Safety examination of some edible plants, Part 2. J Environ Pathol Toxicol 1:71–74

Tilia Species

P.A.G.M. De Smet

Botany

The linden or lime tree belongs to the family Tiliaceae. Its two major officinal species are:

- *Tilia cordata* Mill. (syn. *T. microphylla* Vent., *T. parvifolia* Ehrh., *T. sylvestris* Desf., *T. ulmifolia* Scop.). This species is known in English as small-leaved lime and in German as Winterlinde.
- *T. platyphyllos* Scop. (syn. *T. grandifolia* Ehrh., *T. pauciflora* Hayne). This plant is called large-leaved lime in English and Sommerlinde in German.

The medicinal part of the lime tree is the flower, which is designated as fleur de tilleul in French, flor de tilo in Spanish and Lindenblüte in German [1–7].

Chemistry

Officinal lime tree flowers contain mucilaginous polysaccharides (3%), tannins (2%), and flavonoids (1%) [6–10]. The principal flavonoid is isoquercitrin (= quercetin-3-glucoside) [11].

Fresh blossom samples of *Tilia cordata* and subspecies of *T. platyphyllos* yield approximately 0.2 mg/g of essential oil containing alkanes C_{18-31} (52.1–59.9%), 2-phenylethyl alcohol and its esters (1.0–7.4%), geraniol (0.5–5.9%), eugenol (1.0–2.5%), and *cis-trans* farnesol (0.3–1.6%) [8].

Pharmacology and Uses

Lime tree flower tea is a traditional domestic remedy, which is used as diaphoretic and as an emollient in catharral diseases. It is mildly astringent and is reputed to have antispasmodic properties as well [1,5,6].

Adverse Effects of Herbal Drugs, Vol. 2
(ed. by P.A.G.M. De Smet, K. Keller, R. Hänsel, R.F. Chandler)

Adverse Reaction Profile

General Animal Data

Lanza et al. [12] tested the acute toxicity of dialysed and non-dialysed aqueous extracts from the seeds and sapwood of *Tilia sylvestris* Desf. (= *T. cordata* Mill.) in white Wistar mice, and reported lethal doses in the range of 3–5 g/kg intraperitoneally. These experiments did not involve the official part of the lime tree (viz. the flowers) nor its common form of administration (i.e., an oral beverage).

General Human Data

Lime tree preparations appear to have a good safety record. Apart from rare reports about allergic reactions, there is no well-documented evidence in the literature that these preparations are hazardous.

Allergic Reactions

Picardo et al. [13] recorded allergy to a shampoo containing *Tilia* extract in a patient with a history of seasonal rhinitis. The shampoo induced severe symptoms of generalized urticaria with oedema of the lips, face and mouth, and dyspnoea. Prick tests gave positive reactions to *Tilia* and Compositae, and patch tests yielded localized urticarial reactions to the shampoo, perfume mix and eugenol. Although eugenol was shown to be present in the shampoo, it remained unclear, whether this *Tilia* constituent was responsible for the allergic manifestations. Its patch test concentration (1%) was higher than that in the shampoo, and the patient did not react to other cosmetics, even if they contained eugenol. It is possible, however, that eugenol was released by the hot water used during shampooing, and induced an allergic response through airborne contact.

Falliers [14] reported, from the United States, a case of rhinitis due to a tea infusion prepared from *Tilia*. When requested, this author kindly provided the following details in a personal communication. A 63-year-old female of Greek background had typical seasonal allergic rhinitis associated with tree pollinosis (poplar, aspen, oak, juniper/cedar etc.) and grass pollinosis. She reported recurring rhinorrhoea, sneezing, and congestion after drinking a linden-tea beverage. The possibility of an allergic reaction was supported by a positive intradermal test reaction to a 1:1000 dilution of a *Tilia* extract [15]. Falliers [15] comments that *Tilia* tea is less likely to cause allergy in North America than in Europe, because lime trees in the western hemisphere are primarily insect-pollinated.

Cross reaction between *Tilia* pollen and grass pollen has been described, but this conclusion was challenged by Frankland [17], because *Tilia* pollen is always grossly contaminated with other pollens, particularly grass pollens. Impurity of the test material designated lime pollen is therefore the most likely explanation for the reported cross reaction with grass pollens.

Cardiovascular Reactions

One text book states that too-frequent use of linden flower tea may result in damage to the heart [4], but this statement is not backed up by an original report.

Lanza et al. [12] studied the hemodynamic action of various dialysed aqueous extracts of *Tilia sylvestris* Desf. (= *T. cordata* Mill.) in anesthesized rabbits. Injection into the internal jugular vein produced a hypotensive reaction marked by a drop in diastolic arterial pressure, which was ascribed to vasodilatation. The dialysed seed extract was more active than the dialysed extracts from sapwood, bracts or flowers. It reduced the diastolic pressure by 58%, when 29 mg/kg was injected, whereas a dose of 32 mg/kg of dialysed flower extract resulted in a fall of only 12%. The oral route of administration, which is the most common way of employing a lime tree preparation, was not included in this study.

Central Nervous System Reactions

There is a statement in the literature that tea prepared from very old flowers may produce symptoms of narcotic intoxication, but this claim is not supported by reliable evidence [4].

Dermatological Reactions

See the section on allergic reactions.

Respiratory Reactions

See the section on allergic reactions.

Fertility, Pregnancy and Lactation

No data have been recovered from the literature.

Mutagenicity and Carcinogenicity

No data have been recovered from the literature.

References

1. List PH, Hörhammer L (1979) Hagers Handbuch der Pharmazeutischen Praxis. Vierte Neuausgabe. Sechster Band: Chemikalien und Drogen. Teil C: T-Z. Berlin: Springer-Verlag, pp 180–184
2. Launert E (1981) The Hamlyn Guide to Edible and Medicinal Plants of Britain and Northern Europe. London: Hamlyn Publishing Group, p 48
3. Penso G (1983) Index Plantarum Medicinalium Totius Mundi Eorumque Synonymorum. Milano: Organizzazione Editoriale Medico Farmaceutica, pp 952–953
4. Tyler VE (1987) The New Honest Herbal. A sensible guide to herbs and related remedies. 2nd edn. Philadelphia: George F. Stickley Company, pp 148–149
5. Reynolds JEF, red (1989) Martindale The Extra Pharmacopoeia. 29th edn. London: The Pharmaceutical Press, p 779
6. Willuhn G. Lindenblüten (1989) In: Wichtl M (ed). Teedrogen. Ein Handbuch für die Praxis auf wissenschaftlicher Grundlage. 2. Auflage. Stuttgart: Wissenschaftliche Verlagsgesellschaft, pp 312–314
7. Honerlagen H (1989) Herstellung von Lindenblütentrockenextrakt. Tiliae flos. Schweiz Apoth Ztg 127:130–132
8. Bernasconi R, Gebistorf J (1968) Ein Beitrag zur Kenntnis des ätherischen Lindenblütenöles und zur Chemotaxonomie der Gattung Tilia. Pharm Acta Helv 43:677–688
9. Kram G, Franz G (1983) Untersuchungen über die Schleimpolysaccharide aus Lindenblüten. Planta Med 49:149–153
10. Kram G, Franz G (1985) Structural investigations on the watersoluble polysaccharides of lime tree flowers (*Tilia cordata* L.). Pharmazie 40:501–502
11. Wichtl M, Bozek B, Fingerhut T (1987) Lindenblüten. Isoquercitrin – Hauptflavon der offizinellen Droge. Dtsch Apoth Ztg 127:509–510
12. Lanza JP, Steinmetz MD, Lavaivre-Pierlovisi M, Millet Y, Mourgue M (1982) Action pharmacodynamique et toxicité d'extraits aqueux de tilleul (*Tilia sylvestris* Desf.). Plant Méd Phytothér 16:129–136
13. Picardo M, Rovina R, Cristaudo A, Cannistraci C, Santucci B (1988) Contact urticaria from *Tilia* (lime). Contact Dermatitis 19:72–73
14. Falliers CJ (1989) Pine nut allergy in perspective. Ann Allergy 62:186–189
15. Falliers CJ (Allergy & Asthma Clinic, Denver, United States). Personal communication, September, 1990
16. Jelks M (1986) Allergy Plants. Tampa: World-Wide Publications
17. Frankland AW (1975) The purity of allergenic extracts. Develop Biol Stand 29:101–105

Vaccinium Myrtillus

P.A.G.M. De Smet

Botany

Vaccinium myrtillus L. is a shrubby perennial plant that belongs to the family Ericaceae. Vernacular names include bilberry, blueberry, huckleberry, whortleberry, black whortleberry (E); Heidelbeere, Blaubeere, Bickbeere (G); airelle myrtille, myrtillier (F) [1–5]. Some of the English folk names may produce confusion, as they are also in use for related *Vaccinium* species, such as *V. angustifolium* (blueberry), *V. corymbosum* (highbush blueberry) and *V. vitis-idaea* (mountain cranberry, cowberry, red bilberry, whortleberry, red whortleberry), and for other genera, such as *Gaylussacia* species [1,2,6].

The medicinal parts of *Vaccinium myrtillus* are the leaves and fruit [1,4,5,7].

Chemistry

The **leaves** of *Vaccinium myrtillus* are rich in tannins [4,8–10]. Polyphenolic components are catechins [11], leucoanthocyanes (= hydroxyflavandiols) [11], flavonol glycosides [12,13] and hydroxycinnamic acid derivatives [12]. Non-polyphenolic organic constituents include iridoids [12] and plant acids [9], and trace levels of the quinolizidine alkaloids myrtine and epimyrtine have been recovered from aerial parts [14]. The leaves contain 9 ppm of chromium [15] and their manganese level is also reported to be high [4].

Early phytochemical sources claimed on basis of non-specific analytical methods that the leaves contain arbutin (= hydroquinone-β-D-glucopyranoside). However, in later chromatographical studies this phenolic glycoside was either absent [12,16–18] or present at a trace level not exceeding 0.001% [19]. These chromatographical investigations have also failed to recover the related compounds hydroquinone [12,17,18], hydroquinone monomethylether [18], methylarbutin [16,18], and pyroside (= 6-O-acetylarbutin) [12].

Adverse Effects of Herbal Drugs, Vol. 2
(ed. by P.A.G.M. De Smet, K. Keller, R. Hänsel, R.F. Chandler)

Early research resulted in the isolation of 0.3% of crystalline arbutin from a commercial sample of bilberry leaves [8], and another investigation produced free hydroquinone in crystalline form without detecting arbutin [9]. The reason for these anomalous findings is unknown. One explanation may be the existence of different chemotypes [10]. Another possibility is that the studied materials were contaminated or replaced by leaves of other *Vaccinium* plants [12]. A potential contaminant is *Vaccinium vitis-idaea* L., as it often has the same habitat as *V. myrtillus* [19]. Its leaves contain 3.3–6.6% of arbutin [18,19] as well as hydroquinone [18], pyroside [12,19,20], salidroside [21], and hydroquinone gentiobioside [22]. Another plausible adulterant is *Vaccinium* × *intermedium* Ruthe, which is a hybrid of *V. vitis-idaea* and *V. myrtillus*. Its leaves are almost identical to those of *V. myrtillus* [12] and contain 2% of arbutin, 1.1% of pyroside and 0.15% of salidroside [19]. Contamination with *V. uliginosum* L. is unlikely, as this species yields neither arbutin nor hydroquinone [17–19].

The **fruit** of *V. myrtillus* is also rich in tannins [4,8,10]. It yields derivatives of hydroxycinnamic and hydroxybenzoic acids, flavonol glycosides, monomeric flavan-3-ols (= catechines), dimeric flavan-3-ols (= procyanidins), anthocyanidins and anthocyanins [12,23,24]. Among the non-polyphenolic compounds are iridoids [12], terpenes, pectins and organic plant acids [23]. Arbutin, hydroquinone and pyroside have not been detected in unripe fruit [12].

Pharmacology and Uses

Recent pharmacological research on *Vaccinium myrtillus* has focused on various effects of its anthocyanosides, such as vasoprotective activity [25–27], antiulcer activity [28,29], inhibition of cyclic AMP and cyclic GMP phosphodiesterases [30], and inhibition of platelet aggregation and clot retraction [31,32]. The usefulness of these anthocyanosides as prophylactic treatment of senile cataract [33] and as therapy for diabetic and hypertensive retinopathy [34] is also under study.

The **leaves** of *Vaccinium myrtillus* have been used to prevent and treat a wide variety of medical problems, such as gastrointestinal, renal and respiratory complaints, rheumatism, gout, skin diseases, hemorrhoidal problems, circulatory disorders and functional heart complaints [7]. One of their most common traditional uses has been that of an antidiabetic folk medicine [35,36] but there is no definite proof of their effectiveness in this respect [7,37].

Allen [38] extracted an amorphous substance called myrtillin from botanically unspecified blueberry leaves and reported that intravenous or oral administration diminished the hyperglycemic response to glucose in normal dogs and humans. This activity was not demonstrable in rats or rabbits. Its clinical effect in diabetic patients treated with insulin was feeble and uncertain. Edgars [39] isolated an unidentified glucoside from blueberry leaves and found that this substance possessed hypoglycemic activity when tested in rabbits. However, the blueberry species under study was *Vaccinium corymbosum* and not *V. myrtillus*. Dietering [40] was unable to demonstrate hypoglycemic activity of aqueous leaf extracts in laboratory animals. On the contrary, oral doses corresponding to 0.1–3.0 g of leaves per kg produced moderate hyperglycemia in normal cats. It should be noted, however, that the botanical origin of his test material is not absolutely clear (see the section on general animal data). More recently, a Spanish research group reported hypoglycemic activity of leaf extracts in rabbits [41].

The **fruit** is primarily used as an antidiarrhoeal agent because of its tannin content [4,42]. It may also be used as supportive treatment of pain caused by spastic colon [5] or for local astringent treatment of mild inflammations of the oropharyngeal mucosa [7].

Pharmacokinetics

The pharmacokinetics of *Vaccinium myrtillus* anthocyanosides have been investigated in the rat. The elimination of these substances after parenteral administration was rapid and occurred mostly through the kidneys and the bile [43]. An oral dose gave a bioavailability of only 1.2% with peak plasma levels between 2 and 3 μg/ml after 15 min [44].

Adverse Reaction Profile

General Animal Data

Toxicity studies of *Vaccinium myrtillus* leaves have only been reported by Oettel [45] in 1936 and by Dietering [40] in 1938. Both investigators tested aqueous leaf extracts in the form of dispersed preparations that had been manufactured by the same German firm [40,45].

Oettel [45] studied extracts from "Heidelbeerblättern" (leaves of *V. myrtillus*) and "Preisselbeerblättern" (leaves from *V. vitis-idaea*). Oral administration to cats produced the same toxic symptoms as pure hydroquinone, such as acute agitation, disturbed tonus and hyperglycemia. Doses corresponding to 5 g leaves per kg of cat sometimes produced death with a single dose and were definitely lethal when given repeatedly.

Dietering [40] tested extracts from dried "Heidelbeerblättern" that had been obtained by extraction with cold water and by subsequent extraction with hot water. Acute oral doses up to 0.3 g of leaves per kg did not result in overt problems but 5 g per kg produced hydroquinone-like symptoms, such as restlessness, trembling, copious salivary flow, loss of tonus, dyspnoea and sometimes death. Cats were more sensitive to these effects than rabbits.

Subchronic feeding of cats with doses up to 0.15 g per kg per day did not bring about toxicity. However, daily amounts of 0.6 g per kg for more than 2 weeks gave hydroquinone-like effects (inertia, loss of appetite, loss of weight, anemia), and one susceptible animal reacted with complete loss of muscular tonus, cachexia, icterus and death. Daily treatment with 1.5 g per kg caused severe loss of weight, anemia, icterus, methemoglobinemia, severe dyspnoea, and death.

The effects reported by Oettel [45] and Dietering [40] should be interpreted with caution, as they show a striking resemblance to toxic symptoms of hydroquinone. Oettel [45] claims that he demonstrated about 1% of free hydroquinone in "Heidelbeerblättern" and Dietering [40] states that one of his test extracts was prepared from "Heidelbeerblättern" containing 1.3% of hydroquinone. However, phytochemical evidence for the occurrence of hydroquinone or hydroquinone glycosides in the leaves of *Vaccinium myrtillus* is very scant (see the section on chemistry). Thus the question may be raised whether the studied extracts were prepared from the correct source and not from another *Vaccinium* species or hybrid. Alternatively, the tested materials could have come from a specific chemotype of *V. myrtillus* rich in free or glycosidically bound hydroquinone. However, the available phytochemical evidence for this suggestion is far from sufficient (see the section on chemistry). Another possibility is that the reported toxicity was not due to hydroquinone but to one or more other constituents which still have to be identified [35,46]. If such principles exist they are soluble in ether, because Dietering [40] states that he could administer a special extract, from which "hydroquinone" had been removed by ether, in any amount without observing toxic effects.

All in all, it is impossible to come up with a final verdict on the toxic potential of *Vaccinium myrtillus* leaves without the aid of new toxicological investigations. Such studies are long overdue and should be performed with botanically secured and chemically fully characterized material, so that all present speculations may finally be put to an end.

The toxicity of anthocyane glycosides extracted from the berries of *Vaccinium myrtillus* has been investigated by Pourrat et al. [47]. They found LD_{50} values of 4.11 g/kg i.p. and 0.84 g/kg i.v. in the mouse, and 2.35 g/kg i.p. and 0.24 g/kg i.v. in the rat. No deaths were observed following oral doses up to 25 g/kg in the mouse and 20 g/kg in the rat. Treatment of guinea pigs (for two weeks) and rats (for six weeks) with doses corresponding to five times a human dose of 600 mg per day did not produce toxic effects.

General Human Data

The fruit of *Vaccinium myrtillus* is officially recognized as herbal medicine in France [5] and Germany [7]. The French authorities also permit the medical use of the leaves [5], but the Germans disallow the consumption of this plant part, because therapeutic efficacy remains unproven and because serious toxicity has been observed in animal experiments [7].

As these toxic effects could be due to the use of a *Vaccinium* chemotype, species of hybrid rich in hydroquinone or its glycosides (see the section on animal data), human toxicity data about this compound should be briefly reviewed here. Doses of 300–500 mg of hydroquinone have been ingested daily for 3 to 5 months without apparent ill effects [48]. However, doses of 1 g or more may result in nausea, vomiting, diarrhoea, fibrillations, dyspnoea, cyanosis, delirium and collapse. Hemolytic anemia, cachexia, hepatic steatosis and hair depigmentation have also been reported [49,50]. Fatal human doses range from 5 to 12 g [49–51], and one handbook even reports a fatal dose as low as 2 g [52].

As was pointed out in the section on animal data, daily doses corresponding to 0.6 g of bilberry leaves per kg body weight produced toxic symptoms in cats. If human beings are equally sensitive, daily ingestion of 36 g would be sufficient to endanger persons weighing 60 kg. This amount is higher than the recommended dosage of 1 g per cup 3× per day [4,53]. According to Oettel [45], however, dosages up to 30–50 g per day used to be common in folk medicine.

Drug Interactions

As *Vaccinium myrtillus* has been claimed to reduce insulin requirements, the possibility of an interaction between this traditional remedy and conventional antidiabetic therapy should not be entirely neglected [36].

Fertility, Pregnancy and Lactation

As the reported toxicity of *Vaccinium myrtillus* **leaves** may be due to a chemotype or contaminant rich in hydroquinone and/or its glycosides (see the section on animal data), the reproductive effects of hydroquinone are briefly discussed here. Hydroquinone gives positive results in certain aneuploidy test systems and may therefore represent a genetic risk [54–56]. There are no specific reports in the literature on teratogenic or developmentally toxic potential [57] but inclusion of 0.5 g (total dose) into the diet of female pregnant rats resulted in fetal resorptions [58]. Subcutaneous administration of 100 mg/kg/day (about 0.3 of the LD_{50} value) for a period of 51 days to male rats was reported to interfere with spermiogenesis [57].

Pourrat et al. [47] studied the teratogenic effects of anthocyane glycosides extracted from the **berries** of *Vaccinium myrtillus* in rats, mice and rabbits. They did not observe teratogenic effects from daily doses corresponding to three times a human dose of 600 mg per day. Teglio et al. [59] did not see adverse effects in 51 pregnant women with a mean gestational age of 27 weeks, who took 160–320 mg of anthocyanosides from *Vaccinium myrtillus* per day for a period of three months to treat venous insufficiency or hemorrhoids.

Mutagenicity and Carcinogenicity

As hydroquinone and/or its glycosides may be involved in the reported toxicity of *Vaccinium myrtillus* leaves (see the section on animal data), the mutagenicity and carcinogenicity of this compound are briefly discussed here. Mutagenicity studies involving hydroquinone have shown equivocal results [57,60]. Its carcinogenicity in rodents was recently assessed by Japanese researchers, who treated rats and mice of both sexes at a dietary level of 0.8% for two years. The results suggested potential renal carcinogenicity (increased occurrence of renal adenomas and epithelial hyperplasia of the renal papilla) in male rats and potential hepatocarcinogenicity (increased foci of cellular alteration of the liver and hepatocellular adenoma) in male mice [61].

References

1. Lust JB (1974) The Herb Book. New York: Bantam Books, pp 93, 116–117, 659
2. Launert E (1981) Hamlyn Guide to Edible and Medicinal Plants of Britain and Northern Europe. London: Hamlyn, p 130
3. Van Hellemont J (1988) Fytotherapeutisch compendium. Tweede druk. Utrecht: Bohn, Scheltema & Holkema, pp 627–630
4. Frohne D (1989) Heidelbeerblätter/Heidelbeeren. In: Wichtl M (ed). Teedrogen. Ein Handbuch für die Praxis auf wissenschaftlicher Grundlage. 2. Auflage. Stuttgart: Wissenschaftliche Verlagsgesellschaft, pp 217–221
5. Anonymous (1990) Avis aux fabricants concernant les demandes d'autorisation de mise sur le marché des médicaments à base de plantes. Bulletin Officiel no. 90/22 bis. Paris: Ministère des Affairs Sociales et de la Solidarité
6. Petrides GA (1972) A Field Guide to Trees and Shrubs. Boston: Houghton Mifflin Co, pp 173–177, 277–283, 358–361
7. Anonymous (1987) Myrtilli folium (Heidelbeerblätter)/Myrtilli fructus (Heidelbeeren). Bundesanzeiger nr.76-23.04.87
8. Kröger C (1951) Die Heidelbeere, *Vaccinium myrtillus* L. Pharmazie 6:211–217
9. Ramstad E (1954) Chemical investigation of *Vaccinium myrtillus* L. J Am Pharm Assoc 43:236–240
10. Hegnauer R (1966) Chemotaxonomie der Pflanzen. Band 4: Dicotyledoneae: Daphniphyllaceae – Lythraceae. Basel: Birkhäuser Verlag, pp 89–90
11. Schönert J, Friedrich H (1970) Zur Kenntnis des Gerbstoffs in den Blättern der Heidelbeere (Vaccinium myrtillus L.). Pharmazie 25:775–776
12. Friedrich H, Schönert J (1973) Untersuchungen über einige Inhaltsstoffe der Blätter und Früchte von Vaccinium myrtillus. Planta Med 24:90–100
13. Gerhardt G, Sinnwell V, Kraus L (1989) Isolierung von Quercetin-3-glucuronid aus Heidelbeer- und Rauschbeerblättern durch DCCC. Planta Med 55:200–201
14. Slosse P, Hootelé C (1981) Myrtine and epimyrtine, quinolizidine alkaloids from *Vaccinium myrtillus*. Tetrahedron 37:4287–4292

15. Müller A, Diemann E, Sassenberg P (1988) Chromgehalt von Heilpflanzen gegen Diabetes mellitus Typ II. Naturwissenschaften 75:155–156
16. Wagner G, Böhm M (1957) Über den papierchromatographischen Nachweis von Methylarbutin neben Arbutin. Pharmazie 12:363–366
17. Kraus LJ, Dupáková D (1964) Der derzeitige Stand der Bewertung von Arbutindrogen. Pharmazie 19:41–45
18. Sticher O, Soldati F, Lehmann D (1979) Hochleistungsflüssig-chromatographische Trennung und quantitative Bestimmung von Arbutin, Methylarbutin, Hydrochinon und Hydrochinonmonomethylaether in Arctostaphylos-, Bergenia-, Calluna- und Vaccinium Arten. Planta Med 35:253–261
19. Thieme H, Winkler H-J (1971) Die Phenolglykoside der Ericaceen. 1. Mitteilung: Untersuchungen über Vorkommen und Verbreitung. Pharmazie 26:235–243
20. Friedrich H (1961) Über das Vorkommen von Pyrosid in den Blättern der Preißelbeere. Naturwissenschaften 48:304
21. Thieme H, Winkler HJ (1966) Über das Vorkommen von Salidrosid in den Blättern der Preiselbeere (*Vaccinium vitis-idaea* L.). Pharmazie 21:182–183
22. Thieme H, Winkler HJ, Frenzel H (1969) Über die Isolierung von 4-Hydroxyphenyl-β-gentiobiosid aus Vaccinium vitis-idaea L. Pharmazie 24:236–237
23. Brenneisen R, Steinegger E (1981) Zur Analytik der Polyphenole der Früchte von Vaccinium myrtillus L. Pharm Acta Helv 56:180–185
24. Baj A, Bombardelli E, Gabetta B, Martinelli EM (1983) Qualitative and quantitative evaluation of *Vaccinium myrtillus* anthocyanins by high-resolution gas chromatography and high-performance liquid chromatography. J Chromatogr 279:365–372
25. Lietti A, Cristoni A, Picci M (1976) Studies on Vaccinium myrtillus anthocyanosides. I. Vasoprotective and antiinflammatory activity. Arzneim Forsch 26:829–832
26. Jonadet M, Meunier MT, Bastide P (1983) Anthocyanosides extraits de *Vitis vinifera*, de *Vaccinium myrtillus* et *Pinus maritimus*. I. Activités inhibitrices vis-à-vis de l'élastase *in vitro*. II. Activités angioprotectrices comparées *in vivo*. J Pharm Belg 38:41–46
27. Detre Z, Jellinek H, Miskulin M, Robert AM (1986) Studies on vascular permeability in hypertension: action of anthocyanosides. Clin Physiol Biochem 4:143–149
28. Cristoni A, Magistretti MJ (1987) Antiulcer and healing activity of *Vaccinium myrtillus* anthocyanosides. Farmaco [Ed Prat] 42:29–43
29. Magistretti MJ, Conti M, Cristoni A (1988) Antiulcer activity of an anthocyanidin from Vaccinium myrtillus. Arzneim Forsch 38:686–690
30. Ferretti C, Magistretti MJ, Robotti A, Ghi P, Genazzani E (1988) Vaccinium myrtillus anthocyanosides are inhibitors of cAMP and cGMP phosphodiesterases. Pharmacol Res Commun 20 (Suppl 2):150
31. Bottecchia D, Bettini V, Martino R, Camerra G (1987) Preliminary report on the inhibitory effect of *Vaccinium myrtillus* anthocyanosides on platelet aggregation and clot retraction. Fitoterapia 58:3–8
32. Morazzoni P, Magistretti MJ (1990) Activity of Myrtocyan, an anthocyanoside complex from *Vaccinium myrtillus* (VMA), on platelet aggregation and adhesiveness. Fitoterapia 61:13–22
33. Bravetti GO, Fraboni E, Maccolini E (1989) Preventive medical treatment of senile cataract with vitamin E and Vaccinium myrtillus anthocyanosides clinical evaluation. Ann Ottalmol Clin Ocul 115:109–116
34. Perossini M, Chiellini S, Guidi G, Siravo D (1987) Diabetic and hypertensive retinopathy therapy with Vaccinium myrtillus anthocyanosides tegens double blind placebo-controlled clinical trial. Ann Ottalmol Clin Ocul 113:1173–1190
35. Kraus L, Reher G (1982) Antidiabetisch wirkende Drogen – eine kritische Auseinandersetzung. Dtsch Apoth Ztg 122:2357–2360
36. Bailey CJ, Day C (1989) Traditional plant medicines as treatments for diabetes. Diabetes Care 12:553–564
37. Frohne D (1988) Hydrochinonvergiftung durch Folia Myrtilli? Pharm Ztg 133:522–523

38. Allen FM (1927) Blueberry leaf extract. Physiologic and clinical properties in relation to carbohydrate metabolism. JAMA 89:1577–1581
39. Edgars NK (1936) A new glucoside from blueberry leaf. J Am Pharm Assoc 25:288–291
40. Dietering H (1938) Über die Wirkung von Heidelbeerblättern. Naunyn-Schmied Arch Exp Pathol Pharmakol 188:500–513
41. De Los Angeles Gato M, Calleja JM (1982) Estudio preliminar de la actividad hipoglucemiante del *Vaccinium myrtillus* L. Trab Compostelanos Biol 9:5–14
42. Born C (1990) Hilft bei Durchfall: die Heidelbeere. PTA Heute 4:222
43. Lietti A, Forni G (1976) Studies on Vaccinium myrtillus anthocyanosides. II. Aspects of anthocyanins pharmacokinetics in the rat. Arzneim Forsch 26:832–835
44. Morazzoni P, Livio S, Schilingo A, Malandrino S (1991) Vaccinium myrtillus anthocyanosides pharmacokinetics in rats. Arzneim Forsch 41:128–131
45. Oettel H (1936) Die Hydrochinonvergiftung. Arch Exp Path Pharmakol 183:319–362
46. Thesen R, Braun R (1989) Ganz oder teilweise "negativ" bewertete Arzneistoffe. Pharm Ztg 134:2881–2883
47. Pourrat H, Bastide P, Dorier P, Pourrat A, Tronche P (1967) Préparation et activité thérapeutique de quelques glycosides d'anthocyanes. Chim Thér 2:33–38
48. Lang S, Brewer NR, Carlson AJ (1950) Chronic studies of effect of hydroquinone on man. Fed Proc 9:74
49. Wirth W, Gloxhuber C (1985) Toxikologie für Ärzte, Naturwissenschaftler und Apotheker. 4. Auflage. Stuttgart: Georg Thieme Verlag, p 227
50. Budavari S, red. (1989) The Merck Index. An encyclopedia of chemicals, drugs, and biologicals. Rahway: Merck & Co., Inc., p 699
51. Gosselin RE, Smith RP, Hodge HC, Braddock JE (1984) Clinical Toxicology of Commercial Products. 5th edn. Baltimore: Williams & Wilkins p II–190
52. Dreisbach RH, Robertson WO (1987) Handbook of Poisoning. 12th edn. Norwalk: Appleton & Lange, p 367
53. Chrubasik S, Chrubasik J (1983) Kompendium der Phytotherapie. Stuttgart: Hippokrates Verlag, p 53
54. Parry JM, Parry EM, Warr T, Lynch A, James S (1990) The detection of aneugens using yeasts and cultured mammalian cells. Prog Clin Biol Res 340B:247–266
55. Adler I-D (1990) Aneuploidy studies in mammals. Prog Clin Biol Res 340B:285–293
56. Xu W, Adler I-D (1990) Clastogenic effects of known and suspect spindle poisons studied by chromosome analysis in mouse bone marrow cells. Mutagenesis 5:371–374
57. Anonymous (1985) Hydroquinone: testing requirements. Fed Reg 50:53145–53156
58. Telford IR, Woodruff CS, Linford RH (1962) Fetal resorption in the rat as influenced by certain antioxidants. Am J Anat 110:29–36
59. Teglio L, Tronconi R, Mazzanti C, Guerresi E (1987) Vaccinium myrtillus anthocyanosides in the treatment of venous insufficiency of the lower limbs and acute piles in pregnancy. Quad Clin Ostet Ginecol 42:221–231
60. Devillers J, Boule P, Vasseur P, et al. (1990) Environmental and health risks of hydroquinone. Ecotoxicol Environ Safety 19:327–354
61. Shibata MA, Hirose M, Tanaka H, Asakawa E, Shirai T, Ito N (1991) Induction of renal cell tumors in rats and mice, and enhancement of hepatocellular tumor development in mice after long-term hydroquinone treatment. Jpn J Cancer Res 82:1211–1219

Notes Added in Proof

P.A.G.M. De Smet

Introduction

This book series will be kept up to date by concluding every volume with supplementary notes on monographs that have already been published. These notes are not meant to cover all recent references but focus on new and clinically relevant information about the adverse reaction profile of the herbal drug in question.

Allium Sativum (Volume 1 pp. 73–77)

Rose et al. [1] described a 87-year-old patient with spontaneous spinal epidural hematoma resulting in paraplegia, and attributed this rare event to a transient qualitative platelet disorder, reflected by a prolonged bleeding time despite an adequate platelet count. The only potential cause of the platelet dysfunction that could be detected was the chronic, excessive intake of garlic cloves in average amounts of approximately 2 g per day.

Aloe Species (Volume 2 pp. 119–123)

Photodermatitis to aloe vera was observed in a patch test study that involved the application of an aloe vera product to the back of volunteers. Exposure of the treated area to UVB and UVA radiation resulted in erythema and occasionally oedema and itch in the majority of subjects. Persistent pigmentation was also seen [2].

Cinnamomum Species (Volume 1 pp. 105–114)

The abuse of undiluted cinnamon oil has recently become popular in the United States among school-aged children, because ingestion of even small amounts is said to cause rapid heart beat, lightheadedness, facial flushing, and shortness of breath. The popularity of the cinnamon oil is apparently due to the relative ease, with which it can be obtained from pharmacies and can be carried around with little fear of discovery or chastisement. The principal methods of abuse are: (a) sucking on toothpicks or fingers, which have been dipped in the oil; (b) wrapping a piece of tissue paper or absorbent cotton around toothpicks impregnated with cinnamon oil and repeatedly sniffing the pungent aroma [3,4]. Perry et al. [4] studied 32 cases of such cinnamon oil abuse, most of which involved oral exposure to small amounts. This produced a rush or sensation of warmth, facial flushing, and oral burning. Some children experienced abdominal pain or nausea but no systemic effects were reported. In a few users, dermal and ocular exposures resulted in local irritation.

Serious gastrointestinal, central nervous system and cardiovascular manifestations developed in a 7.5-year-old boy, who intentionally ingested about 60 ml of cinnamon oil after being challenged by a friend [5].

Eleutherococcus Senticosus (Volume 2 pp. 159–169)

Since the preparation of the monograph, important additional data were reported concerning the case of neonatal androgenization that was tentatively associated with maternal use of Siberian ginseng tablets during pregnancy (p. 165). The raw material that was used by the implicated manufacturer in compounding Siberian ginseng tablets during the period when the adverse reaction was observed was submitted to organoleptic, microscopic and chemical analysis. This analysis indicated that the material came almost certainly from *Periploca sepium*, the so-called Chinese silk vine [6]. Administration of this material to rats in oral doses up to 1.5 g/kg (by gavage) did not produce evidence of androgenic potential. This implies that either the neonatal androgenization was not caused by the implicated plant material or the observed effects were specific to humans and possibly related to an undetermined peculiarity of the subjects [7].

***Eucalyptus* Species** (Volume 1 pp. 125–133)

Inhalation of vapors of *Eucalyptus* leaves, which is a common household remedy for respiratory diseases in Spain, can result in abundant *Aspergillus* hyphae in sputum smears [8].

Larrea Tridentata (Volume 2 pp. 231–240)

Further evidence for the hepatotoxic potential of chaparral (*Larrea tridentata*) has been reported from the United States. One individual presented with scleral icterus and diffuse jaundice after the consumption of three 500-mg capsules of chaparral per day for six weeks, while another user complained of abdominal pain and jaundice after taking approximately 150 chaparral tablets over an 11-week period. A causal role of the chaparral products was supported by the temporal relationship between the use of these products and the development of hepatitis and by the rapid improvement of both patients when they discontinued their chaparral use [9].

Pyrrolizidine Alkaloids (Volume 1 pp. 193–226)

A new case of hepatotoxicity associated with comfrey ingestion was reported by Yeong et al. [10]. A 23-year-old man presented with hepatic veno-occlusive disease and severe portal hypertension and subsequently died from liver failure. Light microscopy and hepatic angiography revealed occlusion of sublobular veins and small venous radicles of the liver, associated with widespread hemorrhagic necrosis of hepatocytes. The patient had been on a diet with emphasis on large quantities of fruit and vegetables. In the 1–2 weeks prior to his illness, he consumed steamed young comfrey leaves as a vegetable in reported quantities of 4–5 leaves per day. A causal relationship between the veno-occlusive disease and the intake of comfrey was suggested by the temporal association of events, by the exclusion of other known causes and by the histological changes in the liver, which were compatible with those due to pyrrolizidine alkaloids.

Another human case of poisoning by pyrrolizidine alkaloids was recently reported from Austria, where a 16-month-old boy developed reversible hepatic veno-occlusive disease after being treated regularly since his third month of life with a herbal tea. The herbal tea had been prepared from leaves which his mother had injudiciously mistaken for *Tussilago farfara*. Upon chemical analysis, the incriminated leaf material yielded 0.16% of seneciphyllin and 0.33% of the corresponding N-oxide [11].

***Scutellaria* Species** (Volume 2 pp. 289–296)

As has been pointed out in the Botany section of the *Scutellaria* monograph, skullcap available from British wholesale suppliers was sometimes found to be a *Teucrium* species instead of a *Scutellaria* species (p. 289). This mislabelling of *Teucrium* as skullcap or *Scutellaria* has also been reported from North America [12]. The resulting uncertainty about the exact botanical origin of commercial skullcap could be significant, especially because *Teucrium chamaedrys* has been associated with various cases of hepatitis in France (see below). It is unclear at the moment, whether the hepatotoxic effects that have been associated with preparations containing skullcap should be attributed to *Scutellaria*, *Teucrium* or both.

Teucrium chamaedrys (Volume II p. 81)

In 1992, the French health authorities suspended the marketing licence of herbal preparations containing *Teucrium chamaedrys*, after the use of such preparations had been associated with 26 cases of acute hepatitis, 12 of which were positive on accidental rechallenge [13]. Several cases have been reported in detail [14,15], including a case of fatal hepatitis in a 68-year-old woman [16].

References

1. Rose KD, Croissant PD, Parliament CF, Levin MB (1990) Spontaneous spinal epidural hematoma with associated platelet dysfunction from excessive garlic ingestion: a case report. Neurosurgery 26:880–882
2. Domínguez-Soto L (1992) Photodermatitis to aloe vera. Int J Dermatol 31:372
3. Schwartz RH (1990) Cinnamon oil: kids use it to get high. Clin Pediatr 29:196
4. Perry PA, Dean BS, Krenzelok EP (1990) Cinnamon oil abuse by adolescents. Vet Hum Toxicol 32:162–164
5. Pilapil VR (1989) Toxic manifestations of cinnamon oil ingestion in a child. Clin Pediatr 28:276
6. Awang DVC (1991) Maternal use of ginseng and neonatal androgenization. JAMA 266:363
7. Waller DP, Martin AM, Farnsworth NR, Awang DV (1992) Lack of androgenicity of Siberian ginseng. JAMA 267:2329
8. Vidal C, González Quintela A, Martín F (1991) Eucalyptus vapor causing Aspergillus in sputum smears. Ann Allergy 66:355–356
9. Anonymous (1992) Chaparral-induced toxic hepatitis – California and Texas, 1992. Morbid Mortal Weekly Rep 41:812–814
10. Yeong ML, Swinburn B, Kennedy M, Nicholson G (1990) Hepatic veno-occlusive disease associated with comfrey ingestion. J Gastroenterol Hepatol 5:211–214
11. Stuppner H, Sperl W, Gassner I, Vogel W (1992) Verwechslung von Tussilago farfara mit Petasites hybridus – ein aktueller fall von Pyrrolizidinalkaloid-Intoxikation. Sci Pharm (Wien) 60:160
12. Huxtable RJ (1992) The myth of beneficent nature: the risks of herbal preparations. Ann Intern Med 117:165–166
13. Anonymous (1992) Dossier Technique destiné à la presse profesionnelle médicale et pharmaceutique. Objet: Médicaments à base de germandrée-petit-chêne. Paris: Ministère de la Santé et de l'Action Humanitaire

14. Pauwels A, Thierman-Duffaud D, Azanowsky JM, Loiseau D, Biour M, Levy VG (1992) Hepatite aigue à la germandrée petit-chêne. Hepatotoxicité d'une plante medicinale. Deux observations. Gastroenterol Clin Biol 16:92–95
15. Larrey D, Vial T, Pauwels A, Castot A, Biour M, David M, Michel H (1992) Hepatitis after germander (*Teucrium chamaedrys*) administration: another instance of herbal medicine hepatotoxicity. Ann Intern Med 117:129–132
16. Mostefa-Kara N, Pauwels A, Pines E, Biour M, Levy VG (1992) Fatal hepatitis after herbal tea. Lancet 340:674

Subject Index

Adverse Effects of Herbal Drugs

Volume 1

Edited by P. A. G. M. de Smet (Managing Editor), K. Keller, R. Hänsel, R. F. Chandler

In collaboration with the Pharmaceuticals Programme of the World Health Organization, Regional Office for Europe

With contributions by numerous experts

1992. XIV, 275 pp. 45 tabs.
ISBN 3-540-53100-9

The first volume contains more than 15 monographs as well as an extensive introductory chapter on the quality assurance of herbal remedies.

Contents: Toxicological Outlook on the Quality Assurance of Herbal Remedies. – Allium Sativum. – Aristolochia Species. – Asafetida. – Berberine. – Cinnamomum Species. – Cymbopogon Species. – Eucalyptus Species. – Foeniculum Vulgare. – Gaultheria Procumbens. – Hedeoma pulegioides and Mentha pulegium. – Marsdenia cundurango. – Medicago sativa. – Mentha piperita and Mentha spicata. – Panax ginseng. – Pyrrolizidine Alkaloids. – Sesquiterpene Lactones. – Notes Added in Proof. – Subject Index.

MIX
Papier aus verantwortungsvollen Quellen
Paper from responsible sources
FSC® C105338

If you have any concerns about our products,
you can contact us on
ProductSafety@springernature.com

In case Publisher is established outside the EU,
the EU authorized representative is:
Springer Nature Customer Service Center GmbH
Europaplatz 3, 69115 Heidelberg, Germany

Printed by Libri Plureos GmbH
in Hamburg, Germany